WHAT YOU CAN DO TO PREVENT CANCER

Oliver Alabaster, M.D.

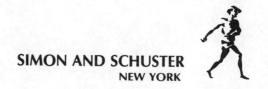

SIMON AND SCHUSTER
NEW YORK

Copyright © 1985 by Oliver Alabaster, M.D.
All rights reserved
including the right of reproduction
in whole or in part in any form
Published by Simon & Schuster
A Division of Simon & Schuster, Inc.
Simon & Schuster Building
Rockefeller Center
1230 Avenue of the Americas
New York, New York 10020

SIMON AND SCHUSTER and colophon are registered trademarks of
Simon & Schuster, Inc.
Designed by Irving Perkins Associates
Manufactured in the United States of America
10 9 8 7 6 5 4 3 2 1

Library of Congress Cataloging in Publication Data

Alabaster, Oliver.
    What you can do to prevent cancer.

    Includes bibliographies and index.
    1. Cancer—Nutritional aspects. 2. Cancer—Diet
therapy. 3. Cancer—Prevention. I. Title. [DNLM:
1. Diet—adverse effects—popular works. 2. Neoplasms—
etiology—popular works. 3. Neoplasms—prevention &
control—popular works. 4. Nutrition—popular works.
QZ 201 A316w]
RC263.A43   1985   616.99'4052   84-27649
ISBN: 0-671-49537-2

To the memory of my father, George H. Alabaster, M.D., F.R.C.S., whose medical career spanned more than sixty years, and whose life continues to inspire me.

Acknowledgments

I wish to thank my colleagues at the National Cancer Institute and the National Academy of Sciences who provided helpful advice, Gabriele Pantucci for his constant encouragement, and Dimitrios C. Rallis for his thoughtful comments.

I would also like to express my appreciation to my wife, to my children—Christina and Clare—and to my close friends for their understanding during the book's seemingly long gestation period.

Finally, special thanks to my editor, Michael Korda, whose advice and constructive criticisms were most helpful, and to the professional staff of Simon and Schuster for their careful review of the manuscript.

Contents

PART ONE

PART TWO

PART ONE

Introduction

First, do no harm.

HIPPOCRATES
460–400 B.C.

Environmental factors such as diet and smoking are now thought to cause as much as 90 percent of all human cancer in the United States (1),* which means that cancer is potentially a *preventable disease.*

Scientists who have studied the effects of diet and cancer have found that about 60 percent of cancer in women and 40 percent of cancer in men could be due to dietary factors (2). Such a remarkable conclusion justifies a complete re-evaluation of our diet to determine which foods we should eat and which we should avoid. This view has recently received a very strong endorsement by an expert committee appointed by the National Academy of Sciences in Washington, D.C., in its 1982 report entitled "Diet, Nutrition and Cancer" (3), by the National Cancer Institute, and by the American Cancer Society in its dietary guidelines issued in 1984 (4).

Since more than a quarter of the total population will eventually develop cancer, this means that about 60 million Americans will be affected. Of these, *approximately 20 million cases might be prevented by relatively simple changes in the national diet (5)!*

Each year there are over 800,000 new cases of cancer in the United States, and nearly every American family will be touched in some way by this dreaded disease. Most of us fear the very word "cancer" because it seems like a death sentence. Worse, it usually conjures up an image of pain and suffering that might last for months, or even years. We feel powerless to prevent cancer—apart from not smoking. We simply live passively, fearfully, wondering if or when cancer will strike. Interestingly, this attitude towards

* These numbers refer to sources which are listed, by chapter, in the "Notes" section at the back of the book.

cancer is very different from our view of heart disease, which is widely accepted as an inevitable consequence of aging or stressful indulgence, and is regarded as a much more "natural" cause of death.

Many of us have had close relatives or friends die of cancer, sometimes quite young or in middle age. As a physician and cancer researcher, I have seen young children deprived of the joy of childhood, and adults full of resentment and bitterness at being singled out for premature suffering and possible death. The loss of a parent can have a devastating effect on the lives of a family. My own mother died from breast cancer when I was twelve, so I have witnessed and felt the full impact of such a family tragedy at first hand.

The development of modern medicine has made a dramatic impact on the survival of patients with some cancers, and has had relatively little impact on the survival of others. The main forms of treatment used today are surgery, chemotherapy, and radiation therapy. All three forms of treatment contribute to the survival of many patients, but I have witnessed the pain and discomfort of surgery, the side effects of chemotherapy, and the debility sometimes produced by radiation. How much better it would be to prevent cancer from developing in the first place.

Virtually everyone knows that smoking can cause cancer, especially lung cancer, yet smokers find it very difficult to stop; their addiction overwhelms all reason. I well remember one of the first cases of lung cancer I saw as a medical student. He was a fifty-one-year-old businessman who lay coughing and breathless in a hospital bed. His face was thin and pale and he looked emaciated. He had lost weight and his uneaten lunch was on a tray nearby. His wife and children were at his bedside, not yet fully aware of the gravity of the situation. As I greeted him I noticed that his hands were stained with nicotine, a sign of his self-destruction. It turned out that his disease was beyond treatment and he died a few weeks later. Today, as a researcher, I would not only consider his smoking habits, but I would also be interested in his dietary habits, particularly his level of consumption of protective factors such as vitamin A and its precursor, beta-carotene.

The inability of a smoker to quit is as understandable as the inability of a compulsive eater to close a box of Swiss chocolate. Yet these forms of neurotic compulsion are not the reason we fail to make sensible adjustments in our diets. What we have always lacked is informed guidance. This situation has now changed. Instead of leaving your fate in the lap of the gods, there is an alternative, a way to lessen your risk of cancer by planned changes in your diet. What is even more encouraging, these changes in your diet will not require you to overcome addictive habits: all that will be asked of you is that you *alter the balance* of many of the foods that you are already eating. In fact, a sensible cancer prevention diet, based upon our present knowledge, uses foods that are readily available in your local supermarket. Once you have understood the importance of various dietary constituents, you will learn how to select food in a healthier way.

Dietary cancer prevention is really much simpler than the absurdly complicated weight-reducing diets that are announced each week. A cancer prevention diet should become the normal diet for everyone. That is not meant to imply that the relationship of diet to cancer is simple, far from it. But a diet that is based upon our present knowledge can be made relatively simple. We need not take into consideration every known food chemical and its possible interaction with other chemicals. This will never be possible, nor is it necessary. Contrary to the impression conveyed by those who sell "health foods," most chemicals are perfectly safe. In fact, our bodies are made entirely of chemicals that are assembled in particular ways. Our whole environment consists of chemicals, many of them absolutely vital to our well-being.

What I want you to understand is the importance of *balance*. The health of the body depends upon maintaining a certain critical chemical balance. An imbalance can often be corrected by the body itself. However, when the balance is disturbed in a way that cannot be corrected, the body may undergo a permanent change that leads to the development of cancer. One of the great challenges of modern cancer research is to understand and control this process.

As you will soon discover in later chapters there is considerable evidence that diets that are high in total fat can increase the risk of certain cancers—one such is breast cancer. Yet each day there are women who endure the physical and psychological mutilation of radical mastectomy (breast removal) for a cancer that may have been caused by excessive fat in the diet. Consider for a moment what such an experience can mean. I have seen such cases many times during my professional life. One immediately comes to mind. An attractive woman, about forty-two years of age, who suddenly noticed a small lump in her right breast. She was naturally apprehensive, but courageously came to see me for advice. After a radical mastectomy had removed all detectable disease, her life changed. She lived each day with great intensity as though it were her last. Her husband fortunately was very supportive. Her children were too young to understand the extent of the ordeal that she had gone through, but their presence gave her great strength. I later learned that she had resolutely decided not to seek further treatment if ever her cancer recurred. This act of defiance was her way of fighting back. Now, ten years later, she is alive and well.

Certain types of cancer have been found to occur more frequently among people whose diet is low in citrus fruits and cruciferous vegetables (cauliflower, broccoli, cabbage, brussels sprouts, for example). Diets like this tend to be low in vitamins A and C, and other vital constituents. One such type is cancer of the esophagus, the passage that conveys food from the mouth to the stomach. Patients who develop esophageal cancer usually have difficulty swallowing solids, but not fluids. The only form of treatment that really offers any hope is surgery. This involves removing the narrowed esophagus, preferably with normal tissue at each end of the removed segment to reduce the chance of any cancerous tissue being left behind. Unfortunately, the cure rate remains rather low. Wouldn't it be far better to avoid this miserable disease by changing our diet? Scientific evidence now available clearly shows that people who regularly eat fresh fruit and vegetables have a lower risk of esophageal cancer as well as other cancers.

Less is known about the influence of different dietary levels of protein intake than of fat intake. Nevertheless, a number of studies by cancer researchers have demonstrated an association of the level of protein intake with cancer of the breast, the colon (large bowel), the rectum, and the pancreas. Colon and rectal cancers are also associated with a high intake of dietary fat, and this illustrates how some dietary constituents (in this case, fat and protein) may act together to increase the risk; a so-called synergistic effect. And some foods may have opposite effects, the relative importance of which may depend upon how much is eaten and how often. Carbohydrates such as sugar and starches have not yet been established as a potential cause of cancer, at least not directly. However, carbohydrates (like fat and protein) contribute to obesity, and evidence already exists that men who are at least 40 percent overweight have an increased risk of colon and rectal cancer; and women who are at least 40 percent overweight have an increased risk of gallbladder, liver, and breast cancer. So stick to your efforts at weight control. Being slim can bring you more than social success—it can reduce your chances of getting heart disease and high blood pressure as well as cancer!

Although most people try to reduce weight for reasons of vanity rather than health, people who take mineral and vitamin supplements do so for their health, not their vanity. Often these supplements are unbalanced and excessive, and the body either excretes the surplus, or stores it. If one takes too much of the water-soluble vitamins, namely the B vitamins and vitamin C, little is stored and most is excreted in the urine. On the other hand, the fat-soluble vitamins such as A, D, E, and K are stored in body fat when taken in excess, and so are more likely to cause side effects.

Considerable evidence exists that vitamins A, C, and possibly E can provide protection against some cancers, but only when taken as part of the natural diet. Although some scientific studies have been initiated by the National Cancer Institute to determine whether vitamin supplements can provide equivalent protection in humans, these studies will take many years to complete. However, some laboratory data indicate a cancer-inhibiting effect of supplemental vitamins A, C, and E in animals, which raises the strong possibility that such an effect may be found in humans too.

This illustrates an important point. When a dietary constituent is suspected of influencing the development of cancer, evidence may be incomplete and a firm opinion consequently unjustified. Nonetheless, the substance in question may one day prove to be of critical importance. Should we wait for all the scientific evidence before deciding to act, or should we act merely on suspicion, on limited evidence? Many doctors did not wait for all the scientific evidence that linked smoking to lung cancer before kicking the habit; the risks were too high. They simply stopped smoking and benefited as a group years before the general public understood the risks clearly. Taking a nutritional supplement, on the other hand, is not giving up something but rather adding something—an action that may have as-yet-unknown long-term side effects. My intention therefore is simply to inform you of the facts as they are known, and to offer you a plan for vitamin or mineral supplements that you can choose to follow if you wish. Within a few years, current research will provide more definitive answers that may confirm or lead to changes in my recommendations.

Along with vitamin supplements, many people take mineral supplements. The role of minerals in dietary cancer prevention has not yet been completely assessed, but some evidence suggests that minerals such as selenium and molybdenum can lower the risk of some cancers. Although there is obviously a need for more research, it is already possible at least to suggest an appropriate intake of cancer-inhibiting minerals such as selenium.

Since the relationship between diet and cancer is not a simple one, you will find that many foods contain various amounts of substances that are both harmful and protective. You may well begin to wonder whether any food can be considered safe. It is therefore important to understand that no diet can eliminate all potentially harmful factors. In the final analysis, there must be compromises, but our goal should be to shift the *balance,* to increase our intake of cancer-inhibiting foods as we learn about them, and to reduce those foods that increase the risk.

While it is possible to achieve a more rational dietary balance when considering only the main dietary constituents, this is much more difficult to achieve when we consider the effects of about 15,000 food additives that are included intentionally or unintentionally in the American diet. Even if they were individually tested, imagine how much testing would be required to find out if they act differently when present in various combinations. An impossible task! And since most food additives are present in very small amounts, many of them are assumed to be harmless—probably a dubious assumption. Over 93% of food additives are made up of sugar, salt, corn syrup, and dextrose, and our exposure to the others is obviously limited, but the story does not end here. Nature has her own "additives." Some foods contain natural inhibitors of cancer formation, while other foods contain natural cancer-causing chemicals such as nitrosamines. And, as if what we eat is not enough to consider, let us not forget that smoking contributes to the development of about one third of all cancer, while excessive alcohol consumption can substantially increase the risk of cancer of the mouth, the larynx, the esophagus, and the lung. It seems that nature makes us pay a heavy price for our pleasures, but at least the choice is largely *ours*.

By choosing to buy this book you have already made a commitment to learn, to understand, and to help yourself in an intelligent way. You would not deliberately choose to eat a quick-acting deadly poison. The risk is clear, and you react rationally. Does it make any sense deliberately to eat foods that could also "poison" your body over the years by inducing cancer? Does it make any sense to smoke? Of course not!

The reaction of the American public to many years of advice about the dangers of smoking is not very encouraging. Of all the known causes of cancer, this is the easiest to understand and to do something about. Yet smoking continues to be directly responsible for more than 30 percent of all cancer deaths, and continues to be a major cause of death and disability from cardiovascular and respiratory diseases. The economic cost of the tobacco habit to the nation runs into the billions and billions of dollars because of both medical and disability expenses, and because of lost industrial production. Yet our taxes are used for tobacco price supports which encourage farmers to continue to produce this deadly drug.

Since the solution to your smoking risk is simply to stop smoking, this really needs little elaboration. How to get rid of an addiction is really beyond the scope of this book. Instead, I will concentrate on the even more important task of explaining the complexities of *dietary* cancer, and how to reduce your chances of getting cancer by understanding and changing your diet. This is a much more demanding goal.

Since approximately 80 percent of cancer stems from either diet or smoking, your diet will control about 70 percent of your cancer risk if you are already a nonsmoker. Clearly, diet must be taken seriously.

Fortunately, there are steps that we all can take today to reduce the risk of cancer and other diet-related diseases. This requires some knowledge and a little determination. We need to be aware of how we live, what we do, and especially what we eat.

Often we marvel at how clever the body is at maintaining itself in proper balance, but there are limits as to how much abuse the body can tolerate. If we expose ourselves to excessive amounts of certain nutrients and nonnutrient chemicals, the body must have a mechanism for getting rid of the excess or the excess will be stored, sometimes as harmful by-products. This can upset the body's delicate balance, eventually producing cancer. Conversely, if we fail to eat enough of certain dietary substances, we can also increase our chances of developing cancer. So it is not simply a question of eating less of everything.

This book will help you to understand how the way you choose to live influences your risk of cancer. The old adage "we are what we eat" now takes on new meaning. After reading brief descriptions of what cancer is, and how it is caused, you will learn how much scientists know about the specific role of diet in causing cancer—knowledge that can be immediately useful to you.

Once you have a simple understanding of the importance of diet as a cause of cancer, I will provide you with dietary guidelines of both a general and specific nature. These guidelines will enable you to understand the basis for safe food selection and preparation using the latest information. This is followed by the detailed Cancer Prevention Diet, which will show you just how easily you can plan your diet to provide you with more whole grain cereals, fruit, vegetables, and fiber—and less fat. To help you on your way to a permanently sensible diet, five sample breakfasts, lunches, and dinners have been created that will automatically provide you with the right dietary balance no matter which breakfast, lunch and dinner you choose to combine. You will also learn how to analyze your diet for the important nutrients, and how to combine this knowledge with a sensible attitude towards weight control. After a three-week introductory program, you will find that your whole attitude to nutrition has changed—for good! And to help you on your way, some selected recipes are included, accompanied by complete dietary analyses.

In case you are beginning to think that you will never be able to eat any of your favorite foods again, let me reassure you that the objective of this cancer prevention diet is to shift the *balance* of what you eat for the rest of your life. That means that any dietary indiscretions on one day can be made up for on other days so that at the end of the week, or the end of the month, the desired balance is maintained.

Although, with time, new information will come along that may lead to changes in my recommendations, the important decision is to use what is currently known to your best advantage. When you have understood how much evidence has been collected over the years, and how compelling much of it is, I think the choice will be obvious.

In the final analysis, I believe that if you act now you can reduce not only your cancer risk but also your risk of other degenerative diseases. And this may be one of the greatest investments in living that you ever make.

CHAPTER 1

The Nature of Cancer

The human body is made of millions of tiny cells, all of which have specialized functions. For example, red cells in the blood carry oxygen to all other cells, while cells of the skin provide a protective covering for the whole body. Normally, cells that form nerves, muscles, and bone are only found in these structures, not elsewhere. *They do not spread beyond their natural boundaries.* Some cells, such as those in the intestine or the skin, are replaced frequently, and therefore these cells multiply at just the right rate to replace those that are spontaneously lost. Normal cell division is therefore very well controlled by the body.

When a cell becomes abnormal in such a way that it cannot recognize its natural boundaries, is able to spread to distant sites in the body, and divides in an uncontrolled way, it has become a cancer cell. In contrast, some cells divide unnecessarily without spreading beyond their natural boundaries. These cells are *benign,* and are found, for example, in a harmless freckle. When these same cells in the freckle change so that they can spread beyond their boundaries and invade other tissues, dividing uncontrollably, they form the *malignant* cancer called melanoma, which is frequently fatal. Cancer cells also usually produce unidentified toxic substances that can make the body generally ill and weak, sometimes producing loss of appetite and loss of weight. The inability of cancer cells to "know their place" leads to these cells invading different organs such as the liver, brain, or bone marrow, so destroying the normal function of these organs. Nearly all cancers occur in normal body tissues where cells have to divide rather rapidly. These tissues are the skin, intestine, the lymphatic system, bone marrow, and bone.

Cancers occur much less frequently in cells that do not normally divide. This is important because cell division provides a great opportunity for cell damage to be passed on to daughter cells. When this damage is of the type that causes cells to escape from the usual limits of growth, these cells acquire the destructive properties that are associated with cancer. It is an unfortunate fact that because the abnormality in cancer cells is always passed from one generation of cells to the next, the development of a single cancer cell in your body might eventually kill you. A sobering thought!

WHY DO WE GET CANCER?

The known causes of cancer are many and complex, while the development of most individual cancers remains unexplained. Our environment exposes us to numerous toxic substances, some of which are known to cause cancer. Examples of these cancer-causing factors are found in our diet, in tobacco smoke, in sunshine, and in industries that expose us to materials such as asbestos, chromium ore, aniline dyes, and polyvinyl chloride. Exposure to ionizing radiation has been clearly established as a cause of cancer, and certain viruses are regarded by some scientists as potential culprits. Heredity, on the other hand, is less frequently implicated directly in the development of cancer. However, a more subtle genetic predisposition to the influence of environmental carcinogens, including those found in diet, could exist, but this is very difficult to prove.

DIET AND NUTRITION

The discovery of cancer-causing chemicals in the environment, though of major importance, does not explain why certain cancers occur more frequently in one country than another; nor does it appear to explain why cancers occur with different frequencies in various parts of the same country. International differences in the incidence of cancer might have remained a mystery but for the migration of large numbers of people to countries such as the United States. African and Japanese immigrants to America married within their own communities for several generations, thus maintaining their genetic (racial) purity while gradually losing their distinctive dietary habits. This has provided the opportunity to compare the incidence of various cancers among these groups with the incidence of the same cancers both in their original countries and here, in native Americans of European stock. What has been learned is one of the most important facts ever to come out of cancer research: namely, that *when people migrate to a new country they gradually acquire the pattern of cancer that is characteristic of their new country,* mostly as a result of losing their original dietary habits and possibly from being exposed to other factors in the environment. This observation means that cancer is potentially a preventable disease that is *not* usually genetically determined, except perhaps through a subtle susceptibility to environmental factors. All that is needed is to identify those factors which increase the risk of cancer and those factors which are protective. Unfortunately, this is not an easy task, but progress has been made.

In a recently concluded twenty-year study of 25,000 Seventh-Day Adventists at Loma Linda University, in southern California, it was learned that the lacto-ovo-vegetarian diet of Seventh-Day Adventists reduced their risk of cancers that are unrelated to smoking—namely cancers of the large bowel, the breast, and the prostate. Furthermore, among those Seventh-Day Adventist males between the ages of thirty-five and sixty-four who *do* eat meat, there was a threefold increase in the risk of dying of a heart attack. Clearly, there is no doubt that what we eat can have a major impact on our risk of developing cancer and heart disease.

Many environmental changes have occurred that have had a substantial influence on human development. Such changes are responsible for the fact that, on average, children of immigrants to the United States are taller and live longer than their parents. This dramatic effect of nutrition on growth is likely to have influenced susceptibility to cancer as well, partly because an abundant diet has tended to make many of us overweight, and partly because the balance of the foods we eat has changed over the past hundred years.

These observations are further supported by the fact that, in laboratory animals, the occurrence of spontaneous cancers in their old age is influenced by diet. A reduction in the total food intake or in specific foods actually *lowers* the cancer risk, even of cancers that are being deliberately caused by exposure to known cancer-causing chemicals. The only exception to this is when a specific dietary deficiency itself causes damage to cells, making them more likely to become cancerous later. The importance of total food intake as a potential cause of human cancer will be discussed in more detail in Chapter 12.

Another more encouraging observation is that some cancers are occurring less frequently. Stomach cancer is now the commonest cancer in Japan, and used to be the most common cancer in the United States. Yet, during the past fifty years, stomach cancer has fallen from first to sixth place in the United States—a change probably brought about by reduced mold contamination of food through better refrigeration and storage. The real difficulty scientists face is how to identify the changes in diet that have proved beneficial. It is easy to remember whether you smoked five, ten, or even fifteen years ago, and even how heavily. It is far more difficult to know what your diet consisted of, let alone the precise chemical composition of the food you ingested. Although you cannot reverse the clock, you should at least understand that the foods which you have been eating all these years have a balance, or imbalance, of naturally occurring carcinogens and cancer-protectors.

SMOKING

You are well aware, of course, that smoking causes lung cancer. What is less well known is that it is also a major cause of other cancers, the misery of chronic bronchitis, and premature death from heart disease.

Although evidence has been found that smoking increases the risk of developing other cancers (such as bladder cancer), the link to lung cancer is the most dramatic. Since it may take a smoker twenty years to develop lung cancer, studies of cigarette smoking that allow for a 20-year delay in its effects have shown a remarkable correlation between cigarette consumption and the development of lung cancer. The evidence, in fact, is so compelling that only those who work for the tobacco industry continue to insist that this correlation is a pure coincidence. Despite the widespread awareness of the risks, however, people continue to smoke, particularly in the lower socioeconomic groups.

This willingness to risk such a precious thing as one's health suggests that addictive pleasures are preferable to a prolonged old age, particularly among the poor. It has also become clear that we should not expect the government to take care of us, because the revenue from tobacco and the economic value of the tobacco industry would be lost if nobody smoked. Furthermore, think of the cost to the government's social security program if the number of people reaching old age increased substantially.

Obviously, we must act to protect our health by taking sensible precautions now.

RADIATION

The importance of radiation as a cause of cancer has been recognized for many years. Exposure to toxic levels of radiation produces genetic damage, and since the genes control cell behavior, this can lead either to cancer or to cell death, depending upon the dose. The usual type of cancer caused by radiation is leukemia, or cancer of the white blood cells. This happened to some survivors of the atomic bombs dropped on Hiroshima and Nagasaki in Japan in August of 1945. The closer the survivors were to the epicenter of the blast, the more likely they were to develop cancer later. Even now there is a higher rate of leukemia among the people of those cities. This illustrates one of the great problems of studying environmental factors. A cancer attributable to exposure to an environmental carcinogen may not develop for twenty years—or even longer. This makes the establishment of cause and effect much more difficult than when the process is rapid.

SUNLIGHT

Sunlight is composed of both visible and invisible radiation. The invisible radiation known as ultraviolet light may cause skin cancer, but only if the exposure is prolonged and intense. This process is therefore quite different from that associated with asbestos, which can increase the risk of lung cancer after only brief exposure. Ultraviolet rays in sunlight may damage cells in the skin, though for most of us who sunbathe moderately, this damage is usually repaired by natural processes. In places like Arizona or Australia, people are sometimes exposed to so much sunlight that cell damage may not be adequately repaired, thus producing a high risk of the serious skin cancer called melanoma. Avoidance of excessive sunlight reduces this risk dramatically, and dietary vitamin A may offer some protection too.

VIRUSES

Another environmental factor that has attracted a good deal of scientific interest is viral infection. There is no doubt that some viruses (one of the three main types of germs; the others are bacteria and fungi) can cause cancer in animals. Their role in the development of human cancer is less clear. The most famous association of a virus with human cancer is that of the EB virus with a common African cancer called Burkitt's lymphoma. But it remains an association. There is no proof that EB virus causes human cancer. The association is complicated by the fact that there is a rare form of lymphoma in the United States that is virtually indistinguishable from African Burkitt's lymphoma, but which is not associated with the EB virus.

More recently, it has become apparent that a form of liver disease known as infective hepatitis can greatly increase the risk of liver cancer, but only if the hepatitis results from infection by a particular one of the three known causative viruses. Even then, the hepatitis must be persistent or chronic for the risk to be present.

Finally, there is some evidence to suggest that certain forms of human leukemia may be due to a virus known as HTLV, but again the precise nature of the causal relationship remains to be established.

One possibility is that viruses insert new genetic material into DNA (more about this later), or activate specific genes called *oncogenes,* which make a normal cell behave as a cancer cell. In fact, it would not surprise me if we eventually discover that dietary factors act on oncogenes too. This very exciting area of modern cancer research is revolutionizing the way we think about cancer.

INDUSTRIAL POLLUTION

Most of us think of industry as the cause of widespread pollution, depositing vast amounts of poisonous chemical waste into the environment. Although this is regrettably true, the commonest form of cancer in the United States today, lung cancer, is caused by smoking rather than industrialization. It is relatively safe to be a nonsmoker anywhere in the United States, but it is dangerous to be a smoker anywhere in the world, even in the pure air and clean environment of a country like Switzerland. Similarly, the next two most common cancers, those of the breast and colon (large bowel) are less common in highly industrialized but poor countries like Czechoslovakia, and much more common in rich agricultural countries like New Zealand.

Industrial pollution therefore does not appear to be an important cause of cancer, but workers in certain industries are exposed to powerful carcinogens that clearly increase their risk of cancer. Asbestos workers, and those who are exposed to asbestos dust even for relatively short periods, have a dramatically increased risk of lung cancer as well as a rare cancer of the pleura—the thin membrane lining the lung and chest cavity—called mesothelioma. Similarly, the mining of chromium greatly increases the risk of lung cancer for those exposed during production and storage. And workers in the rubber industry who handle aniline dyes have a greater risk of bladder cancer. It was noticed relatively recently that automobile workers exposed to polyvinyl chloride have an increased risk of a rare type of cancer of the liver. In the last century, chimney sweeps were found to have a high incidence of cancer of the scrotum, which was even then attributed to coal dust exposure. The discovery of these industrial causes of cancer has been of major importance because it has led to effective prevention through reduced exposure to known carcinogens.

HOW DOES CANCER DEVELOP?

Since about half of all cancer is related to the presence of dietary carcinogens, insufficient dietary anticarcinogens, and too much fat in the diet, and since the rest is mostly due to the presence of environmental chemicals (that is, tobacco smoke) that are taken in by the body, it is worthwhile for us to consider briefly how these substances are responsible for the induction of cancer. The process of inducing cancer is called *carcinogenesis.* Because carcinogenesis takes a long time, cancers are more common in older people and in older animals.

At this point I would like to explain the highly complex process of carcinogenesis in the simplest possible terms. There are early and late stages in this process which are very different.

The Early Stages

In the early stages, cancer-causing chemicals (the carcinogens) interact with the most important part of the cell, the DNA. DNA is deoxyribonucleic acid. This substance is intimately involved in the processes that regulate cell behavior, and it contains the "identity" of the cell, which is passed on from one generation of cells to the next. Permanent damage to the DNA, which is not severe enough to destroy the cell, may change its "identity," and that of its daughter cells as well. For this DNA damage to occur, most carcinogens need to be present for a long time. For DNA damage to be passed to daughter cells, cell division must occur before the cell has had time to repair the damaged DNA.

Because carcinogens are often unstable substances, it is more common for a carcinogen to be made within the body, by the body itself. What happens is this. A toxic chemical, such as aflatoxin B_1 (found in moldy nuts and corn), is normally broken down or detoxified by the liver. During this detoxification process, aflatoxin B_1 is converted into an active carcinogen. This means that certain chemicals (sometimes present as dietary constituents), which cannot cause cancer directly, can be converted into carcinogens in the body. If the body has no way to break down the carcinogen or excrete it, it will persist for a long time, causing damage to the DNA of cells exposed to it. If it is removed from the body fairly quickly, but is replaced by regular exposure of the body to the parent chemical, the effect will be equivalent.

Obviously the only sensible thing to do is to avoid exposing your body to these chemicals rather than to rely on your body to get rid of them.

Although carcinogens that damage DNA are known as *mutagens,*

HOW A CARCINOGEN CAN DAMAGE DNA

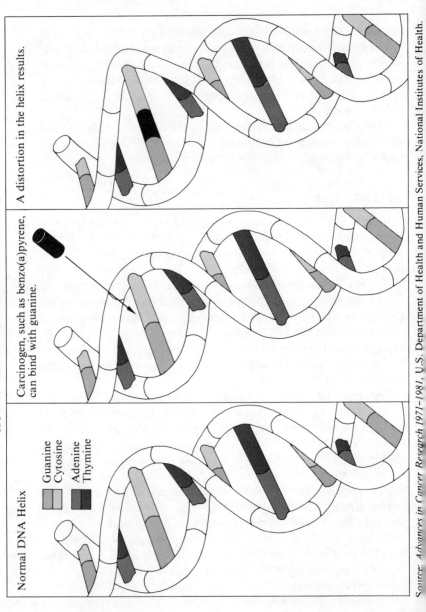

Normal DNA Helix

Guanine
Cytosine
Adenine
Thymine

Carcinogen, such as benzo(a)pyrene, can bind with guanine.

A distortion in the helix results.

Source: *Advances in Cancer Research 1971–1981*, U.S. Department of Health and Human Services, National Institutes of Health.

not all mutagens are carcinogens. Mutagens that initiate the carcinogenic process are called *initiators*. These initiators prepare the way for the next step in the carcinogenic process.

The Late Stage

The late stage is poorly understood even by the experts. The agents involved in this phase of carcinogenesis are called *promotors*. These promotors affect the process by which primitive cells become more specialized (this is called *differentiation*), and they may also encourage cells to multiply. Some scientists believe that promotors encourage the expression of all the DNA damage that developed during the early stage.

The implications of this are clear. If we could remove the early-stage initiators from our environment, we would mostly protect young people; if we could remove the late-stage promotors from the environment, we could protect everyone.

All the experimental evidence so far suggests that diet mostly affects the late stages of carcinogenesis. What is more surprising is that normal dietary components have been shown to increase or lower the incidence of certain cancers initiated by exposure to known carcinogens. The implications of this observation are far-reaching.

Without even knowing the detailed chemical composition of the diet, direct evidence has been found linking obesity with cancer in both animals and man. When laboratory animals are fed unrestricted diets they become more obese than their counterparts in the wild. These obese animals, however, not only suffer the indignity of being overweight, they actually have a much higher chance of developing "spontaneous" cancers. Correlations of this kind have also been made with human cancer (discussed in detail in Chapter 12). But there is an encouraging part to this story. When laboratory animals were placed on a restricted diet and lost weight, becoming more like their wild counterparts, their spontaneous cancer rate dropped to very low levels. Since certain cancers are known to occur with greater frequency in obese people, it is possible that your slimming diet may be helping to reduce your cancer risk—at least a little.

CAN WE IDENTIFY DIETARY CARCINOGENS?

Although scientists are convinced that our diet is responsible for about half of all cancer, and smoking for about one third, it is not going to be easy to identify all the dietary factors that are relevant. The reasons for this are not hard to understand.

In the past, diet-related diseases were discovered by astute observers noticing that one or more nutrients were missing in the diets of people exhibiting the symptoms of the disease. The most famous example is the relationship between scurvy and the lack of vitamin C. Although descriptions of a disease resembling scurvy are found in ancient writings, the first real accounts appear in records of the Crusades. When the great sea voyages of exploration began at the end of the fifteenth century, scurvy became common, and soon was a major cause of disability and mortality among sailors. For more than 250 years this disease remained a mystery. Then in 1747, James Lind, a British surgeon, performed a remarkable experiment. He decided to study the effects of various diets on sailors. One of his dietary treatments consisted of "two oranges and a lemon every day" for sailors with the signs of scurvy. The results were amazing. Not only did the sailors recover, but adding citrus fruit to the regular diets of sailors on long voyages prevented scurvy from developing at all.

The success of this discovery then led to an approach to diet research which concentrated only on defining nutrient requirements in terms of the effects of *deficiencies*. These studies were first done in animals and then in human volunteers. However, it is important to remember that diet-related cancer is caused by either a relative lack of anticarcinogens or a relative excess of carcinogens, and that the process may take many years to occur. Scurvy, on the other hand, involves only one essential nutrient, whose lack is manifested within three months.

After years of studying diet in terms of deficiencies, scientists have recently come to realize something of immense importance: diseases can arise from an abundant and apparently normal diet, consumed over many years! This realization has enormous implications for the control of both cancer and heart disease.

The most obvious ill effect of a "normal" diet is usually obesity.

This is caused in the vast majority of cases by an excessive calorie intake. The harmful effects of obesity have been obvious both medically and socially for many years, and I have already mentioned that obesity carries with it a higher risk of certain cancers. Other ill effects of a normal diet may not be as obvious. For example, it has taken us many years to realize that certain vitamins and most minerals, though necessary in proper amounts, can be toxic when ingested in excess. This is because it is much easier to notice obesity than mineral or vitamin toxicity. Nevertheless, dietary problems such as toxicity and deficiency diseases, manifest themselves fairly quickly, usually within a few months. Imagine how much more difficult it is to find dietary factors that produce gradual, insidious effects over many years. This is the nature of dietary cancer.

Despite these difficulties, however, evidence has been found that vitamin A *deficiency* can increase the risk of cancer of the lung, bladder, and larynx in humans; and that it increases the risk of cancer induced in animals by known carcinogens. Conversely, increasing the intake of vitamin A can inhibit the action of these carcinogens in laboratory animals. Other studies have shown that vitamin C can reduce the probability of developing stomach and esophageal cancer in humans, and this cancer-inhibiting effect has also been supported by experimental studies in the laboratory. Thus, some substances that show toxicity to the body when consumed in excess, may actually have a protective role against cancer when taken in the right amounts.

Scientists usually study the relationship between diet and cancer in the laboratory by observing whether suspected substances can mutate bacteria (that is, damage bacterial DNA) or transform normal cells into cancer cells. Animal studies, which require that the suspected carcinogen be given in large amounts to accelerate the development of cancer, then follow. Obviously, a laboratory test that took twenty years to produce an answer (the time many cancers in humans may take to develop) would be useless, so a rapid test is desirable. Unfortunately, its very rapidity limits its usefulness as a predictor of cancers in humans. High doses of carcinogens over a short period of time may have very different effects from low doses spread over many years. This makes interpretation of data very uncertain. The laboratory tests are also limited because they ignore the way the body reacts to the substance, and whether the presence of other substances in the diet could influence the outcome. And after all this, we are still left wondering whether a carcinogen that causes cancer in rats can also cause cancer in humans. The ultimate experiment that would resolve this issue cannot be done, for obvious reasons, so we are always left with an element of uncertainty. Nevertheless, cyclamate, an artificial sweetener that can cause bladder cancer in rats, has been removed from the American market by the Food and Drug Administration. Many other powerful carcinogens, however, remain in our daily diet, and these must be identified and eliminated.

One very important example of a dietary carcinogen is the pesticide EDB (ethylene dibromide). EDB is one of the most powerful cancer-causing chemicals known, and is a serious contaminant of our grain products and some of our citrus fruit. In early 1984, the Environmental Protection Agency, having been aware of the potential risk for nearly ten years, at last began to take steps to reduce the level of EDB in the nation's food supply, but at a sluggish pace. The result is that all of us will continue to be exposed to this dangerous carcinogen for at least a few more years. In the meantime, the food-growers will find a substitute that probably will not have been thoroughly tested, and which could continue to pose a threat to the nation's health!

Another approach to the study of dietary factors and carcinogenesis has been *epidemiological.* (Epidemiology involves the study of dietary and disease patterns in large numbers of people.) The advantage of this approach is that it avoids the problems inherent in extrapolating experimental evidence from animals to humans. Furthermore, these studies often provide very useful directions for more specific research projects. It is unnecessary to go into detail as to how these studies are usually designed and conducted but, as you can imagine, the accurate measurement of food intake is of fundamental importance. In practice, this is easier said than done.

General information on food intake for a whole country is obtained by measuring the rate of disappearance of food that has been produced or imported, and by measuring the amount of different food products that stock each household. At a personal level, people are asked to describe as accurately as possible what they ate during the previous week, month, or year—perhaps even what their diet consisted of in childhood! The data from these studies are then averaged for each subpopulation or regional group to enable comparisons to be made. The findings have been fundamental to our present understanding of diet and cancer.

Some associations between diet and cancer that have emerged from international studies have not always been confirmed by studies within each country. This is usually because differences in diet between regions within a country are much smaller than the differences between the countries themselves. However, since studies of migrant populations have shown that cancer is predominantly diet-related and not genetic, these international studies provide very strong evidence to support specific dietary factors as being responsible for many types of cancer. In other words, failure to confirm an international study by one that is conducted within a country, is not an adequate reason to ignore the conclusions of the international study. Therefore, *my dietary recommendations may reflect the results of impressive international studies, even when these results have not been convincingly substantiated by national studies or by experiments with laboratory animals.*

I consider this approach justified because dietary recommendations, unlike speculative medical treatment, are unlikely to produce more harmful consequences than the dietary anarchy that currently exists.

My recommendations are also strongly supported by the dietary modifications that have been successfully made by religious communities such as the Seventh-Day Adventists and the Mormons. In both these communities, dietary modifications that were fortuitously similar to the latest scientific recommendations that form the basis of the Cancer Prevention Diet program *have substantially reduced the risk of cancer and heart disease without evidence of harmful effects of any kind.*

This means that you can approach your new diet program with confidence in the knowledge that it is both scientifically sound and of proven value.

What Is Your Cancer Risk?

It is impossible to give you precise statistical odds on your chances of developing cancer. What is possible is to give you a good idea of the scope of the cancer problem, and to discuss the known risk factors in a way that should help you to minimize your own risk of acquiring this fearful disease.

According to the best available estimates, more than 4 million people die each year from cancer, worldwide. In the United States, cancer causes about 20 percent of all deaths, and this percentage rises as the average age increases. However, when the influence of increasing age and population growth is excluded, there is no evidence to suggest that deaths from cancer are increasing—with the exception of cancer of the lung, which continues to increase at an alarming rate.

In 1983, the predicted incidence (number of new cases) of cancer in the United States was 855,000, with an additional incidence of 400,000 cases of treatable, nonmelanoma skin cancer. About 455,000 cancer deaths were also anticipated, despite access to the world's most costly and sophisticated health care system.

Apart from nonmelanoma skin cancer, about 70 percent of cancers arise in the digestive organs (colon, rectum, pancreas, stomach, liver, esophagus); the respiratory system (lung, larynx); the breasts (in women); and the genital organs (uterus, ovary, prostate, testis).

The risk of developing cancer is influenced by a wide range of factors that are summarized in Table 2–1.

To help you to understand the possible influence these factors may have in your life, let us review them in more detail.

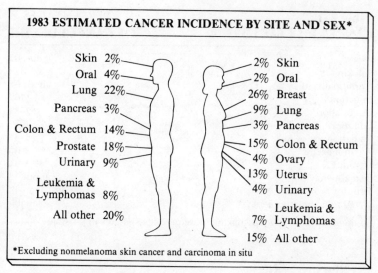

1983 ESTIMATED CANCER INCIDENCE BY SITE AND SEX*

Male			Female
Skin	2%	2%	Skin
Oral	4%	2%	Oral
Lung	22%	26%	Breast
Pancreas	3%	9%	Lung
Colon & Rectum	14%	3%	Pancreas
Prostate	18%	15%	Colon & Rectum
Urinary	9%	4%	Ovary
		13%	Uterus
		4%	Urinary
Leukemia & Lymphomas	8%	7%	Leukemia & Lymphomas
All other	20%	15%	All other

*Excluding nonmelanoma skin cancer and carcinoma in situ

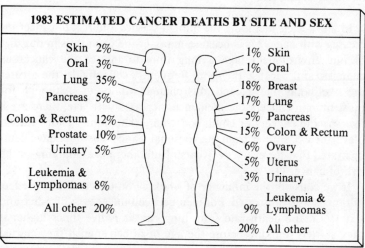

1983 ESTIMATED CANCER DEATHS BY SITE AND SEX

Male			Female
Skin	2%	1%	Skin
Oral	3%	1%	Oral
Lung	35%	18%	Breast
Pancreas	5%	17%	Lung
Colon & Rectum	12%	5%	Pancreas
Prostate	10%	15%	Colon & Rectum
Urinary	5%	6%	Ovary
		5%	Uterus
		3%	Urinary
Leukemia & Lymphomas	8%	9%	Leukemia & Lymphomas
All other	20%	20%	All other

Reproduced with permission of the American Cancer Society.

Figure 2–1

Table 2-1 CANCER RISK FACTORS	PERCENTAGES OF CANCER DEATHS
Diet	40–60%
Smoking	25–35%
Hormonal status	about 6%
Infection	1– 10%
Occupation	2–8%
Pollution	1–5%
Radiation exposure	2–4%
Alcohol excess	2–4%
Heredity	1–3%
Sexual behavior	about 1%
Drugs	less than 1%
Geographic environment	variable

Some risk factors overlap, making more precise estimates impossible.

INCREASING AGE

In all species, including the human species, the risk of cancer increases with age. This is because many of the chemicals in our diet or our environment take a long time to induce the cancerous changes, and because the more frequently cells divide, the greater the likelihood that a cancerous change will occur. Although for most human cancers the incidence increases with age, there are a few specific cancers of childhood where that trend is not evident. Nevertheless, studies from the National Cancer Institute have demonstrated that for every five years of life, there is a doubling of the risk of cancer (1).

If we consider the influence of smoking on cancer risk, the effect of time is well illustrated. For men between the ages of fifty-five and sixty-four, the death rate from lung cancer is five times higher if they started smoking before the age of fifteen than if they started after the age of twenty-five—assuming the same daily cigarette consumption (2). To an extent the reverse is also true. If you stop smoking, there is a progressive decline in your risk of lung cancer, but it takes fifteen years before the risk is equivalent to that of a nonsmoker!

Age is therefore not a direct cause of cancer, but rather it provides the time required for environmental factors to do their worst.

DIET

The National Academy of Sciences, the National Cancer Institute, and the American Cancer Society have now recognized the importance of diet as a major cause of cancer in the United States. It is estimated that as much as 60 percent of cancer in women and 40 percent of cancer in men is attributable to dietary factors (3). It has also been estimated that at least 35 percent of all cancer in the United States could be eliminated by simple changes in the nation's diet, using our current knowledge of dietary risk factors (4).

Some of the factors that you will learn about—and that are of critical importance—include: the amount of dietary fat; the amount of dietary fiber; contamination of some foods with molds such as aflatoxin; the presence of certain food additives; the amount of vegetables and fruit in your diet; your intake of vitamins A, C, E, folic acid and the mineral selenium; and methods of food preparation.

Although it is difficult to obtain a consensus on a subject as sensitive as the nation's diet, and because economic interests sometimes threaten to distort rational debate, it is essential that people be given the opportunity to understand the scientific evidence and to choose for themselves. This book is therefore designed to provide you with both an understanding of the problem of dietary cancer, and a solution that is based upon the latest scientific information—information that will increase and change as a result of continuing cancer research.

SMOKING

Cigarette smoking is *the major single cause of death from cancer* in the United States. About 30 percent of the deaths from cancer could be prevented if tobacco were unavailable. Instead, 129,000 Americans will die unnecessarily of cancer this year because of smoking.

Smoking is directly responsible for 85 percent of lung cancer deaths, 50–70 percent of deaths from oral and laryngeal cancer, more than 50 percent of deaths from esophageal cancer, 30–40 percent of deaths from bladder and kidney cancer, about 30 percent of deaths from pancreatic cancer, and a significant number of deaths from cancer of the stomach and cervix (5).

Since 1910, the annual cigarette production in the United States has increased from 4 billion to 600 billion, bringing with it human tragedy on a grand scale. Despite numerous scientific studies in many countries confirming that cigarette smoking is a major cause of premature disability, disease, and death, our taxes continue indirectly to subsidize the tobacco industry—and people continue to smoke.

Apart from cancer, smoking is also a major cause of premature deaths from heart attacks. The result of combining all the health hazards of smoking is that a twenty-five-year-old male who smokes fifteen cigarettes a day can expect to lose five and one-half years of life! And the more you smoke, the greater the risk.

GEOGRAPHIC ENVIRONMENT

If cancer incidence is examined on an international basis, there is a remarkable variation in the frequency with which different cancers occur. For example, in countries with a high intake of dietary fat, there is usually a higher incidence of cancers of the breast, colon, rectum, pancreas, uterus, prostate, and ovary.

When people migrated from Japan, which has a low fat consumption rate, to Hawaii, which has a much higher fat consumption rate, the pattern of cancer of the breast, colon, and stomach in these migrants resembled that of the indigenous population within one or two generations (6). Intriguingly, studies of first-generation (foreign-born) migrants to the United States have revealed that during their lifetime, stomach cancer mortality is consistent with the country of origin, while colon cancer mortality reflects the country of destination (7).

Such trends have been seen not only among the Japanese migrants to Hawaii (8), but also among Europeans who migrated to the United States and Canada (7).

Table 2–2 summarizes the differences in cancer death rates in various countries around the world. Countries are ranked in order of age-adjusted death rates from all cancers per 100,000 population, based upon information made available in 1976–1977 (9).

Table 2-2
INTERNATIONAL CANCER DEATH RATES

MALE DEATHS per 100,000	FEMALE DEATHS per 100,000
1. Uruguay	Uruguay
2. Scotland	Denmark
3. Belgium	Scotland
4. Netherlands	Hungary
5. Hungary	Ireland
6. France	England and Wales
7. England and Wales	Austria
8. Austria	West Germany
9. West Germany	Chile
10. Singapore	New Zealand
11. Switzerland	Northern Ireland
12. Denmark	Belgium
13. Northern Ireland	Netherlands
14. Hong Kong	Israel
15. Ireland	Sweden
16. New Zealand	Costa Rica
17. United States	Iceland
18. Poland	Argentina
19. Argentina	United States
20. East Germany	Canada
21. Canada	Switzerland
22. Australia	East Germany
23. Chile	Norway
24. Sweden	Venezuela
25. Spain	Australia
26. Norway	Singapore
27. Japan	Poland
28. Greece	Hong Kong
29. Malta	France
30. Israel	Paraguay

Reproduced with permission of the American Cancer Society.

No statistics are available from China or the Soviet Union. But it is thought that the incidence of cancer in China is quite low compared to Western countries.

These countries are listed in decreasing order of cancer mortality. Uruguay, which tops the list for both men and women, had 294 deaths per 100,000 males, and 180 deaths per 100,000 females. With the exception of Venezuela and Honduras, male deaths were significantly higher than female deaths. In the United States, for example, there were 213 male deaths for every 136 female deaths in 1976–1977. However, in 1983, 432,500 new cases of female cancer and 422,500 cases of male cancer were predicted. This may mean that women generally survive cancer better than men.

When one considers the influence of geography *within* the United States there are some interesting regional variations.

Table 2–3
ESTIMATED CANCER INCIDENCE AND DEATHS FOR 1983
WITHIN THE UNITED STATES

	New Cases	Deaths	Death Rate per 100,000
1. District of Columbia	3,200	1,600	260
2. Rhode Island	4,700	2,400	248
3. Florida	51,000	26,600	237
4. Pennsylvania	53,000	27,000	227
5. New Jersey	32,000	16,400	219
6. Maine	4,800	2,500	217
7. Massachusetts	24,000	12,600	215
8. New York	74,000	37,500	212
9. Connecticut	13,000	6,700	210
10. Missouri	20,000	10,500	210
11. Arkansas	9,000	4,700	203
12. Nebraska	6,000	3,200	201
13. Ohio	42,000	21,500	200
14. Iowa	11,200	5,700	199
15. West Virginia	7,700	3,900	199
16. Delaware	2,400	1,200	198
17. Maryland	16,700	8,600	197
18. New Hampshire	3,600	1,900	196
19. Illinois	44,000	22,500	195
20. South Dakota	2,600	1,300	193
21. Indiana	20,000	10,400	192
22. Kentucky	13,600	7,000	191
23. Kansas	8,700	4,600	190
24. Alabama	14,300	7,400	186
25. Oregon	9,800	5,000	186
26. Wisconsin	18,000	9,000	186
27. Tennessee	17,100	8,600	184
28. Oklahoma	11,600	6,000	183

Table 2-3 (*continued*)

	New Cases	Deaths	Death Rate per 100,000
29. Vermont	2,000	950	181
30. Michigan	32,000	16,400	181
31. Mississippi	8,900	4,600	180
32. North Dakota	2,500	1,200	179
33. Minnesota	14,000	7,300	177
34. California	85,000	44,500	175
35. North Carolina	20,000	10,400	170
36. Louisiana	14,800	7,600	167
37. Washington	14,400	7,300	165
38. Arizona	9,000	4,900	165
39. Montana	2,600	1,300	162
40. Virginia	17,200	8,900	158
41. Georgia	17,300	9,000	155
42. South Carolina	9,600	4,900	150
43. Idaho	2,700	1,400	141
44. Texas	44,000	22,400	140
45. Nevada	2,600	1,300	136
46. New Mexico	3,500	1,800	129
47. Colorado	7,600	3,900	124
48. Wyoming	1,300	650	120
49. Hawaii	2,400	1,200	118
50. Utah	3,000	1,500	91
51. Alaska	600	300	69

Reproduced with permission of the American Cancer Society.

Florida has such a high cancer death rate because more elderly people retire there (these data are not age-adjusted). Utah has a lower cancer death rate because the diet of Mormons is much closer to a cancer prevention diet than the diet of the rest of the population. Alaska's low figures are possibly attributable to a diet that is higher in fish.

If you examine Table 2–2 and the map of the United States in Figure 2-2, you will see that the cancer death rate in the northeastern states is double that of Utah, and considerably higher than the states of the Southwest.

The conclusion to be drawn from all this information is that where you live in the world, and where you live in the United States, can make a difference to your cancer risk. But if you bring

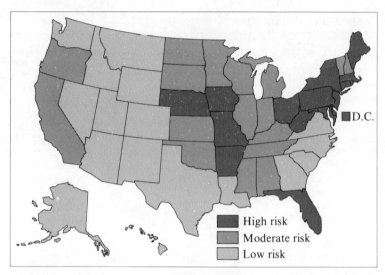

Figure 2-2
GEOGRAPHIC DISTRIBUTION OF
CANCER DEATH RATES—1983

bad habits or risks acquired early in life with you, a low-risk region may not help much. On the other hand, if you move to a high-risk region and bring good habits with you, your risk of cancer may be prevented from rising.

RADIATION EXPOSURE

There is no completely safe level of radiation. And since nearly all forms of cancer can be induced by radiation, the level to which we are exposed is of considerable importance. About 3 percent of human cancer today is caused by radiation (4).

All of us are exposed to what is called "background radiation" every day. Background radiation comes from cosmic rays, and the greater the altitude, the greater the exposure. Some background radiation also comes from the earth itself, but so far no scientific evidence exists that links human cancer to natural background radiation.

The advent of nuclear weapons has resulted in a small increase in background radiation from atmospheric testing, but so far there is no evidence to link this with human cancer, apart from an increase in leukemia among people who lived downwind from the Nevada test site.

Survivors of the atomic bombs that fell on Hiroshima and Nagasaki have shown an increased risk of leukemia, thyroid, breast, and lung cancer.

Most of our radiation exposure comes from medical x-rays, and it is estimated that more than 240 million x-rays annually are performed on the American public. Many of these x-rays were medically justified, but many surely resulted from the pressure on many physicians to practice "defensive" medicine for fear of litigation.

The greatest x-ray exposure come to some of us during the treatment of cancer, and this can increase the risk of second cancers in some patients. In most cases, the benefits of this intense radiation exposure far outweigh the risks of a second cancer. However, when x-ray exposure is not for cancer treatment, the benefits may not always outweigh the risks. Therefore, I suggest that you always discuss the risks with your doctor.

Some occupations have been found to be particularly hazardous. An increased risk of bone cancer has been found in luminous watch dial painters. Radiologists themselves have an increased risk of developing leukemia and skin cancer. Uranium miners, who work with radioactive material, have an increased risk of lung cancer *even if they do not smoke.*

Finally, solar radiation is the main source of ultraviolet radiation, which can cause skin cancer (particularly in fair-skinned people). Avoiding strong sunlight and using strong barrier creams will reduce the risk substantially.

HORMONAL FACTORS

If the ovaries were removed at birth, the risk of a woman developing breast cancer would be virtually eliminated. This illustrates the extraordinary influence that hormones have on the growth and development of cells, and on the risk of their becoming cancerous.

Women who reach the menopause without ever having experienced pregnancy have a higher risk of breast cancer than those who have been pregnant. And the more children a woman has borne, the lower her risk. If her first pregnancy occurred before the age of twenty, the risk is lower still. Women who have never menstruated have three to four times the risk of developing breast cancer after the age of fifty-five compared to other women of the same age who have had normal menstruation. But if menstruation starts late in adolescence, or if the menopause is early, the risk of breast cancer is reduced.

The use of birth control pills that are high in progesterone has been shown to increase the risk of breast cancer, but this risk has probably been eliminated by the reduction in progesterone in low-dose pills. Birth control pills may also help to reduce the risk of ovarian cancer, but it is unclear to what extent the changes in hormone strength and balance will influence these effects.

Finally, the use of DES [diethylstilbestrol] by pregnant mothers has been responsible for the tragic development of cancer of the vagina and cervix in their daughters during childhood. Of course, this risk factor has now been eliminated.

SEXUAL BEHAVIOR

Human attitudes to sexuality can influence the risk of cancer. Early promiscuity is associated with an increased risk of cancer of the cervix (which accounts for approximately 1.5 percent of cancer deaths) (4). Interestingly, this disease is also more common in women who have had several children, and less common in women who have had only one child. In fact, this observation may relate more to the number of sexual partners than to pregnancy and childbirth. It is not known whether the risk for women who have only one sexual partner is increased if that partner previously had multiple partners. In all events, cervical cancer is extremely rare in virgins. Although the precise mechanism by which cervical cancer is induced is not understood, the *nature* as well as the *number* of partners is relevant, for cervical cancer is more common when male partners are uncircumcised. If this observation is coupled with the fact that cancer of the penis occurs only in the uncircumcised, we are led to conclude that hygiene itself plays a role in cervical carcinogenesis; and the most likely culprit is one of the herpes viruses.

The outbreak of AIDS [acquired immune deficiency syndrome] among sexually active male homosexuals in the early 1980s has led to a dramatic increase in the incidence of an otherwise rare form of fatal cancer called Kaposi's sarcoma. Furthermore, because of the breakdown of the body's natural defenses, victims of AIDS have an increased susceptibility to infection, and often die of a life-threatening form of pneumonia called Pneumocystis carinii.

The cause of this immune impairment among homosexuals is now thought to be most likely due to infection with a retrovirus known as HTLV, recently identified at the Pasteur Institute in Paris, and also at the National Cancer Institute in the United States. Having multiple sexual partners also increases the risk of acquiring AIDS, which supports the evidence that AIDS is acquired by the transmission of some kind of infectious agent, notably an HTLV retrovirus. Furthermore, male homosexuals are also at an increased risk of developing cancer of the tongue and the anus (10).

ALCOHOL EXCESS

While a glass of wine each day may actually help to reduce your risk of heart disease, an excessive indulgence in alcohol, especially when combined with smoking, is thought to cause about 3 percent of all cancer in the United States.

Alcohol is known to increase the risk of cancer of the mouth, pharynx, larynx, esophagus, and liver (4). This subject is discussed in greater detail in Chapter 11.

OCCUPATION

Although most occupations do not increase your cancer risk, some do. Current estimates suggest that as much as 5 percent of all cancer in the United States is due to occupational exposure (4).

In 1472, Ulrich Ellenbog, a German physician from Augsburg, published a pamphlet entitled "On the Poisonous, Evil Vapors and Fumes of Metals." This was the first study of occupational hazards, and it described the irritating effect of fumes of lead and mercury experienced by goldsmiths.

The first clinical report of an occupational cancer hazard was made by Percival Pott in 1775. In this report he described the increased risk of cancer of the scrotum among chimney sweeps. His observations illustrated typical characteristics of carcinogen exposure. However, it was his grandson, Henry Earle, who observed in 1823 that only a small proportion of the exposed chimney sweeps would actually go on to develop cancer, and that this might take as long as twenty years to develop. His observations stimulated ideas about environmental causes of cancer, differences in individual susceptibility, differences in the susceptibility of different body tissues, and the long latency period before cancer develops.

Occupational cancers mostly result from exposure to toxic chemicals in manufacturing industries, or from exposure to certain types of dust in mining. The degree of risk can range from minor to major. For example, as much as 20 percent of male bladder cancer has been attributed to occupational chemical exposure! Some of the better-known occupational cancers are listed in Table 2–4.

Since there are over 50,000 known chemicals (with new ones joining that list every week), and since only about 500 have ever been tested for their cancer-causing potential, it is obvious that we do not have a clear idea of the risk posed to us by their existence.

Table 2–4
SOME OCCUPATIONAL CANCERS

Occupation	Type of Cancer
• Rubber workers, dye manufacturers, coal gas workers	Bladder
• Asbestos workers and anyone exposed to asbestos	Lung, mesothelioma, esophagus, stomach, colon
• Glue and varnish workers	Leukemia
• Cadmium workers	Prostate
• Workers exposed to chromium	Lung
• Uranium miners, luminizers, radiologists (radiation exposure)	Lung, bone, marrow
• Manufacturers of isopropyl alcohol, hardwood furniture makers, leather workers	Nasal sinuses
• Nickel refiners	Lung, nasal sinuses
• Farmers, seamen, and anyone exposed to ultraviolet light	Skin
• Makers of polyvinyl chloride (PVC)	Liver

The only sensible attitude is to avoid exposure to known toxic chemicals whenever you have a choice.

INFECTION

Infection can occur with bacteria, viruses, fungi, or parasites. Bacteria and most parasites can usually be destroyed by treatment with antibiotics or other drugs. Viruses cannot yet be treated effectively.

Infection may involve selected parts of the body. For example, bacteria may infect the lungs (pneumonia), viruses can infect the liver (hepatitis), and parasites called schistosomes may infect the bladder. The importance of these examples is that hepatitis increases the risk of liver cancer and schistosomes increase the risk of bladder cancer; fortunately, bacteria do not directly increase your risk of lung cancer. Although some viruses are also suspected of causing some other types of cancer, there is no evidence implicating bacteria in carcinogenesis. However, bacteria normally residing in our intestines often play an important role in the breakdown of dietary carcinogens.

Viruses have excited a great deal of scientific interest, yet there is still very little evidence that they play a direct role in the causation of human cancer, despite intensive study during the past twenty-five years. One intriguing observation resulted from the study of a child whose leukemia had been eradicated, but who developed leukemia again after a transplant of normal marrow cells from a healthy relative. In that case it was possible to prove that the leukemic cells were those of the donor. This meant that the normal donor cells had been converted to leukemic cells by some other factor in the body, possibly a resident virus.

In daily life there is little that we can do to control our exposure to viruses, or any effect that they might have.

POLLUTION

The air we breathe, the water we drink, and the food we eat are all contaminated to some extent with the products of our civilization.

Air pollution at its most severe can drastically reduce visibility, irritate the eyes, and precipitate pneumonia in the elderly. The London fog of 1952 killed thousands of Londoners, but not from cancer.

It has been noted that although lung cancer is more common in our cities than in the countryside, it still remains very low among urban nonsmokers. This observation suggests that air pollutants may work in conjunction with the chemicals in tobacco smoke to cause lung cancer, rather than as a direct cause of lung cancer. Yet, if one compares the death rate from lung cancer in Maine with that in New Jersey, the rates appear comparable. Evidently, at least with respect to lung cancer, the pure air in Maine does not confer any benefits over the more polluted air in New Jersey.

Nonetheless, one particular air pollutant which cannot be ignored is asbestos. Even small amounts of asbestos on the clothes of factory workers have been held responsible for the increase in the incidence of mesothelioma (usually a rare form of cancer) among family members. Furthermore, many school buildings around the United States still have asbestos insulation, which is probably putting the lives of our children at risk.

Water pollution, on the other hand, is still the cause of a great deal of disease around the world. The availability of clean water and proper sanitation has probably done more to improve our health than anything else. In the industrialized countries, we believe that we have the finest, cleanest water available. But this precious resource is being slowly destroyed by industrial pollution.

Although anxiety about water pollution as a possible cancer risk has been expressed for twenty-five years, the number of carcinogenic substances appearing in our drinking water continues to rise. Over 700 synthetic organic chemicals have been identified in the American water supply, and about 40 of these are either known or suspected carcinogens! Apart from asbestos fibers, which often contaminate the water supply near large cities, other cancer-causing chemicals such as polyvinyl chloride, benzene, and chloromethyl ether have also been found.

Some minerals are present in our water supply. Probably the one which has the most certain association with cancer is arsenic. For example, in Taiwan, water contaminated with arsenic has caused skin cancer (11).

Despite the fact that there is relatively little evidence that water pollution has directly caused human cancer in the United States, this is not a reason for complacency. As the concentration of pollutants increases, the risk of cancer will surely increase too. The new epidemic of cancer in the fish population should be a warning to us all.

In 1984, twelve years after the Clean Water Act, it was noticed that the fish which were returning to once polluted waters, such as the Hudson River and Michigan's Torch Lake, were suffering from a very high cancer rate. And the fish that were most affected were those that lived nearest to the bottom, where the concentration of chemical contaminants is highest.

In the Hudson River, for example, more than 80 percent of the Atlantic tomcod that are more than two years old have liver cancer. And in Everett Harbor, Washington, more than two thirds of the English sole have damaged livers that are usually cancerous.

When water pollutants were concentrated and painted onto the skin of bullheads, many of those fish developed cancer within a year. Although the implications are rather alarming, some fish, such as striped bass, do not develop tumors in the way bullheads do; so other factors also influence the effect of chemical pollutants.

What has happened to fish may not happen to man. But alarm over the increased risk of cancer among people whose homes are built on chemical waste dumps, and the implications that this surely has in terms of water pollution, should make us determined to act now rather than wait for human tragedy to manifest itself.

From a nutritional point of view, fish should be one of the best forms of "meat" protein; however, eating fish rich in chemical contaminants hardly constitutes sound dietary advice. Any dietary recommendation that I make is therefore based on the assumption that you will seek out sources of food that are not polluted. This may not always be easy!

HEREDITY

Not everyone is at the same risk of developing cancer, no matter what the cause. This is also true for animals that are studied in the laboratory. When you expose a group of inbred laboratory mice to a carcinogen, some of them develop cancer and some do not. If you increase the dose of the carcinogen, more of them are affected. Why? The most important reason is that there are subtle genetic differences which influence individual susceptibility to carcinogen exposure. The same principle holds true for humans.

Human cancer is caused by a variable mix of hereditary and environmental factors. Heredity is pot luck. The environment you can partially control. Consider a fair-skinned woman living in Arizona who develops nonmelanotic skin cancer. Her fair skin increased her risk of reacting to the ultraviolet rays in sunlight which can cause skin cancer. By often exposing herself to the strong sunlight of the Arizona desert at midday without protective clothing or sun screens, this woman greatly increased her risk of skin cancer. In this example, her inherited fair skin—over which she had no control—reacted to the environment, over which she had some control. This principle applies to many different types of cancer. However, except for differences in some specific cancer risks for men and women, we usually do not know which inherited characteristics provide vulnerability or protection.

There are also a few rare diseases which are inherited and which predispose to certain cancers. There are also a few families in which, for no apparent reason, there is an abnormally high cancer risk. In these families there is usually an increased risk of cancer in general rather than a preponderance of a particular type of cancer.

However, there are some types of breast cancer, colon cancer, and brain cancer that can be inherited. Some individuals with stomach cancer and lung cancer may also have an inheritable form. For example, the risk of colon cancer or breast cancer can increase as much as twenty- to thirtyfold in these families. I remember hearing of one tragic family in which the risk of breast cancer was extraordinarily high. The mother of three daughters had breast cancer, and two of the daughters had developed breast cancer by the age of twenty-two. The third daughter was twenty when I heard of this, and her physicians were debating whether she should have both breasts removed as a preventive measure. A horrifying decision for both the young girl and her physicians.

In a few instances, racial differences appear to protect against a specific cancer. For example, dark-skinned races are protected from the harmful effects of sunlight and seldom develop melanoma [except on depigmented palms and soles]; Orientals very seldom develop chronic lymphocytic leukemia, wherever they happen to live. Obviously, these differences must be the result of some genetic rather than environmental difference.

I do not wish you to be left with the impression that cancer is an inherited disease. Family risks apply to very few cancers, and the vast majority are brought about by environmental factors that must be identified and controlled. By the same token, you should not feel that inherited factors will *protect* you from cancer. Just as some laboratory animals appear genetically protected at low levels of carcinogen exposure and vulnerable at high levels of carcinogen exposure, so humans are also more vulnerable when carcinogen exposure increases. Never has this been more clearly shown than in the relationship between the number of cigarettes smoked and the risk of lung cancer.

STRESS AND EXERCISE

A great deal has been written about the harmful effects of stress and the virtues of regular exercise. The difficulty in relating either to cancer risk is that the evidence at best is only circumstantial. The problem is similar to the question of whether disturbed childhoods cause criminal behavior. If you choose to think that everyone has had some problems in childhood, then criminals are no different from anyone else. Alternatively, you can look only at the childhoods of convicted criminals, and since many of them reveal problems, you can conclude that these problems were the cause of their criminality.

In the case of cancer patients, many of them will reveal some stress in their lives. But stress is also part of the lives of many people who do not have cancer. If we extend the discussion to include the risk of other diseases, especially heart disease and high blood pressure, then the evidence that stress is harmul to health is much stronger. As with so many other aspects of life it is probably a question of degree. A little stress is beneficial because the stimulus is needed to prevent one from losing interest in life. On the other hand, too much stress places an intolerable burden on *any* organism. Sooner or later something will give way. In an attempt to explore the relationship of stress to cancer, some experiments have been carried out with mice, but the stress imposed on mice (electric shocks) has little to do with human stress, and I personally do not think that any difference in their cancer rates can be extrapolated to humans.

When it comes to exercise, there is no evidence that regular exercise influences cancer risk per se, but there is a great deal of evidence that it contributes to general health and well-being.

SOCIOECONOMIC STATUS

The evidence linking socioeconomic status to cancer is limited. Of course, dietary differences between different social and economic groups certainly exist in the United States and elsewhere, but we have relatively little precise dietary information about the differences.

Studies of two relatively uncommon forms of cancer, Hodgkin's disease and testicular cancer, have revealed that they occur more commonly among those with above-average education who are in higher socioeconomic groups. Certain more common cancers—cancer of the colon, the skin cancer called melanoma, and cancer of the uterus—are also found with greater frequency in higher socioeconomic groups. Although there is no explanation for these intriguing observations, I do not mean to suggest that you should drop out of college to avoid these cancers!

In contrast, both esophageal and stomach cancer are more common in lower socioeconomic groups in virtually all countries of the world. This is most probably the result of a combination of smoking, alcohol, and a poor diet that lacks an adequate amount of fruit and vegetables.

Now that you are familiar with the main risk factors, how do they relate to the common cancers that may have already afflicted close friends or members of your family?

Table 2–5 summarizes some of the important risk factors associated with the more common types of cancer. The estimated number of new cases for 1983 are included to give you an idea of how often different cancers occur.

The term "geographic environment" is used in this table to mean

Table 2-5
COMMON CANCERS AND SOME OF THEIR RISK FACTORS

Cancer Type	Some Risk Factors	New Cases 1983
SKIN	Race (fair skin); strong sunlight; radiation; arsenic in water.	400,000
MELANOMA	Latitude, strong sunlight; fair skin; family tendency; Irish descent; soles of feet in blacks; upper socioeconomic group.	17,500
LUNG	Smoking; diet (low vitamin A and beta-carotene); asbestos; radiation; exposure to nickel and chromium. Pathologists have increased risk.	135,000
BREAST	Diet (high fat, meat; ? low selenium); obesity; no pregnancy; late pregnancy; early menarche; late menopause; high-dose birth control pill;* geographic location; upper socioeconomic group; urban areas.	114,900
COLON/RECTUM	Diet (high fat, high cholesterol, meat, beer, nitrosamines, low fiber, lack of vegetables, low vitamin A and C); some occupations; asbestos exposure; some bowel diseases; obesity; urban areas; upper socioeconomic group.	126,000
PROSTATE	Diet (high fat, lack of vitamin A, lack of vegetables); smoking; geographic location; race (blacks); family tendency; ? higher sexual activity; cadmium exposure; ? dietary zinc; previous venereal disease; some occupations.	75,000
PANCREAS	Smoking; diabetes; diet (? fat, ? coffee, ? alcohol, ? meat, ? eggs); increased risk among Jews and Polynesians; reduced risk among Mormons and Seventh-Day Adventists; urban areas.	25,000
LEUKEMIA	Radiation; race (less in Orientals); heredity; some drugs; some chemicals; ? viruses.	23,500
STOMACH	Diet (smoked and salt-pickled foods; lack of vegetables rich in vitamin A and C; nitrite and nitrate levels; obesity; smoking; nitrates in drinking water; lower socioeconomic status.	24,500
ESOPHAGUS	Diet (low intake of green vegetables, fruit, trace minerals, fish and animal protein, vitamins A, B_1, C; high intake of very hot beverages, pickled or moldy foods); smoking; alcohol; urban areas; lower socioeconomic status.	9,000

* Most current birth control pills are not high-dose; if you are in doubt, consult your physician.

Table 2-5 (*continued*)

Cancer Type	Some Risk Factors	New Cases 1983
UTERUS	Diet (high fat, meat); factors similar to breast cancer; high socioeconomic status; postmenopausal treatment with estrogens; obesity; low-dose birth control pill reduces risk	39,000
UTERINE CERVIX	Diet (lack of fruit, ? excess protein); promiscuity; uncircumcised male partners.	16,000
OVARY	Diet (high fat, meat); risks similar to breast cancer; asbestos exposure; risks reduced by pregnancy and low-dose birth control pill.	18,200
BLADDER	White males at greatest risk; smoking; occupations such as house painter, chemical worker, hairdresser, truck driver, textile worker, printer; diet (? lack of dietary vitamin A, ? coffee, ? artificial sweeteners, high fat).	38,500
KIDNEY	Smoking; diet (? coffee, milk, meat); obesity; cadmium exposure.	18,200
LIVER	Infection with hepatitis virus; moldy food contaminated with aflatoxin; urban areas.	13,300
MOUTH/ PHARYNX	Smoking, especially combined with alcohol; betel chewing in India; prolonged mouthwash use; "dip snuff" use in the South; lack of vitamins A and B complex; asbestos exposure; occupations such as printer, leather worker, bartender, waitress.	27,100
LARYNX	Smoking; alcohol.	11,000
HODGKIN'S DISEASE	High socioeconomic groups; higher education.	7,100
LYMPHOMAS	Urban areas; upper socioeconomic status; after kidney transplants.	23,600
MULTIPLE MYELOMA	Radiation; race (blacks); family tendency; occupations such as printing (exposure to lead vapors) and radiology.	9,600
THYROID	Radiation exposure; more common in females.	10,200
BRAIN	White males at greatest risk; occupations such as oil refinery worker, chemists, embalmer, farmer; exposure to pesticides. Can affect children: lead exposure; epilepsy in siblings; diet (nitrates); high-dose x-rays; barbiturate drugs taken by mother during pregnancy.	12,600
BONE	Radiation; race (rare in blacks and Orientals).	1,900

The question marks placed in front of certain items means that these are suspected to be a risk factor, but that the association has not been proved.

Table 2–6

DO ANY OF THESE RISK FACTORS APPLY TO YOU?

Above age fifty-five
Smoker
Typical American diet
Occupational exposure to carcinogens
High alcohol intake
Lived many years in high-risk area
Overweight
Radiation exposure
Blood relatives with cancer
Chronic infective hepatitis
Strong sun exposure
Urban environment
Upper socioeconomic group (colon)
Lower socioeconomic group (esophagus and stomach)
Early onset of menstruation
Late onset of menopause
Never been pregnant
First pregnancy after age thirty
Early promiscuity (females only)
Uncircumcised male

the effect of living in a different state in the United States or in a different country.

For readers who like facts and figures, the message should be clear. There are many cancer risk factors that have been identified, and some that have not. Perhaps the easiest way to remember them is to see how many of these risk factors apply to you. Of course, if you do have some of these risk factors it does not mean that you have cancer or will necessarily get it. It means that your chances are increased to some degree.

Some of these risk factors can be changed, others cannot. Diet is clearly one factor that is in need of major improvement, especially since it is thought to account for about 60 percent of cancer among women and 40 percent of cancer among men in the United States.

Other risk factors should also be reduced whenever possible. The sensible approach to reducing your chance of developing cancer is summarized in Table 2–7.

The next chapter will introduce you to the current American diet, and give you some idea of how it has evolved as a result of the

Table 2-7
WHAT YOU CAN DO TO REDUCE YOUR CANCER RISK

- Stop smoking!
- Adopt a cancer prevention diet!
- Reduce your exposure to radiation!
- Reduce your exposure to strong sunlight!
- Moderate your alcohol consumption!
- Avoid an occupation associated with an increased cancer risk!
- Maintain an ideal weight!
- Live in a low-risk area if possible!
- If you are over thirty-five, consult your physician annually!

power of the food industry and the manipulative power of advertising.

However, before we leave this chapter, you must be made aware of the eight warning signs of cancer; so here they are. Try to commit them to memory.

Table 2-8
THE EIGHT WARNING SIGNS OF CANCER

- A lump or thickening in the breast
- A change in a wart or mole in the skin
- An ulcer or sore that does not heal
- A change in your bowel or bladder habits
- A persistent cough or hoarseness of the voice
- Constant indigestion or difficulty in swallowing
- An unusual bleeding or discharge
- A recent unexplained weight loss of 10 pounds or more

Note: The existence of any one of these warning signs does not mean that you definitely have cancer, only that you should visit your doctor for a checkup.

Source: The American Cancer Society.

CHAPTER 3

What on Earth Are We Eating?

About 35 percent of cancer in the United States could be eliminated by relatively simple changes in the nation's diet. However, before we make constructive changes in our diets, we have to know as much as we can about the food that we expose our bodies to each day. Most of us either eat what is placed before us or choose foods on impulse. It has sometimes amazed me to see scientists who are experts in nutrition choose from a menu. They may pick items with some of the very worst ingredients, completely ignoring all that they have learned from years of study. This is the dietary equivalent of doctors who smoke without regard for risk. Obviously the desire to gratify our senses can completely overwhelm our common sense—if we let it!

Finding out exactly what is in our total diet is not easy, especially when you realize that even a simple potato is made of over 150 different chemicals. In recent years there has been an increase in the willingness of manufacturers to list some of the ingredients in their food products—mostly as a result of laws forcing them to do so. But this is only part of the story. Often the actual amount of each constituent is not revealed, and some ingredients remain quite obscure. Terms like "natural coloring" and "artificial color" can mean almost anything to the consumer, and most of us have little knowledge of what these substances are or what they may do, particularly when combined with all the other natural chemicals that we eat. Many manufacturers are reluctant to reveal the nature of nonnutritive food additives. Some of these compounds have been shown to be involved in either causing or inhibiting the development of cancer. Although most food additives are in fact useful because they can improve the nutritional value and flavor of food while preventing spoilage, others may be harmful and should be avoided.

Possibly the whole idea of foods being classified only by their nutritive value may need to be revised, and changes in the chemical composition of our food supply must be adequately monitored and regulated.

HAS OUR DIET CHANGED MUCH?

Between 1909 and 1976, there was little change in the food supply and the total consumption of nutrients in the United States. (However, there is a considerable difference between the total consumption of nutrients by all Americans, and the *balance of nutrients consumed by an individual.*) Nevertheless, some changes did occur. These were detected by measuring the rate at which certain foods "disappeared." These studies indicated that there was a small decline in the consumption of total calories, with no change in total protein, and a modest decline in carbohydrates. Total consumption of most vitamins and minerals remained unchanged, but that of iron, Vitamin B_1, Vitamin B_2, and niacin was increased, while that of magnesium was decreased. The increases were almost entirely due to the enrichment of refined flour and the popularity of white bread, while the loss of magnesium occurred during the process of refining whole wheat grains.

The relative stability of the American diet between 1909 and 1976 is deceptive, however. During this period the use of pesticides and fertilizers increased enormously, while the addition of hormones and antibiotics to animal feed by farmers became commonplace. Although these changes in farming methods were very effective ways to increase food production, nobody really knows what effect these changes have had on the chemical composition of the American diet.

Often food grown in one region is transported or exported to another before it is eaten. For example, a typical New York supermarket may be stocked with local produce, fruit and vegetables from California, beef from Texas, potatoes from Idaho, and bread made from wheat grown in the Midwest. This apparently simple fact complicates any attempt to analyze the relationship between what people eat and their cancer risk, because the frequency of cancer varies a good deal from one region to another within the United States. Evidence already exists that differences in the vitamin and mineral content of vegetables may result from the way they are grown, transported, and stored. Consequently, it is likely that regional variation in the chemical nature of food contributes to regional variation in cancer incidence.

Let us now review some examples that will serve to illustrate the extent to which the American diet has changed over the years. Any of these examples could influence your chances of getting cancer, depending on how much your own diet is typical of these national trends.

- Food color additives increased tenfold between 1940 and 1977. Since some coloring agents were found to be carcinogenic, the thirty coloring agents now in use have been extensively tested for carcinogenicity. (This does not apply to artificial flavorings, some of which have never been tested.)
- Soft drink consumption increased by 50 percent between 1960 and 1977. This included diet soft drinks that increased our intake of saccharin, known to be capable of causing bladder cancer in laboratory animals. Saccharin is now sold only with a warning label.
- The intake of fresh potatoes has declined by 66 percent since 1900, whereas the intake of processed potatoes has increased 4,400% in the past thirty years. The total intake of potatoes is now less than half that consumed in 1900; this is a major change in the intake of one of our most basic dietary constituents.
- The intake of fresh fruit and vegetables has declined by about 30 percent since 1909, but this has been matched by a comparable increase in the consumption of processed fruit and vegetables (though much of the fruit consumption is now in the form of fruit juices). This trend has altered the natural fiber content in our diet, formerly supplied by these foods. And there may well be adverse effects resulting from the use of various preservatives, artificial flavorings, and other chemicals in processed vegetables and fruits.
- The intake of canned and bottled tomato products increased by 500 percent between 1920 and 1976. As with other foods, this processing not only alters the composition of food, but it also eliminates the natural seasonal variation in dietary intake that occurs with fresh vegetables.

- Vitamin C production in United States in 1960 was 2,392 metric tons. This increased to roughly 14,800 metric tons in 1982. Since vitamin C can be used as a food preservative as well as a nutrient, it is not always recorded among the listed ingredients on food products. So sometimes we do not know when we are eating it. This increase in vitamin C consumption is desirable, however, because there is evidence that vitamin C can reduce the risk of cancers such as those of the esophagus and stomach.
- Consumption of butter and lard (both of which are saturated fats) has fallen by about 80% since 1950, but this has been accompanied by a very significant increase in the intake of margarine and vegetable oil (unsaturated fats). While these changes in fat consumption should help to reduce the development of heart disease, the persistence of excess fat in the diet unfortunately increases the risk of certain cancers. This situation is aggravated by the fact that the total amount of fat eaten by the average American has actually gone up by 27 percent in the past thirty years! What makes this development even more surprising is that this increase in fat consumption has taken place during a period of social history when nobody wished to be fat.

  The number of calories derived from fat in the modern American diet has increased by a staggering 35 percent since the beginning of the century. Fat now accounts for over 40 percent of America's total calorie intake, bringing with it an increased risk of cancers such as those of the breast and prostate. Reducing fat consumption is therefore a major goal in dietary cancer prevention.
- Until recently, fiber was thought to be unimportant and was largely removed from our "civilized" diet. In fact, it was considered a real nuisance, possibly preventing the absorption of some minerals, and definitely preventing bread from being "pure" and white! Fortunately for all of us, a British scientist, Denis Burkitt, made an astute observation: certain African tribes whose "primitive" diets were high in fiber had a very low incidence of typical Western diseases such as colon cancer, heart disease, varicose veins, and obesity—diseases that have only become common in Western societies during the twentieth century.

  Most of us still eat far too little fiber, even though there is evidence that a high-fiber diet could help to reduce our total calorie intake, limit the damaging effects of dietary fat, possibly reduce the risk of colon cancer, and reduce the incidence of other diseases such as diverticulitis.
- Food is not always what it used to be! Mass-produced food items such as pizza, TV dinners, or smoked meats may not be made with the same ingredients as were used ten years ago. Food substitutes, fillers, preservatives, and artificial flavorings can change the composition of

food products without any of us realizing it. And who knows what effect these changes will have on our health?

- Artificial sweeteners such as saccharin have been deliberately added to our diets, and have consequently been consumed freely. Since they are promoted as a way to slimness and health by keeping calorie intake low, most of us give little thought to the harm these substitutes could cause. In fact, cyclamates have been banned because of their cancerous effects on animals, and saccharin is sold with a warning label for the same reason. Only time will tell whether Nutra-Sweet will suffer the same fate.
- The number of food products available to consumers in the United States has increased from around 1,000 in 1945, to nearly 10,000 in 1980! The full impact of this change is quite unpredictable, but most of us blindly support this trend just for convenience.
- In 1979, the comptroller-general of the United States reported that, of the 143 drugs and pesticides present as residues in raw meat and poultry, *forty-two were known causes of cancer!*
- Since 1909, it has been estimated that the consumption of french fried potatoes has increased by about 500 percent. Preparation of french fries requires extreme heat. This cooking process produces many chemicals that are mutagenic; that is, they have been shown to cause damage to the DNA of bacteria in laboratory tests. Similar products are formed during the frying or broiling of meat or fish! So not only may foods contain carcinogens, but also the method of *preparing* foods may itself create carcinogens.
- Consumption of fresh dark-green vegetables and deep-yellow vegetables has declined significantly. These vegetables contain many valuable nutrients such as beta-carotene (a precursor of vitamin A) and nonnutritive fiber, both of which have protective properties against some cancers. The role of vitamin A is of special interest and is discussed in detail in Chapter 8.

CAN WE MAKE SENSE OF ALL THIS?

These examples illustrate some of the major changes that have taken place in the American diet since the turn of the century. And these changes are continuing at an accelerating rate as more food products seduce us from overstocked supermarket shelves. What are we really doing to ourselves while we indulge our impulsive appetites? Does this changing diet actually make any difference to our chances of getting cancer later in life? How certain is our present knowledge? Do we know enough to propose definite changes in the balance of our daily diet, or has modern research only revealed the tip of a very large iceberg? Should we wait and wait for all the facts to be in, or should we make a start now, knowing that today's dietary recommendations may need to be modified in the light of tomorrow's research?

At the present time we do not know for certain whether changes in the total food supply in the the United States have increased or decreased our individual risk of cancer. Obviously, the balance of our own diets is much more important than changes in the nation's food supply. Yet the studies of nations, regions, and large groups of people have produced statistics from which certain trends have emerged. These trends can be used to infer risks or benefits to individuals.

Many changes in our diet have occurred at the same time. Some of these changes may work together, and some may cancel each other out. During the past seventy years, the American diet has dramatically shifted from vegetable to animal protein (see Chapter 5), from complex to simple carbohydrates (Chapters 6 and 7), and from animal to vegetable fats (see Chapter 4). It would be astonishing if such a sudden shift in the balance of the human diet had no effect on our susceptibility to many diseases, including cancer.

Epidemiologists have studied the diet of large groups of the American population to probe these mysteries. Most of their studies have analyzed diets in terms of the *presence* of certain nutrients. What they have found so far is fascinating. *The amount of fat, vitamin A, vitamin C, and protein in the diet appears to influence the development of cancer.*

These epidemiological studies correlate well with what would be predicted from the result of laboratory studies with animals. This is particularly true for fat, vitamin A, and vitamin C, but the evidence is rather less substantial for total protein intake. Remember, however, that lack of evidence may be the result of either negative scientific data, or the lack of scientific interest in the subject in the past. Nonetheless, there is now evidence that vitamin A and possibly vitamin C can reduce the occurrence of several common cancers, while excessive fat and possibly excessive amounts of protein can increase the risk of other cancers.

However, it is not easy to separate these effects from those that might be caused by the coexistence of other dietary factors. For example, the presence of citrus fruits in the diet indicates the presence of vitamin C, but these fruits also contain *flavonoids,* which may be equally important. Milk contains vitamin A, but *dairy products other than milk* (which have less vitamin A than milk does), are associated with an increased risk of breast cancer, suggesting that vitamin A may have a protective role. This view is supported by a study published in Japan in 1977, which showed that two glasses of milk each day could substantially reduce the risk of stomach cancer, the most common cancer in Japan (1).

Sometimes the association between a dietary substance and the risk of cancer is hard to analyze. It is possible, for example, that the protective effect of certain vegetables is due to the presence of natural chemicals such as *indoles* or *isothiocyanates,* because these substances can prevent carcinogenesis in the laboratory. Yet, how can these effects be distinguished from those produced by the simultaneous presence of vitamin C, vitamin A (or its precursor, beta-carotene), fiber, or minerals such as calcium? Clearly much is not yet understood.

The balance between meat and vegetables is also very important. As the meat component of the diet declines, it results in fewer nutrients such as fat, protein, vitamin A, and zinc; fewer mutagens that might be produced during cooking; and fewer pesticides (contaminating grains used in animal feed) or other chemical residues that may be carcinogenic. On the other hand, an increased consumption of vegetables that contain fiber, minerals, vitamins, and starches (complex carbohydrates) will also lower the cancer risk, making it difficult to determine which dietary change is most significant. If you stop to think of the incredible number of chemicals the body takes in each day, it is really remarkable that some of the associations of dietary factors with cancer have been so well identified.

As you continue to read this book you will learn of the importance of various foods that are in your present diet, could easily be added to it, or should be subtracted from it. But before any dietary modifications are made, it would be useful to know what you have been eating all these years, and what you are actually eating now.

HOW TO ANALYZE YOUR DIET

Your dietary habits of five, ten, or twenty years ago may be a vague memory, but they certainly could be influencing your chances of getting cancer today, especially since the carcinogenic process may take as long as twenty years to develop. However, before we go any further let me make on thing clear: *if you have developed good dietary habits in the past you may not need to change them.* But if you are an ordinary mortal like the rest of us, the chances are that your diet is in drastic need of revision!

The first step in this process is to make a serious attempt to analyze your own diet. This is easiest to do with the help of the questionnaire that follows. It should reveal the strengths and weaknesses of your present diet. Ideally, details of your diet in childhood, adolescence, and young adulthood would be an advantage, but the possibility of an accurate assessment is so small that it is probably worthless. In any case, the diet that you can change is your present one, not the one you enjoyed (or were subjected to) ten or twenty years ago.

Another advantage of this questionnaire is that it will enable you to reevaluate your progress at periodic intervals. In this way you can keep a close eye on your dietary digressions, and correct them appropriately.

The dietary questionnaire is scored so that you have a way of assessing your dietary habits on a regular basis. It is also designed to teach you the basis of a healthier diet. The scoring system should not be the cause of intense anxiety or depression. Your score will indicate whether you are on the right track or the wrong track. That is all. A bad score does not mean that you are about to develop cancer, nor that all hope is lost! In fact, since some of the terms used here will be clarified later, you may want to answer this questionnaire again after you have finished the book.

Regular self-assessment should reinforce good dietary habits, and I hope that after three weeks on the Cancer Prevention Diet you will see your score improve dramatically!

The perfect score is 140—and nobody gets that! If you score above 100, your dietary habits are excellent!

If your score is above 60 you are on the right track, but your diet could be modified to your advantage.

If you score between 30 and 60, you have plenty of reading ahead of you! And you should be prepared to make major changes in your diet.

If you score below 30, you will have to do more than "make

major changes." You would be well advised to empty your refrigerator, pantry, and cupboards and plan your diet (if not your life!) all over again.

The nutritional questionnaire can be used to recall your typical diet over the past month, the past year, or the past five years. Another way to use it would be to consider which answer is most applicable to half your lifetime. The accuracy of your answers is obviously important but the questionnaire will be most useful as a means to monitor the development of good diet habits. Once you have completed the introductory cancer prevention diet program, your score should steadily improve. And you will find it a very reassuring trend!

Some people have diets that are different in structure from the one on which the questionnaire is based, and in this case some of the questions may not apply. The only solution to this problem is to eliminate those questions from the questionnaire initially, but restore them once you have begun your new diet.

Now, if you are feeling curious, why not explore some of the evidence that links your diet to your risk of cancer?

NUTRITIONAL SELF-ASSESSMENT		SCORE
1. If your diet of whole grain bread averages 2 or more slices:	daily	+4
	5 days/week	+3
	3 days/week	+2
	1 day/week or less	0
2. If your diet of whole grain breakfast cereals averages the equivalent of 1 serving:	daily	+4
	5 days/week	+3
	3 days/week	+2
	1 day/week or less	0
3. If your diet averages 1 serving of rice, pasta or equivalent:	daily	+4
	5 days/week	+3
	3 days/week	+2
	1 day/week or less	0
4. If your diet averages 2 pieces of fruit:	daily	+6
	5 days/week	+4
	3 days/week	+3
	1 day/week or less	0

NUTRITIONAL SELF-ASSESSMENT		SCORE
5. If you regularly (when in season or available) eat any of these fruits 2 days/week, or more:	citrus fruits	+4
	apples	+2
	peaches	+2
	apricots	+2
	cantaloupe	+2
	If you have not eaten any of these fruits in the past month.	−4
6. If your diet averages 2 or more vegetables:	daily	+6
	5 days/week	+4
	3 days/week	+3
	1 day/week or less	0
	If you have not eaten green or yellow vegetables for one week or more	−5
7. If, on average, you eat any of these vegetables 1 day/week or more:	broccoli	+3
	brussels sprouts	+3
	cabbage	+3
	cauliflower	+3
	spinach	+3
	carrots	+3
	soybeans	+3
	lima beans	+3
	winter squash	+3
	If you have not eaten any of these vegetables for two weeks or more	−5
8. If you average 1 serving of red meat:	every day	−5
	5 days/week	−3
	3 days/week or less	0
9. If you average 1 serving of poultry (without skin):	every day	+4
	5 days/week	+3
	3 days/week	+2
	1 day/week or less	0
10. If you average 1 serving of fish:	every day	+4
	5 days/week	+3
	3 days/week	+2
	1 day/week or less	0

NUTRITIONAL SELF-ASSESSMENT		SCORE
11. If your fish comes from:	polluted freshwater lakes or rivers	−5
	the ocean	0
12. If you average:	2 or more eggs [egg yolk]/day	−5
	1 egg/day	−2
	3 eggs/week or less	+5
13. If your average milk intake is equivalent to one or more glasses/day of:	skim milk	+3
	1% milk	+2
	2% milk	0
	whole milk	−5
14. If you average:	more than 1 ounce of cheese every day	−3
	less than 1 ounce of cheese every day	+2
15. Select the two sources of fat that you choose most often:	butter	−4
	soft margarine	+3
	corn oil	+3
	olive oil	+1
	soybean oil	+4
	coconut oil	−4
	safflower oil	+3
	other saturated oils	−4
16. If your daily *added* fat (used in cooking, dressings, on bread, etc.) averages the equivalent of:	2 tablespoons of soft margarine/oil	+5
	4 tablespoons	+3
	6 tablespoons or more	−5
17. If you average 1 glass or more of orange juice: [or other fruit or vegetable juice]	every day	+5
	5 days/week	+3
	3 days/week	+2
	1 day/week or less	0
18. If you cook 2 or more days/week by any of these methods:	frying	−3
	barbecuing	−5
	baking	+3
	broiling	+1
	steaming	+5
	microwave	+5

NUTRITIONAL SELF-ASSESSMENT		SCORE
19. If you eat smoked foods on average:	2 or more times/week	−5
	once/week	−2
	twice/month	−1
	once/month or less	+5
20. If you eat salt-cured foods (which contain nitrates) on average:	2 or more times/week	−5
	once/week	−2
	twice/month	−1
	once/month or less	+5
21. If you eat pickled foods on average:	2 or more times/week	−5
	once/week	−2
	twice/month	−1
	once/month or less	+5
22. If you eat processed foods containing nitrate preservatives on average:	every day	−5
	5 times/week	−4
	3 times/week	−3
	once/week	−1
	once/month or less	+5
23. If you eat hamburgers on average:	4 or more times/week	−3
	1–3 times/week	0
	less than once/week	+3
24. If you eat french fries on average:	4 or more times/week	−3
	1–3 times/week	−2
	less than once/week	0
25. If you average 1 serving* of "junk" food such as potato chips, candy bars, or high-calorie snacks (ice cream, for example):	4 or more times/week	−5
	1–3 times/week	−3
	less than once/week	0
26. Do you regularly remove fat or skin from meat or poultry?	yes	+3
	no	−3
27. Do you regularly look for low-fat products when you shop?	yes	+4
	no	−2
28. Do you use artificial sweeteners?	daily	−3
	3 days/week	−1
	1 day/week, or less	0

* For details of what constitutes 1 serving, consult Chapter 15.

NUTRITIONAL SELF-ASSESSMENT		SCORE
29. If you drink wine, beer, or hard liquor, is your daily average equivalent to:	1 glass [4 ounces] of wine?	+3
	1 can [12 ounces] of beer?	−2
	1 ounce liquor?	−2
	more than double this daily average?	−3
	Less than this daily average?	0
30. If your weight is:	normal for your height	+5
	10% above your ideal weight	0
	20% above your ideal weight	−3
	40% or more above your ideal weight	−5
	TOTAL SCORE:	

CHAPTER 4

Dangerous Fat

Fats provide about 40–45 percent of the energy in the affluent American diet. In contrast, the economically deprived people of Africa and the Orient consume about 10 percent of their calories in the form of fat. Considerable evidence has accumulated that associates a high fat intake with cancer of the breast, cancer of the prostate, cancer of the colon, cancer of the liver, and cancer of the pancreas. Furthermore, a high dietary fat intake, particularly of saturated fats, clearly increases the risk of developing cardiovascular disease, the major cause of premature death in Western societies. Other diseases such as diabetes and obesity are also associated with a high fat intake. Not surprisingly, all these diseases are much less common in poorer countries where dietary fat intake is low.

Even within the United States, there is variation in the types of fats consumed by people in different income groups. The rich tend to consume more salad oils and cooking oil, whereas the lower income families consume more lard. But estimates of fat consumption have their limitations. These estimates are based on purchase figures or the disappearance of supplies, and they cannot adequately account for the wastage of fats that occurs during cooking or eating. These estimates also give no indication of the range of individual variation of fat intake that inevitably exists among the U.S. population. Nevertheless, there is no escape from the fact that the American fat consumption is among the highest in the world. This ignoble distinction detracts greatly from the general health and well-being of most Americans. So much so, in fact, that it has led to the development of a multibillion dollar diet and health industry.

Of course, you are aware that in the United States body fat is considered unsightly and is a distinct social disadvantage, but have you really been aware of the medical importance of fat in your daily diet? There is an obvious distinction between body fat and dietary fat. Some understanding of this relationship would be helpful before we explore the evidence that links dietary fat to cancer.

BODY FAT

The human body is made up of various kinds of cells, some of which are called *adipose* or *fat-storage cells.* These act as the storage depot for body fat, and this fat depot actually serves some very useful functions. The most important function of fat is to provide a concentrated source of energy for all the metabolic processes that are necessary to sustain life. Each gram of fat (one tablespoon weighs about 14 grams) provides 9 calories, more than twice as much as that provided by either carbohydrates or proteins, each of which provides only 4 calories per gram.

Unfortunately, the fact that fat is such a potent calorie source is a mixed blessing. As a source of energy, stored fat is unsurpassed. However, the body stores excess calories derived from *any* source (including surplus proteins, surplus carbohydrates, and even alcohol) in the form of body fat. There is no other way for the body to get rid of excess calories. Once stored, fat is very difficult to remove. One pound of fat is equivalent to about 4,000 calories. This means that you would have to reduce your calorie intake by about 500 calories below what is needed to meet energy requirements each day for over a week to lose even one pound of body fat. The alternative is to increase your calorie requirements by greatly increasing your physical activity, a tough choice for most of us. Interestingly, increasing your mental activity will not make any difference to calorie consumption from body fat since the brain is the one organ that is unable to use fats as a source of energy. Instead, it requires carbohydrates such as glucose to meet its energy needs.

Fat has other functions apart from supplying and storing energy. It cushions vital organs, providing essential support and protection as well as insulation. Fat also has a metabolic role; it is necessary for the formation of special regulatory hormones such as the prostaglandins and sex hormones, as well as for the storage of fat-soluble

Table 4–1
ESSENTIAL FACTS ABOUT BODY FAT

- A surplus represents stored energy from excess calories.
- Fat provides the body with insulation.
- Fat provides support for vital organs.
- Fat is used for the production of sex hormones.
- Fat stores vitamins A, D, E, and K.
- Fat is equivalent to about 4,000 calories per pound.
- Fat is hard to lose!

vitamins such as A and E. A more familiar role of fat is to provide the oils that lubricate the skin. Additionally, fat is the major component of internal organs such as the brain and the liver. It will also not have escaped your notice that it contributes to certain distinctive features of the female form! In fact, nature has provided women with at least 20 percent more fat than men. Women should therefore not spend their lives trying to lose all of it.

DIETARY FAT

Our diet contains many kinds of fats which vary in their chemical composition and consequently in their taste. They can be of animal or of vegetable origin. Fats, or lipids as they are known scientifically, are made up of substances called fatty acids. The fatty acids are the building blocks of fats just as the amino acids are the building blocks of proteins. Think of fatty acids as the various beads that are used to make up a necklace.

The different fatty acids are composed of varying amounts of carbon, hydrogen, and oxygen. Most fatty acids can be synthesized by the body but linoleic acid cannot. It must in consequence be derived from our diet and is therefore considered an *essential fatty acid*. Fortunately it is present in most foods that originate from plants and animals.

Linoleic acid is used by the body to make vital components of cell membranes—the outer "skin" of each cell. Apart from linoleic acid, the two other fatty acids that are considered essential are *arachnidonic acid* and *linolenic acid,* and these are usually well supplied in a reasonably balanced diet.

More than 90 percent of dietary fat is in the form of *triglycerides.* These are built of fatty acids that come in three types: saturated, monounsaturated, and polyunsaturated. Other associated substances are cholesterol and phospholipids.

These different fatty acids are important because their presence in the human diet can influence the development of cancer, as well as cardiovascular diseases such as heart disease, atherosclerosis (narrowed blood vessels), and stroke (a blocked or bleeding artery in the brain). To help you to understand how these fatty acids differ from each other, let us consider a fatty acid as a straight chain of carbon atoms that are joined together and which have the capacity to attach a certain number of hydrogen atoms. This is similar to an open bracelet which is made of loops that are joined together, and to which you can attach varying numbers of charms.

When the full quota of hydrogen atoms is attached, the fatty acid is *saturated.* When some hydrogen atoms are attached, but there is still space for two more, then the fatty acid is considered *monounsaturated.* If only a few hydrogen atoms are attached, and there is space for four or more hydrogen atoms, then the fatty acid is *polyunsaturated.*

For example, *palmitic acid* (shown below) is a saturated fatty acid with a chain of 16 carbon atoms. *Oleic acid* (also shown below) is a longer-chain monounsaturated fatty acid with a chain of 18 carbon atoms, two of which are unsaturated—that is, they have space available for a hydrogen atom. These two fatty acids are typical of the fatty acids which, in varying amounts, make up our dietary fats. When the majority of fatty acids in a fat are saturated, the fat is called a saturated fat; if most of the fatty acids that make up a fat are unsaturated, then the resulting fat is called an unsaturated fat.

Apart from the three types of fatty acids, there is another associated chemical that is very important from a health standpoint: *cholesterol.* Individuals who have a high level of circulating cholesterol in their blood are at an increased risk of developing cardiovascular diseases such as heart attacks and strokes.

The level of blood cholesterol is influenced by the combined dietary intake of fat and cholesterol, as well as by the amount produced by the body itself (mainly in the liver and the intestines). Although a low cholesterol intake is usually beneficial, changing dietary cholesterol levels for some people seems to have little effect on their blood cholesterol levels. What does seem to make a difference

EXAMPLES OF FATTY ACIDS

PALMITIC ACID

```
HO   O
  \ //
   C
   |
H—C—H
   |
H—C—H
   |
H—C—H
   |
H—C—H
   |
H—C—H
   |
H—C—H
   |
H—C—H
   |
H—C—H
   |
H—C—H
   |
H—C—H
   |
H—C—H
   |
H—C—H
   |
H—C—H
   |
H—C—H
   |
   H
```

OLEIC ACID

```
HO   O
  \ //
   C
   |
H—C—H
   |
H—C—H
   |
H—C—H
   |
H—C—H
   |
H—C—H
   |
H—C—H
   |
H—C—H
   |
   C—H
   ‖
   C—H
   |
H—C—H
   |
H—C—H
   |
H—C—H
   |
H—C—H
   |
H—C—H
   |
H—C—H
   |
H—C—H
   |
   H
```

is the type of fat that is eaten with dietary cholesterol. In general, more cholesterol is absorbed into the bloodstream in the presence of long-chain than of short-chain fatty acids. From a practical point of view, this means that *more cholesterol is absorbed by your body when your diet also contains more saturated fat.*

Another important concept to understand is how cholesterol is transported around the body. Cholesterol is insoluble in water and it is carried in the bloodstream by specialized proteins called *lipoproteins.* These proteins occur in three main forms: high-density lipoproteins (HDL), low-density lipoproteins (LDL), and very-low-density lipoproteins (VLDL).

The HDL are beneficial since they carry cholesterol away from cells in the arterial walls; the LDL and the VLDL are potentially harmful, since their role is to *supply* cells with cholesterol.

Cells regulate their need for cholesterol by producing receptors on their surface to which the lipoproteins can attach, facilitating absorption of cholesterol. When a cell has produced enough of its own cholesterol, it cleverly turns off the production of these special receptors. Failure of this sophisticated control system leads to the development of heart and blood vessel disease.

Certain factors can influence the level of lipoproteins in our blood:

- A diet that is high in saturated fats will tend to increase the levels of harmful LDL and VLDL by encouraging their production in the liver.
- In contrast, dietary polyunsaturated fats tend to reduce the harmful effects of "bad" LDLs and increase the beneficial effect of "good" HDLs.
- Regular strenuous exercise can raise the levels of protective HDLs, and there is evidence that prolonged jogging, long-distance running, or other forms of *vigorous* physical activity will substantially reduce the risk of dying prematurely from a heart attack. Moderate physical activity that uses up about 2,000 calories per week (one hour's brisk walk uses up 450 cal.) is also sufficient to reduce the risk of death from heart disease nearly as much. However, a complete lack of physical activity does increase the risk of death from heart disease by as much as 85 percent! (1)
- Obesity is associated with lower levels of HDLs, but these can increase after losing weight.
- Premenopausal women have a greater proportion of HDLs than men, and so tend to resist the harmful effects of cholesterol better than men.

Table 4–2
SOME EPIDEMIOLOGICAL EVIDENCE

- Countries with high-fat diets have more cancers of the breast, colon, prostate, pancreas, ovary, uterus (endometrium), bladder, and stomach.
- Husbands of women with breast cancer eat more fat.
- A high-fiber diet may prevent fat-induced colon cancer.

This is associated with a lower risk of heart disease for women below the age of fifty. After fifty, women begin to catch up with men as they lose their natural hormonal protection following the menopause.

THE EVIDENCE THAT FAT CAUSES CANCER

Of all dietary ingredients, fat has shown the greatest association with the development of cancer. Evidence has been obtained from epidemiological studies and from laboratory studies tht clearly links fat intake with certain cancers.

Cancers of the breast, ovary, uterus, bladder, prostate, colon, liver, and pancreas have all been shown to occur more frequently in people who consume diets high in fats. Of course, high-fat diets are associated with other dietary nutrients, and this makes the study of the precise role of fat difficult. Nonetheless, the association with cancer is strong enough to justify a complete reevaluation of our need for dietary fat.

Epidemiological Evidence Linking Dietary Fat to Human Cancer

Breast Cancer   Comparisons of statistics between various countries that have relatively high or low per-capita fat intake have revealed striking differences in either breast cancer incidence or mortality (2). The total fat intake appeared to be the main culprit, since no evidence was found that could identify specific oils or fats.

Gaskill and his colleagues compared per-capita fat intake between states in the United States and found a significant correlation between total fat intake and the risk of breast cancer (3). In this study, dairy products appeared to increase the risk.

Similar results were found in England, where the mortality trend for breast cancer correlated best with the intake of total fat, sugar, and animal protein consumed ten years earlier (4). Of course, such a study depended heavily on the accuracy of the dietary analysis over a long period of time, but since it is likely that similar "reporting errors" were made by those questioned who did not have breast cancer, the results of these studies must be taken seriously.

Examining statistical trends is one thing, but going directly to cancer patients can be even more revealing. When the diets of breast cancer patients were looked at, several studies found good evidence that a high dietary fat intake increased the cancer risk. One study compared the diets of breast cancer patients to others among Seventh-Day Adventists in California (5). These two groups were matched for age, sex (breast cancer also occurs, rarely, in men), number of children, age at first pregnancy, breast-feeding, and so on. Then dietary differences were assessed. (In a study of this sort, the disease-free group is called the "control group.") The results revealed a direct association between the consumption of high-fat foods and the existence of breast cancer.

One study did not look only at fats, but rather examined specific foods as well. The results showed an increased risk of breast cancer with increasing consumption of beef and other red meats, pork, and even sweet desserts (6).

Finally, a study of the Japanese in Hawaii compared the diets of husbands whose wives either had, or did not have, breast cancer (7). Not surprisingly, the husbands of women with breast cancer had a much higher fat intake. It was assumed, probably correctly, that the wives of these men had followed a similar eating pattern, and had paid a heavy price.

Gastrointestinal Cancer   Cancer of the stomach, pancreas, colon, and rectum are the most important forms of gastrointestinal cancer. Between 1940 and 1970 there have been dramatic changes in the frequency with which these cancers occur in the United States. And no one really understands why. For example, the incidence of stomach cancer has fallen by about 60 percent, the incidence of colon cancer has increased by about 35 percent, and the incidence of rectal cancer has fallen by about 15 percent.

Dietary fat has been associated with gastrointestinal cancer in a number of studies. Colon cancer has been studied the most, but not all studies are in complete agreement. The most convincing evidence linking colon and rectal cancer to fat intake comes from international studies that contrast one country with another (2). The least convincing studies have been conducted within countries, comparing one region with another. Regional variations are less striking than international differences, and the design of many studies could not determine the extent to which people vary in their individual fat intake.

A provocative study was carried out in Scandinavia (8). Diet diaries were kept by two groups of people with different risks of developing colon cancer: high-risk Danes from Copenhagen and low-risk Finns from Kuopio. The results were fascinating. Fat intake was about the same, but the fiber intake was significantly higher in the low-risk group. It thus seems reasonable to conclude that a high intake of dietary fiber can modify the effect of dietary fat.

The same low-risk Finnish group was then compared to a high-risk group in New York. Although their total fat intake was similar, the New Yorkers derived more of their fat from meat than the Finns, who got most of theirs from dairy products (9). Although this suggests that we may be better off if we eat less meat, there is little doubt that the Finns consumed more fiber.

From this study and other studies we must conclude that the total fat intake is not the only consideration. The *source* of fat and the *amount of dietary fiber* is important too.

Despite the fact that there appears to be an association between dietary fat and cancer of the stomach and pancreas, the results with stomach cancer are really conflicting. Only one case-control study showed a link to dietary fat, particularly the frequent eating of fried foods and the use of animal fats in cooking (10).

On the other hand, cancer of the pancreas was associated with dietary fat in one international study (11), and in Japan it has increased in conjunction with a rising fat intake (12).

Prostate Cancer   The prostate gland is situated at the base of the bladder in men. It is sensitive to hormonal influences, a feature that seems to increase the sensitivity of cells to high dietary fat.

International comparisons of mortality from prostate cancer, including one study that examined statistics from forty-one countries (13), showed a strong correlation with total dietary fat intake. A similar conclusion was drawn from a study of four ethnic groups in Hawaii, implicating both animal and saturated fat (14). This means that in countries with a high dietary fat intake, the deaths from prostate cancer are also high.

Other scientists looked at deaths from prostate cancer in white Americans county by county, carefully correlating these statistics with variations in diet (15). The conclusion was essentially the same. A high fat intake again correlated with deaths from prostate cancer.

This observation might make you wonder what would happen to the mortality from prostate (or any hormone-related) cancer if a country that had a traditionally low fat consumption changed to a high fat consumption.

Well, this is just what has been happening in Japan. The past thirty-five years have provided an opportunity to study the effect of a major dietary change on a relatively stable population. The impact of this change on prostatic cancer suggests a direct relationship; as the fat intake has risen, so has the mortality from prostatic disease (12).

The last major piece of evidence consists of two studies which found prostatic cancer patients had a higher fat intake than comparable men who appeared free of disease (16,17).

You may have noticed during this discussion that I have stressed the word "mortality," not "incidence." This distinction has intriguing implications. You see, malignant cells are found in the prostates of most men over seventy years of age, but only some of these men actually develop widespread, life-threatening prostatic cancer. Possibly, and this is only speculative, a high level of dietary fat intake may cause a local cancerous change to progress into an extensive, devastating illness.

Experimental Evidence Linking Dietary Fat to Cancer

Breast Cancer   As long ago as 1930, two scientists, Watson and Mellanby, reported the first link between dietary fat and cancer (18). They found that the addition of butter (12.5–25%) to the low-fat (3%) diet of mice increased the incidence of coal-tar–induced cancers from 34% to 57%!

Table 4-3
A SUMMARY OF THE EXPERIMENTAL EVIDENCE

- High-fat diet increases breast tumors in mice.
- Fat mice develop more tumors than normal ones.
- Diets high in unsaturated fat increase animal cancers.
- Polyunsaturated fats make animal breast tumors grow faster than saturated fats.
- Rat colon cancers grow faster on high-fat diets.
- Animal liver cancer is more likely when the diet is low in lipotropes such as choline, methionine, vitamin B_6, vitamin B_{12}, folic acid.
- Rat pancreatic cancer risk is increased by a high-fat diet.
- A low-fat (20 percent) diet balanced between polyunsaturated and saturated fats can lower cancer risk.

In another study, scientists found that the addition of 15% fat (shortening) to the diet increased the production of skin tumors in laboratory animals from 15% to 83% (19). This effect was greatest when the fat was added about six to twelve weeks *after* the carcinogen. These experiments were also the first to suggest that the degree of unsaturation might be important.

In 1942, it was shown that dietary fat could increase breast tumors in mice (20). When the high-fat diet was started early (at 24 weeks of age), the effect was greater than when it began later (at 38 weeks). This suggested that prolonged exposure to a high-fat diet from a relatively early age was more likely to be harmful—an observation that we should remember when we thoughtlessly feed our children french fries or potato chips!

Later, in 1957, more tumors were found to develop in obese mice than in normal ones, and a reduction in calorie intake was shown to prevent the development of breast tumors in these mice (21). But it was not that simple. This relative protection could in fact be overwhelmed by simply increasing the dose of the chemical carcinogen, suggesting that it was not just excess calories that were the problem.

Further experiments have shown that when mice were fed diets which were equal in calories but unequal in fat content, those fed the high-fat diet developed many more tumors (20). However, there is more to the story than simply "fat." Many studies have suggested that this tendency of fat to encourage the formation of cancers in animals is actually due to the presence of *unsaturated* fats, and in particular to the presence of the essential fatty acid *linoleic acid.* For a while this raised concern that a diet which might be good for heart disease might also be bad for cancer.

Then, in 1971, scientists demonstrated that if the fat content was high enough (above 20 percent), then it did not matter as much which type of fat was in the diet (22).

Subsequent studies have shown that if a small amount of unsaturated fat (3 percent) is added to a larger amount of saturated fat (17 percent), then the animals respond to a carcinogen as though the diet were made up entirely of unsaturated fat (23).

Further experiments were then performed using animals that had been exposed to other carcinogens and to radiation (24), and the results confirmed that a high-fat diet encouraged the formation of radiation-induced breast tumors.

Although a high-fat diet obviously enhances the process of carcinogenesis, what effect might such a diet have on the growth of an existing breast cancer? Experiments designed to answer this question produced some rather complex results, and if you like brain-teasers, try to find your way through this maze!

Initial experiments indicated that the *rate of growth* of established breast tumors increased in animals that were fed a diet of 20 percent polyunsaturated fat compared to those receiving a diet of 20 percent saturated fat. This was true even if an 18 percent saturated fat diet was supplemented with 2 percent linoleic acid (25). Interestingly, a group of animals that received only 2 percent linoleic acid, and no other fat, had a much lower tumor growth rate. So it appears that linoleic acid cannot act alone, but requires the presence of a critical amount of total fat.

Are you confused? It is not easy to understand what these complex research results mean. How do they relate to human breast cancer? Well, the answer is being sought by the National Cancer Institute in a study designed to examine the influence of a low-fat diet (20 percent) on the life expectancy of a group of women with breast cancer who have also received standard therapy. Their cancer recurrence rate will be compared with that of a control group of women who have also received standard therapy but whose dietary fat intake has not been restricted. This is a good example of experimental work leading to a clinical trial. But let us not wait years for the results of this study before acting to minimize our risks!

Colon Cancer   Dietary fat is not only associated with breast cancer in animals. There is evidence of an association with cancer of the colon, the liver, and the pancreas as well. Using a rat model of colon cancer in which the cancer is induced with a chemical carcinogen, scientists have found dramatic evidence that a high intake of dietary fat (35 percent beef fat) increased both the number of rats with colon tumors and the frequency of tumors within each rat (26).

Similar studies examined the different effects of saturated and unsaturated fat, and found that when the total dietary fat was reduced to 5 percent, unsaturated fat had the greatest effect on tumor formation. This difference did not hold up, however, when the dietary fat intake was increased to 20 percent of dietary calories (27). The importance of this observation is that it suggests that *unsaturated fats are relatively safe when part of a diet limited to 20 percent fat.*

Further experiments with various strains of mice and rats have confirmed that colon cancer occurs more frequently when the animals are fed high-fat diets (28), but some studies have indicated that—as with breast cancer—even with relatively low-fat diets, the development of tumors can be enhanced by increasing the dose of the carcinogen. So clearly more than fat alone is involved in the carcinogenic process.

What was of great interest in some of these experiments was the finding that, as with skin cancer, dietary fat only made a difference if it was given *after* initiation by the carcinogen, and not before. In the human context, this means that if we have been exposed to a significant dose of a carcinogen in the past, *our present fat intake could make a real difference to our future cancer risk.*

Cancer of the Liver and Pancreas   The liver seems to be particularly vulnerable to a deficiency of dietary substances called lipotropes, which have an affinity to fat. The most important ones are choline and methionine; others are folic acid, vitamin B_{12}, inositol, and vitamin B_6. In experiments using the powerful carcinogen azaserine, scientists have shown that the development of tumors is greatly increased in rats fed on lipotrope-deficient diets (29). Not only that—the carcinogenic effect was also greater when the diet was high in fats, particularly polyunsaturated fats. Using another known carcinogen, aflatoxin B_1, it was clearly demonstrated that unsaturated fats were even more effective (that is, *increased* the incidence of liver tumors) when they were given before the initiation phase of carcinogenesis than afterward (30). This means that even if you have not yet been exposed to a carcinogen, a high level of unsaturated fat in your diet could make the effect of any future exposure to a carcinogen worse.

Pancreatic cancers in animals are also influenced by dietary fat. Studies using rats exposed to the same carcinogen, azaserine, revealed that the level of saturated fat in their diets determined the number of rats that developed pancreatic tumors (31).

The studies discussed above are typical of the type of research experiments that have been used by scientists to understand the relationship between dietary fat and cancer. What is of vital importance, of course, is to know whether what happens in animals is similar to what happens in humans.

It is impossible to plan experiments with people in the way they are planned with rats. But the epidemiological studies are generally very well supported by laboratory studies, and this makes the conclusions more convincing. In my judgment, there is compelling evidence for reducing fat consumption to very low levels.

Table 4-4
WHAT TO REMEMBER ABOUT DIETARY FAT

- Fat contributes 40–45 percent of U.S. dietary calories.
- 90 percent of fats are triglycerides made from fatty acids.
- Fatty acids are: saturated (bad),
                monounsaturated,
                polyunsaturated (better).
- Other dietary fatty substances are:
                cholesterol, and
                phospholipids.
- Cholesterol is carried in the body by special proteins:
                high-density lipoproteins (HDL),
                low-density lipoproteins (LDL),
                very-low-density lipoproteins (VLDL).
- HDLs reduce the risk of heart disease.
- HDLs can be improved by diet and exercise.
- A high-fat diet increases your risk of cancer of the breast, colon, ovary, uterus, bladder, prostate, liver, and pancreas.
- A low-fat diet would reduce your risk of these cancers.

IS THERE A CASE AGAINST CHOLESTEROL?

High-fat diets have been condemned by heart specialists for years, especially diets that are high in saturated fats and cholesterol. Measurement of cholesterol intake has provided us with information about more than heart disease; it has enabled scientists to see whether cholesterol levels in either the blood or the diet can influence the development of cancer.

Analysis of the per-capita food intake in twenty industrialized countries has strongly associated dietary cholesterol intake with death from colon cancer, while demonstrating that dietary fiber affords some protection (32). Such epidemiological evidence encouraged scientists to examine the diets of patients with gastrointestinal cancer. This has not been as enlightening as we would hope. Blood cholesterol levels have been found to be either high (33) or low (34).

This probably seems confusing, but what almost certainly happened was that the abnormally low cholesterol levels were created by the debilitating disease, rather than the other way around. In short, the evidence linking cholesterol levels to heart disease is clear, but the association with cancer remains ambiguous. Present evidence suggests that if your blood cholesterol is in the range of 180–200 milligrams per milliliter, you should have less cancer risk. However, do not be misled by this. There are many factors associated with cancer, and cholesterol is but one factor among many!

HOW DO FATS ACTUALLY CAUSE CANCER?

If scientists knew how fats actually "cause" cancer, we would have a clearer understanding of the whole process of cancer formation. At this stage in the war on cancer, we only have some interesting ideas and some interesting theories, but no certainties.

One of the ideas which has been proposed is that a high-fat diet acts on the endocrine [hormone-producing] glands, and that this is why a high-fat diet is associated with cancers of endocrine-sensitive tissues like the breast, ovary, uterus, and prostate (35). The mechanism for such an effect is still far from clear, however. One possibility is that the cells change the character of their membranes, thus altering the expression of hormone receptors on their surface. Hormones usually cannot act without cell receptors, so an increase in receptors could result in increased sensitivity and an abnormal cell response, leading to malignancy. There is some evidence to support this idea.

A diet that contained 20 percent corn oil was compared to one with only 0.5 percent corn oil for its effect on a certain type of hormone receptor (36). The result was that many more hormone receptors were found in breast cancer cells taken from the rats that had received the high-fat diet. Food for thought!

More recently, some studies at the Massachusetts Institute of Technology have addressed the relationship between certain types of dietary fat and the development of cancers in rats (37). Experiments were designed to find out just which fats are really important, and which play only a minor role. This distinction may eventually turn out to be crucial to successful dietary cancer prevention. After all, since we cannot stop eating fats completely, we must find out which fats are safe to eat.

The results of these experiments were very interesting. Some fats, such as corn oil and sunflower seed oil, influence the formation of breast cancers, but only if fed after exposure to the carcinogen. Lard, on the other hand, had an effect if it was fed to the animals both before and after carcinogen exposure, but no effect if fed only after carcinogen exposure.

These kinds of experimental results help scientists and, for that matter, everyone else to understand that fats act in different ways, even though the end result may still be an increased cancer risk.

WHAT YOU SHOULD DO ABOUT FAT

Excessive dietary fat is dangerous to our health. Only about a tablespoon a day is necessary for a healthy body! The evidence clearly suggests that you should drastically cut down your fat intake, and I strongly advise you to reduce your fat intake to a *daily average of 20 percent of total calories.*

Nutritionists have felt the need to reduce the fat content of the American diet for several years, and indeed their recommendation to reduce fat intake to 30 percent of calories found its way into the U.S. government report called "Dietary Goals of the United States," published in 1977. Of course, since this was a government report it erred on the side of caution. But when you consider the deplorable state of the American diet, just what were the government nutritionists afraid of?

In fact they were not afraid of anything. Rather, there was a general fear that any dietary policy that went beyond this recommendation would result in the outright hostility of the food industry, and would stand little chance of being followed by the American public. Even in the 1982 report of the National Academy of Sciences on Diet, Nutrition and Cancer, the 30 percent dietary fat figure was chosen by the scientific committee as a compromise. In fact, several scientists on the committee felt that the scientific evidence indicated that fat in the American diet should be cut to 20 percent of total calories.

HOW EASY IS IT TO CUT YOUR FAT INTAKE?

Reducing your fat intake is one of the most important aspects of your new diet. It will not be easy. Fat is everywhere in your diet, and is often well hidden. Even "lean" meat has a high fat content, sometimes as high as 60 percent! When you buy milk you probably think that "2% milk" means that 2 percent of the nutrients are fat. Not so! The 2 percent figure is arrived at by including the water content in the calculation, which is very misleading. In fact, in whole milk, 48 percent of the calories come from its fat content, while 2% milk contains 30 percent "fat" calories! These figures should be printed in bold letters on every carton.

At present, you probably eat excessive amounts of high-fat meat such as beef, pork, ham, bacon, and lamb, and inadequate amounts of low-fat meat such as fish, chicken, and turkey. So adjustments in both the amounts and the nature of your meat intake will be essential.

Some rich sources of dietary fat include other dairy products such as butter and cheese, as well as foods that are as diverse as nuts, ice cream, margarine, cookies, pastries, salad dressings, and potato chips. Fat is present in many of the foods we have acquired a weakness for because it often improves both the texture and the flavor. These temptations will have to be controlled if you are to succeed.

To make your transition from a high-fat diet to a low-fat diet as painless as possible, the Cancer Prevention Diet is designed to teach you how to regulate and monitor your fat intake as part of your daily diet planning. This is discussed in detail in Chapter 15.

CHAPTER 5

Protein—Is More Better?

The word protein comes from the Greek word *protos,* meaning "first." Since 1838, when the Dutch chemist G. J. Mulder recognized the significance of dietary proteins, we have learned a great deal about their importance in the human body and in human nutrition. In many ways proteins are the most important of all nutrients. However, the importance of dietary protein in the development of human cancer is uncertain.

Proteins are associated with all forms of life, playing a critical role in the body's structure and function. Although the human body is more than 60 percent water, the "solid" 35–40 percent is mostly protein. Most of this protein is used to make our bones, muscles, nerves, and other tissues. Some specialized proteins, such as enzymes and hormones, influence body chemistry; other specialized proteins, antibodies, defend us against infection and cancer.

Proteins are built up from small components called *amino acids.* The number of different amino acids, and the order in which they are arranged, influence the final structure that is formed. After all, why is a bone different from a muscle?

Altering the number and arrangement of amino acids can also determine whether the resulting protein becomes a hormone, an antibody, or an enzyme. The control of this process is regulated by the specialized genetic material within each cell, using other special proteins to carry out the instructions.

The amino acids that are used to make proteins are of two main types: essential and nonessential. The *essential* amino acids are literally indispensable dietary constituents because they cannot be made in our bodies. The *nonessential* amino acids differ only because they can be made within our bodies, and we therefore do not have to include them in our diet.

The essential amino acids are very similar in all animals, and humans are no exception. All of the essential amino acids are present in every protein in the body, while an additional nine nonessential amino acids are present in most human proteins.

When you eat protein from any source, it is broken down in the digestive system into amino acids, which are then absorbed into the bloodstream, where they mix with amino acids coming from body tissues. This mingling of amino acids derived from body tissues with amino acids derived from dietary sources occurs all the time as our proteins are continually broken down and rebuilt.

Not all amino acids are used to build proteins; some may be converted into fat, and some provide energy if other sources are insufficient. Whatever the fate of your dietary protein, it is important that your diet contain the proper *balance* of amino acids for the protein to be used effectively. This means that you must eat enough of the right proteins. Proteins that contain all the essential amino acids are called *complete proteins,* while those that do not are called *incomplete proteins.* Failure of the body to make sufficient complete protein will gradually produce signs of protein deficiency. Frequently, foods that contain only some of the essential amino acids can be combined with other foods that contain the missing amino acids to provide complete protein. Fortunately this usually happens automatically with any sensibly balanced diet.

Table 5-1
AMINO ACID CONSTITUENTS OF PROTEIN

Essential Amino Acids	Nonessential Amino Acids
Histidine	Alanine
Isoleucine	Arginine
Leucine	Asparagine
Lysine	Aspartic acid
Methionine	Cystine
Phenylalanine	Glutamic acid
Threonine	Glutamine
Tryptophan	Glycine
Valine	Proline
	Serine
	Tyrosine

THE FUNCTION OF PROTEINS

The principal uses of proteins are to develop, maintain, and rebuild body tissues throughout life; to regulate the body chemistry; to influence body function and development; to resist infection; and to help to maintain water balance.

As every parent knows, protein is required for growth. Most body tissues also require repair, and this uses up proteins too. In body tissues like the bone marrow, in which cells are replaced frequently, there is a great demand for protein. On the other hand, tissues like the brain change little and therefore do not use much protein. Most of the protein that is broken down releases amino acids that can be used over and over again to make new protein. Perhaps conservation is not such a new idea after all.

Proteins are used by the body to make hormones such as thyroxine and insulin. Other hormones, such as the sex hormones, are carried around the body by proteins. The role of hormones is to control the rate of the chemical reactions that are involved in all vital bodily processes. Small shifts in the balance of hormones have profound consequences for our inner sense of well-being. For example, an excess of thyroxine causes severe weight loss, a deficiency of insulin causes diabetes, and most of us can guess what might happen when the sex hormone level increases and decreases. (Do not imagine, however, that changing your level of dietary protein will influence your sex hormone level or its effects!)

The body regulates its total water balance mainly through sophisticated control of kidney function. But the amount of water in individual cells is controlled to a considerable extent by the level of intracellular protein and the level of proteins in the blood stream. When the level of proteins is low in the blood, water leaves the blood and enters the tissues, causing swelling. This problem arises from certain diseases that are associated with low levels of protein and it is often seen in starving people who are severely protein-deficient.

You may have noticed that some shampoos are described as "pH-balanced." In fact the body is pH-balanced too. This simply means that there is a balance between acidity and alkalinity. The normal pH of arterial blood is between 7.36 and 7.44. When the body is exposed to stress that threatens the stability of the pH, there are some very clever mechanisms in the body to maintain the pH

Table 5-2
SOME FUNCTIONS OF PROTEINS

Growth
Tissue repair
Resistance to infection
Production of hormones
Control of water balance
Control of body pH
Control of body chemistry

within these narrow limits. One of these mechanisms involves *buffers,* which are chemicals that react in such a way that the pH remains almost unchanged. Buffering is also provided by blood proteins, and thus in this way they also play a vital part in maintaining our inner well-being.

Finally, proteins are vital for the production of antibodies, those specialized proteins that prevent us from dying rapidly of overwhelming infection. Antibodies are proteins that are tailor-made to destroy specific invaders such as bacteria or viruses. Consequently, there is an enormous variety of them. Some persist for only a short time, others may persist throughout life. Antibodies are deliberately produced by vaccination, and vaccination programs have lead to the virtual elimination of smallpox and polio—diseases that have been the scourge of mankind for centuries.

EVIDENCE LINKING DIETARY PROTEIN TO CANCER

There is a conviction in the minds of many people that the more protein we eat, the better. This is not true. In fact, the National Research Council recommends only 0.8 grams per kilogram of body weight per day for healthy adults. This amounts to only 56 grams (2 ounces) every day for a man weighing 70 kilograms (154 pounds), or 44 grams (1.5 ounces) every day for a woman weighing 55 kilograms (121 pounds). Most of us eat more protein than this every day. This is not difficult, since, for example, only 3 ounces (85 grams) of lean steak will provide 27 grams of protein.

A number of cancers in humans have been associated with diets that are high in protein. The evidence for this association, however, is not nearly as convincing as for dietary fat. The cancers associated with excessive protein intake are of the breast, uterus, prostate, colon, rectum, pancreas, and kidney.

Some Epidemiological Evidence

Breast Cancer   Cancer of the breast is the commonest cause of cancer deaths among women. You already know that fat is a very important dietary cause, but a comprehensive study that was published in 1975 found evidence that protein is a danger too (1). This study examined people who had developed twenty-seven types of cancer (the incidence) in twenty-three countries, and the number of people who died of fourteen types of cancers (the mortality) in thirty-two countries. In this massive piece of research, a wide range of environmental and dietary factors were examined, and it was concluded that national prosperity and protein intake not only tend to go together, but also increase the cancer risk. And of all the cancers looked at, breast cancer showed the most convincing association with a high protein intake. Other studies came to the same conclusion even though different techniques were employed (2,3,4,-5). In all these studies, the association was with protein of animal origin rather than vegetable origin.

Another way of studying the effect of a dietary nutrient is to analyze the diets of patients who have developed cancer, and then to compare their diet history with a comparable group of people who do not have cancer. The validity of this case-control approach is dependent in large part on the accuracy of human memory. In three studies of this type (6,7,8), only one established a clear link between dietary protein and breast cancer (8).

Colon and Rectal Cancer   Unlike breast cancer, these cancers affect men and women more or less equally, but like breast cancer they have shown a remarkable relationship to human nutrition. The first report of a direct correlation between intestinal cancer and protein intake was made in 1969 (9). This study measured the intake of animal protein and the mortality from intestinal cancer in twenty-eight countries. Although the basic conclusion was also supported by other studies (1,10,11,12,13), these studies mostly looked at specific foods such as meat, sugar, beer, and eggs.

This illustrates a fundamental difficulty with studies that associate specific foods with cancer. Let us look at eggs, for example. Eggs are rich sources of fat, cholesterol, and protein. Since we already know that fat increases the cancer risk, how can we tell which actor is the principal villain? The answer is that it may not be possible from epidemiological studies, but it may be possible if we use laboratory experiments that have been designed to answer specific questions.

Within the United States the findings have not always been consistent. Both Mormons (beef-eaters) and Seventh-Day Adventists (vegetarians) have about 30–40 percent less colorectal cancer than other Americans (14). This can only be rationalized if one invokes other causes of colon cancer or a protective effect of other dietary constituents.

On balance, I find that there is a suggestion that a high-protein diet may increase the risk of colorectal cancer, but it is not a major risk factor.

Pancreatic Cancer   Few epidemiological studies of pancreatic cancer have been carried out. The first suggestion of an association of pancreatic cancer with animal protein intake was made in 1967 (15) and was later confirmed in a study in 1975 (1). These studies were conducted on a large scale and examined many different cancers in many countries.

More specific studies were conducted in Japan. One, published in 1968 (16), was somewhat unusual. Specially designed questionnaires were sent to relatives of patients who had died of pancreatic cancer. Subsequent dietary analysis revealed an association between the disease and the consumption of high-meat diets by men. Of course, since high-meat diets are not only high in protein but are inevitably high in fat too, the conclusions are not clear-cut.

Another large Japanese study was designed to follow the fate of 265,118 people and to examine the diets of those who went on to develop pancreatic cancer. The conclusion was that a high-meat diet increased the risk of pancreatic cancer two and a half times (17).

If we choose to call a high-meat diet a high-protein diet—which it certainly is—then this supports the association of a high-protein diet with pancreatic cancer. On the other hand, there is no direct evidence that a high-protein diet in which the protein is derived from sources other than meat is equally risky. And the problem of separating the effects of fat from the effects of protein remains unsolved. Probably the full story has yet to be told, and I think the case against protein in this context is incomplete.

Cancer of the Kidney   Evidence that dietary protein can increase the risk of cancer of the kidney is scant. Although a strong positive correlation between animal protein and the incidence of renal cancer was reported in 1975 (1), when patients who had kidney cancer were questioned about their diets, no link could be found to protein intake (18). With so little to go on it is difficult to draw a firm conclusion, yet small pieces of evidence such as this add up, encouraging a policy of moderation in protein intake.

Cancer of the Uterus (Endometrium)   Two studies have suggested a link between uterine cancer and total protein intake (1,19). However, uterine cancer is sometimes associated with breast cancer, which perhaps is not surprising since they are both hormonally dependent tissues. Whether the association with each other is dietary or is linked to some other body imbalance remains unclear. Yet both these cancers are associated with a high protein intake as well as a high fat intake. Once again, these are foods that often go together, and we are left wondering whether to blame fat or protein. Perhaps studies of patients with uterine cancer will provide the answer, but they have yet to be done.

Prostate Cancer   We have already reviewed the evidence that a high fat intake increases the risk of prostate cancer. As before, this association makes it harder to define the role of protein, because fat and protein so often go together.

The most impressive study done so far still leaves this dilemma unresolved. This was carried out in Japan in 1977 (17). Since 1950, there has been a steady increase in meat consumption in Japan. This has been accompanied by a steady increase in prostate cancer. Whether this change is due to meat protein or fat or both, the evidence lends support to the idea that meat consumption should be reduced along with fat consumption.

Some Experimental Evidence

The scientific approach to exploring the mysteries of Nature involves logic, intuition, imagination and serendipity. In the search for understanding and wisdom, each observation and each clue must be scrutinized and used to build that great edifice which is human knowledge.

This process has never been more evident than in our relentless desire to conquer cancer. Each piece of evidence uncovered by epidemiological studies is used to plan experiments that can examine specific questions with greater precision in the laboratory. When laboratory results support the epidemiological data I feel that the conclusions deserve to be taken seriously. When they fail to support epidemiological results, judgment must be withheld pending further investigation.

There have been far fewer studies of dietary protein than of dietary fat. Most of the earlier studies focused on the effect of either a specific amino acid restriction, or on the effect of high versus low intakes of dietary protein. Sometimes the calorie intake was inadequately controlled, which made interpretation difficult since calorie restriction can itself limit tumor growth (20,21). Sometimes there was inadequate control of fat intake, which made interpretation of the results virtually impossible (22).

Even when there does appear to be an effect of dietary protein on tumor growth, it is important to determine whether the effect is due to a specific amino acid or to a more general effect of protein. In a number of animal experiments, scientists have found that low-protein diets that have been supplemented with specific amino acids result in an increased risk of cancer. And this increase may be just as great as that produced by an increase in total dietary protein (23,24,25). This observation was dramatically illustrated by some experiments with animal breast tumors (26). In these experiments, female mice failed to develop the expected breast cancer when they were fed a casein (a milk protein) diet that was deficient in the amino acid *cystine*. For twenty-two months they remained protected; then the same diet was *supplemented* with cystine. Within no time they developed breast cancer! This provides dramatic evidence that the amino acid balance can influence cancer formation.

Cystine is not the only amino acid that has been shown to influence cancer development. A deficiency of the amino acid *lysine* has also been shown to inhibit breast tumors in mice (27), and the addition of lysine but not of cystine has been shown to increase leukemia in mice that were on casein diets (28).

Many studies have examined protein intakes that usually ranged

from 5 percent (the minimum required for normal growth) to about
20 percent of dietary calories (the amount most mammals consume). Diets that are close to the 5 percent minimum suppress the
growth of most tumors, although there have been one or two exceptions in which growth is increased. Diets that contain about 20–25
percent protein can enhance the development of tumors, while
higher amounts of protein have shown paradoxical effects—actually reducing tumor growth instead.

In general, there is a lack of information about the specific effects
of animal as opposed to vegetable protein. It is also difficult to be
certain of the interplay between protein and other dietary factors.
Nevertheless, there is an underlying suggestion that the dietary
protein may make a difference. Further research is needed to un-
ravel this mystery.

HOW DOES DIETARY PROTEIN INFLUENCE
CANCER DEVELOPMENT?

Unfortunately, we know very little about how dietary protein influences the development of cancer. During carcinogenesis, there
are a number of changes that must take place before a cancer develops. Some of these changes are influenced by the level of dietary
protein. Numerous experiments have shown that cancer is more
likely to develop when the diet is high in protein. For example, this
has been shown in rats, which developed liver cancer after exposure
to the notorious mold carcinogen aflatoxin B_1 (29). In this instance,
one possibility is that a low-protein diet suppresses the activity and
development of certain liver enzymes that are involved in the metabolism of aflatoxin B_1, thereby increasing the carcinogenic effect.

HOW DO WE ASSESS OUR PROTEIN NEEDS?

The evidence that protein intake in general makes a significant
difference to the risk of getting cancer is not yet conclusive. It is also
unknown whether there is any difference in the effects of protein
derived from animal as opposed to vegetable sources.

Yet evidence has been presented to you which does suggest the possibility that a high-protein diet could be harmful. So we must face the question, How much protein do we really need?

Protein is required to provide us with the animo acids that we need. Excess amino acids are broken down into metabolic waste products that are excreted by the body. It is not yet clear how an *excess* of amino acids could actually be harmful, nor how any particular amino acid could specifically increase our cancer risk.

The National Academy of Sciences has published nine editions of Recommended Dietary Allowances (RDA) for nutrients, the most recent being in 1980. Their recommendations for dietary protein requirements are based upon certain important assumptions that do not include an assessment of cancer risk.

When the diet contains no protein at all, the total excretion of protein by the body (in the form of breakdown products of tissue protein) is a measure of the amount of protein we need in order to repair tissues damaged through normal wear and tear. Yet life is not quite that easy. Simply replacing the exact amount that is lost is not good enough, because not all protein is equally absorbed or equally utilized.

All foods do not necessarily provide the full range of essential amino acids that we need. Some proteins provide less essential amino acids than others. Since *utilization* of protein by the body is limited by the essential amino acid that is supplied in the *smallest* quantity, we may not meet our body's minimum requirements if we choose our sources of protein unwisely.

Some people have increased protein requirements due to a variety of causes. For example, pregnant and lactating mothers, growing children, and manual laborers all have increased protein needs. The elderly, on the other hand, may have reduced protein needs. If you are in doubt, you should consult your personal physician for advice.

Since dietary protein must satisfy our need for essential amino acids, it is important to realize that only 20 percent of the adult body's protein requirement needs to be supplied by essential amino acids—although in children it is higher. In 1975 the Food and Nutrition Board of the National Research Council published a guide to minimum essential amino acid requirements for man. This is summarized in Table 5–3.

In assessing the protein value of foods, we have to measure the

Table 5-3
ESTIMATED AMINO ACID REQUIREMENTS

| Amino acid | MG/KG BODY WEIGHT/DAY | | | Ideal amino acid balance (mg/g of protein) |
	Infant (4-6 months)	Child (10-12 years)	Adult	
Histidine	33	?	?	17
Isoleucine	83	28	12	42
Leucine	135	42	16	70
Lysine	99	44	12	51
Methionine and Cystine	49	22	10	26
Phenylalanine and Tyrosine	141	22	16	73
Threonine	68	28	8	35
Tryptophan	21	4	3	11
Valine	92	25	14	48

Source: Food and Nutrition Board, 1975.

It should be noted that 2 grams per kilogram of body weight per day of protein *whose quality reflects the ideal amino acid balance* shown above would be sufficient to meet the daily needs of an infant.

effect of the amino acid composition in order to assign a nutritional score. Nutritionists have employed a variety of methods to do this. One method involves the use of a biological assay. Growing rats are given known amounts of different proteins and the relative effect of each type of protein on weight gain is measured.

Using this system, whole egg or milk protein is scored at 100, while wheat gluten scores only 20. This means that five times as much wheat gluten must be fed to the growing rat as egg or milk protein to achieve the same growth effect. It also means that all the protein in egg and milk is utilized, but all the protein in wheat gluten is not.

There are three other points that I want you to understand. First, any method of assessing the protein effect ignores the highly complex interaction with other foods, and may therefore be rather misleading in terms of the human diet.

Second, it has been found that the efficiency with which protein is utilized declines as the total protein intake approaches the minimum requirement. The lack of information about the efficiency of protein utilization in complex human diets has led most nutritionists to recommend more protein than may be needed, in order to compensate for this effect.

Third, it is also important to recognize that estimates of protein requirements are only valid if the body's energy needs (calorie requirements) are satisfied. An inadequate energy supply prevents the body from making full use of dietary protein—but this is hardly a problem in our obese society.

You now should have some basic understanding of proteins. The next step is to know how much should be in your diet. Remember, your needs will be influenced by your age (growing children need more; the elderly need less), your level of physical activity, pregnancy, and lactation. Stress does little to increase your protein needs, although protein requirements are increased by some diseases and reduced by others.

Disabilities that *increase* protein requirements are those caused by severe injury, severe burns, fractures, prolonged bed rest, reduced intestinal food absorption, and cancer.

Diseases that *reduce* the need for protein are liver and kidney failure.

DIETARY RECOMMENDATION

The American people consume huge amounts of protein. In fact, they consume more protein per capita than any other nation on earth, and much more than they need.

After careful dietary analysis, the Food and Agricultural Organization and the World Health Organization published a report in 1973 which concluded that the average healthy adult needed 0.45 grams of protein per kilogram of body weight per day (equivalent to ¾ ounce/100 lbs.).

To achieve this in practice, the report suggested that the daily allowance be increased by 30 percent to compensate for inefficient utilization of protein. This recommendation raised the allowance to 0.6 grams per kilogram of body weight per day (equivalent to 1 ounce/100 lbs.).

Even this was not enough. Since our diet contains protein of mixed quality (in terms of the balance and availability of essential amino acids), it is impossible for any of us to have more than a vague idea about the amino acid quality of the food we eat. Information such as that presented in Table 5–3 is a statement of fact that is almost useless in practice. To compensate for this, the official recommended dietary allowance for protein was raised to 0.8 grams per kilogram of body weight per day (about 1 ounce per 80 lbs.).

This represents an average allowance of 56 grams (2 ounces) of protein per day for a 5'10" man weighing 70 kilograms (154 pounds), and 44 grams (1.5 ounces) for a 5'4" woman weighing 55 kilograms (121 pounds).

Despite these recommendations, you may well be wondering how much protein the average American actually eats each day. Without considering the relative nutritive value of the different sources of dietary protein, most estimates indicate that the average American eats *twice* as much protein as the recommended daily allowance!

This means that we could reduce our protein intake by half and still be conforming to current dietary policy. And since protein is often accompanied by fat, reducing our protein intake would help us to reduce our fat intake—a vital goal of the Cancer Prevention Diet.

Although the average protein content of the indulgent American diet has remained at 12 percent of an excessive calorie intake since record keeping began in 1909, there has been a change in the source of this protein. In 1909, our dietary protein was derived equally from animal and vegetable sources. Now only about a third of our protein is derived from vegetable sources. To what extent this shift in the balance of protein intake has influenced our cancer risk is uncertain, but a diet high in animal protein usually increases blood cholesterol levels and is associated with atheroma (narrowing of the arteries) and with atherosclerosis (hardening of the arteries), and so is obviously less desirable from a health standpoint.

Clearly, a reduction in animal protein should lower our risk of heart disease and stroke; and a reduction in animal protein (and total protein) *may* reduce our cancer risk as well.

To illustrate just how easily we consume large amounts of protein—often in response to effective advertising—let's look at a typical day's food intake in Table 5–4.

Table 5-4
TYPICAL SOURCES OF DAILY PROTEIN

Food	Amount	Complete Protein	Incomplete Protein
Lean meat	5 ounces	44 grams	
Fish	3 ounces	22 grams	
Chicken	1 leg	12 grams	
Milk	1 glass	8 grams	
Egg	1	6 grams	
Cheese	1 ounce	7 grams	
Peas	1 cup		5 grams
Rice	1 cup		4 grams
Potato	1 baked		4 grams
Peanuts	1 tablespoon		3 grams
Bread	1 slice		3 grams
Cereal	1 bowl		4 grams
Corn	1 ear		2 grams
Carrot	1 average		1 gram

Remember, all the protein required by someone of average height and weight (male: height 5'10", weight 154 pounds; female: height 5'4"; weight 120 pounds) is provided by eating about 60 grams of protein per day. This is easily supplied in your daily diet if you eat *some* meat.

Although the percentage of our dietary calories provided by protein has been stable over the years, the *total amount* of food that we eat has increased to such an extent that we are eating far too much. As we reduce the total calorie content of our diet, so we will bring down our protein intake to levels that are much more appropriate to our needs. If every American followed this advice, the effect on the nation's diet would be enormous. What is more, any tendency for excess protein to increase our cancer risk would be removed.

Although I think that a reduction in total protein intake to levels that are closer to those recommended by the National Research Council would be worthwhile, it is interesting to note that the levels of protein recommended in most European countries are considerably higher than in the United States. In fact the recommended levels are fairly close to the elevated levels of protein in the present American diet. But we must not forget that these recommendations completely ignore any relationship between dietary protein and cancer risk. As so often happens in life, there is plenty of room for disagreement among the experts!

At the present time there is no need to change the *percentage* of dietary calories provided by protein. Maintain your protein intake at 12–18 percent of total calories. This is particularly important when most of your protein is of vegetable origin.

The Cancer Prevention Diet will train you to reduce your protein intake from meat and to increase your intake of vegetable protein. This will automatically reduce the chance of overindulging in protein, because you have to eat a lot more vegetables than meat to achieve your daily protein allowance.

Now that you have a good idea of the importance that you should attach to protein in your daily diet, and how you should moderate your protein intake, let us move on to the carbohydrates—those foods that have been so misjudged for so long.

Table 5–5
WHAT TO REMEMBER ABOUT PROTEIN

- Proteins are made of essential and nonessential amino acids.
- Proteins are either complete or incomplete.
- Incomplete proteins do not have all the essential amino acids.
- Essential amino acids are needed for normal body function.
- Americans eat twice as much protein as they need.
- A high protein intake may increase your cancer risk.
- Protein intake must be between 12–18 percent of total calories.
- You must double your protein intake from vegetable sources.
- You must reduce your intake of protein from meat.
- Your protein intake must remain regular and balanced.

CHAPTER 6

The Safe Carbohydrates

Everyone has heard of carbohydrates, usually being criticized unfairly as the dietary villain responsible for all our weight problems. To correct this impression, we will review the various kinds of carbohydrates so that you can understand what they are, what they do for us or to us, and where they occur in our diet. You will discover how some types may actually lower your cancer risk; how they usually do *not* make you fat; what other diseases are associated with them; and why you should expand their place in your diet.

First, you must get rid of any prejudices that you may have against carbohydrates. Most of us think of protein as "high-class" food that is the most desirable in our affluent society, and carbohydrates as "low-class" food that is undesirable (associated with the Third World and poverty). We are really quite wrong! Our very affluence seems to encourage us to eat foods that are worse for our health. This tendency must be avoided. Many carbohydrates are in fact excellent sources of nutrients, and constitute some of our *safest* foods. Only by understanding the nature of your diet and what effect it is having on you will you be motivated to make the changes that are so vital to your future well-being.

Carbohydrates are made from carbon, hydrogen, and oxygen. To most of us, however, they are *sugar, starch,* and *fiber.* The three basic elements—carbon, hydrogen, and oxygen—can be linked together with varying degrees of complexity. Not surprisingly, this has led to carbohydrates being classified as "simple" and "complex." Simple carbohydrates are the sugars that are known scientifically as *monosaccharides.* The safe complex carbohydrates are the starches known scientifically as the *polysaccharides.*

Examples of simple sugars are glucose, fructose and galactose. Two simple sugars can also be linked together to form what is called a *disaccharide*. A well-known example of this is the combination of glucose and fructose to form sucrose, or table sugar. Incidentally, there is no nutritional difference between white sugar, brown sugar, or honey—contrary to popular myth.

Complex carbohydrates, such as glycogen, can be broken down by the body to form glucose, while other complex carbohydrates, such as fiber, are mostly indigestible. Since fiber is a very important component of some complex carbohydrates that may give protection against some cancers, it will be considered separately in the next chapter.

Another carbohydrate that has influenced human existence since well before Biblical times is alcohol. Since this particular carbohydrate is associated with the development of certain cancers, it will also be considered separately in a later chapter.

THE FUNCTION OF CARBOHYDRATES

Carbohydrates have been the main source of energy in the human diet since the dawn of time. Long before our ancestors began to cultivate the cereals that have provided dietary starch for over 10,000 years, primitive man ate tubers, wild fruits, nuts, and honey. These foods provided the energy he needed to survive. It is estimated that carbohydrates supplied early man with a very high proportion of his calorie needs.

In the modern American diet, carbohydrates supply roughly 45 percent of dietary calories, while in the Caribbean they supply about 65 percent, and in Africa nearly 80 percent. When carbohydrates are taken in the form of ordinary sugar, absorption is rapid because little digestion is required. Complex carbohydrates, such as starch, require more digestion, yet still provide a readily usable source of energy. Once absorbed by the body, unused carbohydrates are stored as glycogen in the liver and muscles, for later conversion to glucose as needed.

Without an adequate amount of carbohydrate in the diet, the body uses body fat and protein as alternative energy sources. But this is not a satisfactory way to burn up body fat because without carbohydrates, the body cannot metabolize fat properly. Instead, fat is only partially broken down, and forms dangerous toxic acids called *ketones*. Moreover, since the brain can only use glucose as a source of energy, fat and protein have to be converted into glucose before they can be used by the brain—a very inefficient process.

Glucose itself liberates 60 percent of its energy as heat and 40 percent in potentially usable form. Of course the heat is not entirely wasted, since it helps to maintain the body at the right temperature, while the remaining energy enables the body to carry out all its essential functions.

Energy is also required for cell growth and tissue repair, and for the synthesis of chemical compounds. However, any variation in the amount of energy required by individuals of the same body weight is mainly caused by differences in their respective levels of muscular activity. For example, walking requires four times as many calories as lying down.

Another important function of carbohydrates is to spare the destruction of normal body proteins, leaving them available for growth and tissue repair. If dietary carbohydrates are too low, this inevitably leads to the breakdown of our proteins to provide energy (although considerable protein breakdown only occurs when fat stores are exhausted). Not only do carbohydrates save our proteins but, if the diet is deficient in certain amino acids, carbohydrates can also be used to make these amino acids. This helps the body to rebuild vital proteins.

Failure to eat enough carbohydrates can also lead to dehydration. What happens is this: the low levels of dietary carbohydrate lead to the incomplete breakdown of fat, which in turn causes an increase in the urinary excretion of sodium (salt) and ketones. This excretion of salt and ketones cannot occur without an increased water loss. If this water is not adequately replaced, dehydration is inevitable.

Table 6-1
IMPORTANT FUNCTIONS OF CARBOHYDRATES

- Provide the body with energy.
- Preserve body protein.
- Help to maintain fluid balance.
- Provide indigestible fiber.

On the other hand, if you eat far too much carbohydrates, the surplus calories are eventually stored as fat. This is not a feature unique to carbohydrates, however; it occurs with a surplus of dietary fat or protein too.

These normal functions can be satisfied by a daily intake of as little as 50–100 grams of digestible carbohydrate (1).

CARBOHYDRATES AND OUR CANCER RISK

Very few epidemiological studies have examined the role of carbohydrates in the development of cancer. Of the few that have, none provide any evidence that diets which are relatively high in complex carbohydrates are harmful. (However, certain specific carbohydrates, namely indigestible fiber and alcohol, do influence the development of cancer. These carbohydrates are considered separately in Chapters 7 and 11 respectively.)

Let us now take a look at some of the epidemiological and experimental evidence so that you will understand why complex carbohydrates deserve the prominent place they have in the Cancer Prevention Diet.

Some Epidemiological Evidence

Only a few studies have examined the association of various types of carbohydrates with either cancer incidence (how many people get it) or cancer mortality (how many people die from it).

A weak association has been found between dietary carbohydrate and cancers of the pancreas, the liver, the breast, the stomach, and the esophagus. Let us look briefly at the evidence, some of which is rather difficult to interpret.

Cancer of the Pancreas and Liver   In 1975, scientists reported a significant correlation between sugar intake and death from pancreatic cancer. At the same time, they failed to demonstrate any relationship between the incidence of the disease and sugar intake. Moreover, this limited observation was confined to women (2). The same study also found a weak association between the incidence of liver cancer and the intake of potatoes (a rich source of starch). To my mind, these limited findings do not amount to a significant case against carbohydrates, although they deserve further study.

In this type of situation, one must remind oneself that diets that are rich in one particular nutrient may also be deficient in others, and that it may be the deficiency which makes the real difference. The absence of adequate dietary information from patients in studies of these diseases, however, reduces the importance of these findings.

Breast Cancer   In 1978, there was an interesting report of dietary factors associated with breast cancer (3). In particular, it was noticed that the development of breast cancer was associated with a high intake of refined sugar. This observation supported a study carried out in 1973 (4), in which it was reported that there was a direct correlation between the development of breast cancer and the intake of simple carbohydrates. This was one of the more significant findings because it was supported by laboratory experiments.

In a 1975 study (5), researchers found that there was actually an *inverse* correlation between the incidence of breast cancer and the level of another dietary carbohydrate—starch. That is, the *higher* the level of starch intake, the *lower* the incidence of breast cancer. This means that a high intake of starch may in fact *protect* you from developing breast cancer.

The lesson to be drawn from this evidence is that while certain refined carbohydrates such as sugar may be harmful in excess, the unrefined, complex carbohydrates may be beneficial.

Cancer of the Stomach   After studying mortality rates for stomach cancer in sixteen countries, it was found that there was a rather striking direct correlation between the intake of cereal in the form of flour and the risk of death from stomach cancer (6). However, only one other study of patients with stomach cancer has revealed an above average intake of starch (7). But since this observation has not been made in other studies, it must be regarded as preliminary. Furthermore, no laboratory studies have succeeded in substantiating either of these two observations.

Cancer of the Esophagus   Most attempts to demonstrate an association between dietary carbohydrate and cancer of the esophagus have failed. However, there has been one study which evaluated the dietary patterns of patients in Singapore who had esophageal cancer (8). Their diets were compared with those of a comparable group of patients who had other diseases. The results suggested that the patients with esophageal cancer had a higher consumption of carbohydrates such as bread and potatoes. Of course, they may also have had a higher consumption of something else too, and were never asked. Alternatively, there is always the possibility that these patients were eating fewer protective fruits and vegetables *because* they ate more bread and potatoes. Conceivably, the problem could have nothing to do with starch at all.

Although such a study remains rather provocative, it is not possible to draw any conclusions from an isolated study that has not been substantiated elsewhere.

Some Experimental Evidence

A few attempts have been made by scientists to study the effects of different carbohydrates on the development of cancers in laboratory animals. These studies were unfortunately rather poorly designed, so the effect of a sugar such as sucrose or glucose could not be separated from differences in total calorie intake, nor from the effects of other carbohydrates in the diet.

In any case, the results do not reveal any convincing association between dietary carbohydrate and cancer formation. Only one study has suggested that animals fed sucrose have a greater risk of chemically induced cancer than do rats fed starch (9). Since there are many types of carbohydrate, more research is clearly needed.

OTHER DISEASES ASSOCIATED WITH CARBOHYDRATES

Obesity and diabetes are the only diseases that are related to dietary carbohydrate. Obesity is mainly the result of excessive calorie intake, and many of those excess calories come from foods that are overloaded with *refined* carbohydrates such as sugar.

The problem starts early. Baby-food manufacturers have been criticized because they deliberately raised the sugar content of baby foods, both to increase their appeal and to create in children a long-term dependence on sweet foods. The importance of this policy as a way to create sweet profits cannot be underestimated. The manufacturers responded to criticism by lowering the amount of added sugar; instead, they let the fruits ripen longer so that the natural sugar content would increase sufficiently to compensate for what they had left out. Hardly a responsible response to the knowledge that they were directly contributing both to the nation's future obesity and to tooth decay. You see, people who were fat as children find it very difficult to be slim as adults. This is because a high-calorie diet in infancy and childhood is directly responsible for the production of an excessive number of fat cells in the body. Once formed, these fat cells remain forever—waiting to store fat if given the chance. Furthermore, habits acquired in childhood are also the hardest to change later.

The other serious disease associated with carbohydrates, though not caused by them, is diabetes. This disease is commonly associated with an inadequate production of insulin by the pancreas (an endocrine gland behind the stomach). Patients with this disease often have to take injections of insulin to help them to control blood sugar levels. The insulin helps the sugar to enter the cells, where it is used for energy. Without enough insulin, the sugar cannot be utilized, and its level in the blood rises. This causes major problems in some people: premature heart disese, blood vessel disease, and even blindness.

In the past, diabetics had to follow rigorous diets that involved careful regulation of their carbohydrate intake. The simple carbohydrates such as glucose and fructose were especially important to regulate since it was assumed that they were absorbed rapidly. In contrast, the complex carbohydrates were assumed to be absorbed slowly. It was feared that rapid absorption of simple carbohydrates would lead to a sudden rise in blood sugar, with serious consequences. This view has recently been challenged at the University of Colorado, where it was found that the absorption of simple and complex carbohydrates is far from predictable—in diabetics or anyone else (10).

In fact, these studies showed that some simple carbohydrates such as fructose do not affect blood glucose levels, and some complex carbohydrates act like simple ones. For example, a potato causes a rapid rise in blood sugar, even though it is made of complex carbohydrates. On the other hand, ice cream has virtually no effect at all despite the presence of simple carbohydrates.

You may be wondering why this matters. Well, a rapid rise in blood sugar makes normal people sleepy, which is hardly a very serious problem. Much more significant, however, is the belief held by some scientists at the University of Toronto, who think that people whose diets tend to cause a slow rise in blood sugar are the ones who avoid heart disease, some cancers, and diabetes (11). If this is indeed true, then we have an incentive to identify the influence of various carbohydrates on blood sugar so as to ensure that the dietary balance of carbohydrates limits rapid increases in blood sugar.

Interestingly, both refined and natural cereals cause the blood sugar to rise rapidly, while starches such as pasta and beans have hardly any effect at all. Sometimes the combination of carbohydrates makes an important difference. For example, when bread is combined with beans, the blood sugar rises little, just as you would predict from beans alone. But when bread is eaten with cheese, the blood sugar rises rapidly, just as you would expect from bread alone!

Despite these inconsistencies, cereals such as bread provide us with natural nutrients and fiber, and are very important components of our diet. So the real implication of these findings is that *as the relative amount of carbohydrate in our diets is increased, the balance of different carbohydrates becomes increasingly important.* For the moment, it would seem reasonable to try to balance your intake of cereals and starches to minimize these effects as far as possible. In practice, this means adding more foods like beans, rice, and pasta to those carbohydrates (bread, sugar, potatoes, cereals) that rapidly increase the blood sugar.

WHAT ARE REFINED CARBOHYDRATES?

The refining of foods such as sugar and flour is a relatively recent development in human history. In yet another attempt to improve on nature, it was decided that brown sugar and brown bread were coarse and uncivilized, and so ways were found to make them both white. At first, little if any thought was given to the nutritional consequences of this action. In fact, the refining process removes most of the nutrients from food, some of which have to be deliberately replaced. An absurd exercise! To illustrate this process, let us consider what refining does to the ordinary, natural flour made from wheat.

A grain of wheat consists of three basic parts, and each contains valuable nutrients.

- The outer part is known as *bran*. Bran contains very useful indigestible fiber, the B vitamins (niacin, B_6, riboflavin, thiamin, and pantothenic acid), and nearly 20 percent of the grain's protein. All of these components are lost during the refining process.
- At one end of the inner grain is a small part called the *germ*. The germ contains some polyunsaturated vegetable oil, B vitamins (thiamin, niacin, B_6, and pantothenic acid), as well as vitamin E and nearly 10 percent of the protein. This is removed from milled wheat.
- The main body of the wheat is called the *endosperm*. The endosperm is composed mostly of starch, which would normally provide energy for the sprouting germ. This contains almost 75 percent of the protein, and large amounts of two B vitamins (pantothenic acid and riboflavin). In addition, there are small amounts of other B vitamins as well. You'll be glad to hear that the endosperm mostly survives the refining process.

When wheat is stone-ground, however, nearly all the nutrients survive. This is a most efficient milling process, because it causes losses of only 5–10 percent of the grain, and then mostly the nonnutritive part of the bran. Other refining methods are more destructive, and so less desirable.

White flour consists only of the endosperm, with only about 25 percent of the nutrients remaining. Nearly 75 percent of the vitamin E is lost, and over 90 percent of the fiber. The only possible advantage that results from this processing is the removal of phytic acid, a substance that can limit the absorption of the important minerals calcium, iron, and zinc.

Other lost vitamins and minerals are at least partly replaced in white bread, but none of the fiber is restored: a major loss to dietary cancer prevention. Incidentally, if you like rye flour, make sure you use the dark rye since this is derived from the whole wheat kernel.

THE MAIN SOURCES OF CARBOHYDRATES

Carbohydrates, more than any other food group, can be found in forms that are either nutritionally rich, or nearly worthless. So it is really worth knowing the nutritional value of what you are eating.

Plants are the world's original source of carbohydrates. Using sunlight, they form glucose which, in turn, is used to form the complex carbohydrates such as starch and fiber. Fiber provides the structural strength of the plant, while the starch is stored to provide energy.

The main sources of carbohydrates in our diet are whole grains, cereals, sugar, syrup, honey, nuts, vegetables, and fruit. Seeds are often the richest source of nutrients, including carbohydrates, for they must possess enough nutrients to support the growth of a new plant. Wheat, oats, rice, peas, corn, beans, potatoes, yams, sweet potatoes, and casava are some of our most nutritious sources of complex carbohydrates.

The simple carbohydrates such as sucrose are found mainly in sugar cane, sugar beets, and maple syrup. Fruit provides a good source of fructose, which turns into glucose as the fruit ripens.

Bread is still our commonest source of carbohydrate. Often it is enriched with milk, honey, and fiber—all of which provide even more carbohydrates. Remember, however, that adding simple carbohydrate like sugar or honey does nothing to increase the nutritional value of any food! Keep this in mind when buying breakfast cereals that boast of their nutritional value.

Don't forget that one of the best ways to obtain good carbohydrates and the most nutrients for the least calories is to eat stone-ground, whole wheat bread.

Pasta, another wheat product, deserves special mention. It is not only a favorite of all Italians, but also a favorite of everyone who is young at heart. Pasta is made from a hard wheat called durum, which is refined into a flour called semolina.

In all its forms, pasta is actually a rather good source of starch because it also contains about 12 percent of good-quality protein. Since there is little fat, the calorie content is also relatively low. The benefits of using pasta in a high-carbohydrate diet are supported by observations that the blood fats were much lower in southern Italians (who live on a 55–60 percent complex carbohydrate diet) than in northern Italians or Americans, who live on a 40–45 percent mixed carbohydrate diet, and who eat more saturated fat (12).

Cereals are another common source of good carbohydrate in our diet. Again, it is the whole grain cereals that are the most nutritious. Oatmeal, a form of wheat that is "rolled" least, is also excellent, and can lower cholesterol levels. Ideally, cereals should be eaten with skim or low-fat milk.

Cold breakfast cereals, often presented as God's answer to our call for the ultimate health food, are sometimes very poor nutritional value for the money. It is a measure of the power of advertising that we buy so much of them. To increase their appeal, particularly to the young and defenseless, some manufacturers coat their cereals with sugar, thus greatly reducing the *nutrient density* (the amount of nutrients in relation to the number of calories). The best way to remedy this is first, to avoid sugar-coated cereals and second, to add ripe fresh fruit that is naturally sweet. This can be very appealing to children, particularly if they are trained from an early age to accept fruit.

You should also understand that the vitamins added to cereals are often only a fraction of the RDA (Recommended Daily Allowance)—and many nutritionists believe that the RDA values are too low. Despite the low vitamin levels, let me urge you to eat the high-fiber bran cereals, which have the greatest anticancer value (as you will learn in Chapter 7).

Rice is the staple food for nearly half of the world's population. It is the most widely eaten source of carbohydrate in the world, although not the most commonly eaten source in the United States. (It is interesting that the British sent all our rice to England during the Revolutionary War, but Jefferson fortunately restored rice to the American continent by smuggling some rice kernels out of Italy in 1787).

Rice is most frequently eaten in its less nutritious "polished" form. This form of preparation strips the rice of some of its protein, half its riboflavin (vitamin B_2) and pryridoxine (vitamin B_6), two thirds of its niacin (part of vitamin B complex), and four fifths of its thiamin (vitamin B_1)—a considerable waste when you consider that half the world is malnourished, if not starving!

Another method of processing rice is known as parboiling. Parboiled rice is derived from steamed brown rice that is polished to produce converted rice. This process retains more nutrients than direct polishing of milled rice, which have lost the bran and the germ. However, no method of processing can provide the natural nutrition of brown rice. Because of the natural bran covering, it takes much longer to cook brown rice (about 45 minutes instead of the 20 minutes required for converted rice, or 5 minutes required for "instant" precooked rice). You may be reluctant to endure this inconvenience, but think carefully about the missing nutrients when you buy that expensive packet of "minute" rice.

Corn, which is both a grain and a vegetable, is part of the diet of the New World. First cultivated by Indians throughout North and South America, it is now a dietary staple in Mexico. In the United States, corn is either grown as sweet corn (about 20 percent sugar) that is eaten as corn on the cob, or as field corn, which contains less sugar and more starch, and which is used mainly for making hominy grits or corn meal (both of which lack the germ and the bran of the whole corn kernel). Although the early American settlers ate large amounts of sweet corn, most corn grown in the United States today is used for cattle feed, and thus converted into protein and harmful animal fat. Both sweet corn and field corn are available in white and yellow varieties, and the only nutritional difference is that yellow corn has more vitamin A. One type of corn that remains popular, of course, is high-fiber, low-calorie popcorn, but popcorn can hardly be said to play a major role in our diet.

Barley is a grain with a long history. In biblical times, before the discovery that wheat and rye could react with yeast to produce raised breads, barley was used to make flat bread. In fact, there is even a story of 5,000 people being fed with five loaves of bread made from barley. Without invoking the thought that barley has miraculous powers, there is no doubt that it is an excellent grain, delicious in soups, popular as a breakfast cereal (in Scotland), and long used in the production of beer and whiskey.

Other grain sources of carbohydrate that are popular in different parts of the world include *bulgur* and *cous-cous* in Middle Eastern and North African countries, and *millet* in parts of Africa, China, and India.

The last major source of complex carbohydrates is the wide variety of fruit and vegetables available at every supermarket. The *legumes,* a class of vegetable that includes lentils, pinto beans, kidney beans, soybeans, blackeyed peas, and navy beans, represent particularly good sources of carbohydrate—and are also good sources of protein. What's more, these vegetables are also low in calories. Weight for weight, soybeans provide nearly as much protein as beef but only half the number of calories, little fat, and no cholesterol.

Among the wide choices of fruit, the greatest emphasis should be given to the citrus fruits and those that contain higher concentrations of vitamins A and C. (More specific food choices are discussed in greater detail later.)

DIETARY RECOMMENDATION

Selected sources of carbohydrates are some of our safest sources of energy and anticancer nutrients. Foods containing complex carbohydrates also provide us with fiber, which is of great value in reducing cancer of the bowel and limits our desire to eat calorie-rich foods. By reducing our need for harmful fatty foods, a high-carbohydrate diet can also give protection against both cancer and heart disease.

Unfortunately for the American people, there has been a steady downward trend in carbohydrate consumption and an upward trend in fat consumption since the beginning of this century. What is worse, the carbohydrate consumption shows a marked shift away from starch, and towards the nutritionally dubious simple sugars. These trends mean that a sizable part of the American diet provides us with calories and little else—except an increased risk of developing cancer, obesity, and heart disease!

This trend must be reversed if you are to reduce your risk of cancer. I therefore recommend that you *increase your intake of complex carbohydrates and natural sugars to 60 percent of your total calories, while reducing your intake of refined sugars to 10 percent of total calories.* This means that your total carbohydrate intake will rise from the present average of about 45 percent of total calories to 70 percent of total calories, a level still below that found in African diets.

If you remember that carbohydrates provide only 4 calories per gram, while fat provides 9 calories per gram, you can see that the shift in your diet away from fat towards carbohydrate will bring you a real reduction in calories for the same amount of food intake.

What is most reassuring is that there is no evidence that a relative increase in complex carbohydrates is harmful in any way to a healthy individual, and the benefits come not only from the accompanying anticancer nutrients and fiber, but also from the displacement of dietary fat.

CHAPTER 7

Protective Fiber

Fiber is the indigestible part of fruit, vegetables, and whole grain cereals. It has now become a household word, thanks to the pioneering efforts in the 1960s of a brilliant British surgeon, Dr. Denis Burkitt, and later to popular journalism and the food industry.

While in Africa twenty to thirty years ago, Denis Burkitt made some very original observations. He discovered the existence of a special form of cancer, which he called Burkitt's lymphoma and which he found was curable with drug therapy. He also observed that African tribes having diets that were very high in roughage (dietary fiber) had very few of the diseases that are common in the United States and in other affluent Western societies. The gastrointestinal diseases that are conspicuously rare in African tribes and other primitive societies are: cancer of the colon and rectum, diverticulosis, appendicitis, hemorrhoids, constipation, hiatal hernia, and gallstones. Other diseases that are also greatly reduced in these people include diabetes and the degenerative disorders of blood vessels that cause varicose veins and coronary heart disease.

The potential importance of these observations can be understood when you realize that in the United States degenerative heart disease is the leading cause of death, and cancer of the colon is the leading cause of death from cancer.

Although of course there are differences in genetic susceptibility between individuals exposed to the same risk factors, it is the influence of the environment that is the most important cause of the development of most diseases. All that is now required is to establish just what aspect of the diet or life-style of these African peoples contributes most to their freedom from our diseases. In Burkitt's opinion, the level of dietary fiber was the critical factor (1), while other scientists suggested that the benefits also stemmed from the low levels of dietary fat, refined sugar, and salt that accompanied the high intake of fibrous dietary starch (2).

While Denis Burkitt was making his observations about the potential value of fiber as a dietary constituent, the actual amount of fiber in the American diet was steadily declining. In fact there has been about a 25 percent decline in the average consumption of fiber since the beginning of this century. This decline is due mostly to the increased consumption of refined carbohydrates and fat, which have displaced fruit, vegetables, and whole grain cereals from our diet. This deplorable change must be reversed! I should point out, though, that even before this decline, the American diet did not contain enough fiber, in terms of potential cancer protection.

In order to get the best out of your dietary fiber it is helpful to understand what dietary fiber is, what kinds there are, where to find them, and why they may improve your health while possibly reducing your risk of developing colon cancer and other degenerative diseases.

WHAT IS DIETARY FIBER?

Unfortunately, too many people advocate increasing total fiber intake without realizing that the benefits of fiber may not depend upon the total intake, but rather upon the intake of *certain types* of fiber.

Although some benefits will result from a general increase in dietary fiber, it is looking more and more likely that the greatest protection against disease may depend upon our ability to define the right balance of the different types of fiber in our diet. However, although scientists have not been able to define the perfect balance of dietary fiber, it is clear that the poor people of Africa and Asia are doing something right.

All fiber is derived from the cell walls of plants, and it is fiber that gives plants their firmness. Plant fiber consists of several components; the major ones are lignin, cellulose, hemicellulose, and pectin. In addition, the plant cell wall also contains other nonfibrous substances such as proteins and fats.

Other sources of dietary fiber include natural carbohydrate food additives known as gums and mucilages.

Although all components of dietary fibers except lignin are complex carbohydrates, this does not mean that they all act in the same way. If someone tells you that "fiber always prevents constipation," or that "fiber always reduces cholesterol," they are misleading you. By acquiring some understanding of what different fibers do, you will be able to use them more effectively to protect your health.

Fibers produce their most beneficial effects by absorbing water. This increases stool bulk and causes softening. What is even more important, this increase in stool bulk stimulates the intestine to move undigested food residues and other waste much faster. This is how most fibers exert their laxative effect.

By the way, not all fibers absorb water equally. Hemicellulose and cellulose absorb the most water and so these are the best at preventing constipation. In contrast, lignin absorbs little water, reduces bacterial digestion of other fibers, and sometimes actually contributes to constipation. Pectins, gums, and mucilages are soluble in water. This means that they cannot absorb water, and are consequently unable to exert any beneficial effect on bowel function.

Another difference between the fibers is the way they are digested. Cellulose, hemicellulose, and pectin are *partially* degraded by the fermenting action of intestinal bacteria. This produces gases that can cause flatulence. This potentially troublesome problem can be minimized if the change to a high-fiber diet is made gradually.

Now that you have some idea of the different components of dietary fiber, how can you relate this knowledge to the kind of information that is sometimes found on food labels?

You may have noticed that fiber content is often presented as "crude fiber," or just "fiber." In fact this is quite misleading. Crude fiber consists only of cellulose and lignin, and the other fibers are ignored. Even the U.S. Department of Agriculture publishes analyses of food constituents that include only crude fiber values, and these are currently being completely revised.

The basic problem of estimating our real fiber intake is this. Crude fiber is whatever remains after boiling food with solutions of acid and alkali. This is a very different form of digestion from that which takes place in our own digestive systems. Obviously, our bodies attack food less viciously. The result is that the food you eat may contain anywhere from four to seven times more dietary fiber than the crude fiber estimate suggests (3).

However, more accurate methods of analyzing dietary fiber have recently been devised. Consequently, the fiber content of the foods listed in this book will represent the best available estimates of true dietary fiber. This will enable you to estimate your daily fiber intake much more accurately than is now possible using conventional "crude fiber" tables. It also means that the recommended levels of dietary fiber in the Cancer Prevention Diet will appear substantially higher than the levels discussed in most nutritional literature.

THE EFFECTS OF DIETARY FIBER

Before we explore the intimate relationship between dietary fiber and colorectal cancer, you should know a little more about the effects of fiber. In this way you will develop an understanding of your new diet that will make you welcome the necessary food changes rather than resent them. It is also important to understand that when you increase your fiber intake you may increase your requirement for other vital nutrients such as calcium, zinc, iron, magnesium, and copper. These may need to be taken as supplements if your dietary fiber intake is always very high (consistently more than 40–50 grams per day).

The extraordinary ability of cellulose and hemicellulose to absorb water, which results in a softening and enlargement of the stool, produces a laxative effect that is of immediate benefit to the many people who suffer from diverticular disease (areas of weakness in the bowel wall) or from spastic colon (bowel cramps). Before becoming interested in cancer research, I treated many patients who were suffering from these conditions with a high-fiber diet, and had gratifying success.

The entire basis for this treatment depends upon the influence of a natural high-fiber diet on the "gut transit time." In one study, African villagers on their typical high-fiber diet, were found to average only 36 hours for the time it takes food to travel from mouth to rectum. In contrast, the gut transit time for a group of British men on a typical low-fiber Western diet averaged 77 hours. Even more impressive was the fact that the daily fecal output of the Africans weighed about four times as much! Not surprisingly, Africans do not suffer from diverticulosis or spastic colon.

Now this may not sound very important. After all, you may say, so what? Spastic colon or diverticular disease aren't that important (unless you suffer from them). Well, these are not the only benefits. A number of other side effects come from this change in bowel habit. And some of these side effects are the vital ones that actually reduce your risk of cancer and heart disease.

A high-fiber diet based upon whole grains and vegetables causes a change in the nature of the bacteria that normally live in the gut; a change in the composition of the stool so that it contains less harmful bile acids; an increased binding of carcinogenic chemicals by fiber, making them less harmful; and a reduction in the absorption of harmful fats and cholesterol. All these changes are tremendously important to the cancer-protecting effect of fiber. Yet not all types of fiber will produce all these effects, or work in the same way.

For example, when you look at the effects of fibers from bran, carrots, and cabbage, you find that they produce a similar result in dissimilar ways. Bran resists digestion, so it increases stool bulk by its very presence, and by its capacity to absorb water when in the bowel. On the other hand, carrots and cabbage are both fully digested, and this process stimulates tremendous growth among bowel bacteria; it is these multiplying bacteria that increase the stool bulk (4).

Elimination of Cancer-Causing Chemicals

No matter how stool bulk is increased, it is thought by scientists that the increase dilutes the harmful effects of any chemicals that have been ingested or that have been formed in the bowel itself. As you can imagine, this increase in bulk lowers the concentration of any cancer-causing chemicals in your bowel and reduces the time that they would have to cause damage to the cells lining the bowel wall.

If you stop to think about it, this natural effect of fiber is far superior and infinitely preferable to taking one of the more than seven hundred laxatives that are sold across the counter in the United States.

Reducing the Absorption of Dangerous Fat

As you are now well aware, a major goal in dietary cancer prevention is to reduce your intake of fat. It is also one of the hardest things to give up. But one of the great things about increasing your dietary fiber is that it should help to reduce the absorption of any excess fat that may have crept furtively into your diet (4).

Unfortunately, not all fibers are equally good at this. Bran, one of the most popular fibers, has little effect on fat absorption, so this fiber will not compensate for a sudden dietary indiscretion.

The best fibers for this are pectins, which are found mostly in fruit; guar gum, which is found in beans; and the fibers that are found in carrots and rolled oats. These fibers can also lower blood cholesterol substantially, including the especially harmful LDL cholesterol.

This effect of fiber is really good news because it means that we can reduce the risks of both cancer and heart disease simultaneously.

CAN DIETARY FIBER HELP YOU TO CONTROL YOUR WEIGHT?

As if reducing the risk of cancer and heart disease is not enough, fiber has one more ace up its sleeve.

Obesity rivals democracy as a national obsession—and with good reason. There are more overweight people in the United States than in any other country in the world. Each week there is a new diet, launched with much fanfare, that promises an easier way to lose weight. These fad diets usually fail. In fact, long-term weight reduction and weight control using the high-fiber Cancer Prevention Diet offers you a much better chance of success.

When you increase your fiber intake you will be eating cheaper foods such as fruit and vegetables that are lower in calories. The fiber itself will absorb water in the stomach, and this will make you feel that you have had a substantial meal—even though you will have had fewer calories. An added bonus is that the low-calorie starchy foods containing fiber usually have very little high-calorie fat.

Certain bulk-producing fibers (such as those in bran) also help to reduce the number of calories that you absorb by hurrying food through the intestines after the delay in the stomach. This shortens the time available for digestion and absorption of any calorie-rich food that just happens to be alongside. Fiber also traps some fat and a little protein. These are then excreted, denying the body those extra calories too.

FIBER IS GREAT IN THEORY, BUT DOES IT WORK?

I am quite convinced that nearly everyone would benefit from a substantial increase in dietary fiber. There is so much evidence that our low-fiber diet contributes to the present epidemic of chronic degenerative diseases that we can ill afford not to increase our daily fiber intake.

It is a commonly held view among scientists that scientific theories are never proved, only disproved. In this sense, it remains to be "proved" that a diet high in fiber will protect us from colon cancer and possibly other cancers, either by inhibiting the cancer-promoting effect of fat or by reducing the effect of carcinogens. Despite this semantic distinction, there is a great deal of epidemiological and experimental evidence to indicate that a high-fiber diet will reduce our colon cancer risk.

Having suggested that you increase your fiber intake, I should point out that the scientific efforts to prove that a high-fiber diet does indeed reduce the risk of colon and rectal cancer have met with mixed results.

While most scientific studies showed that people at high risk for colon cancer had diets that were low in total fiber (3,5), a few studies have failed to demonstrate a beneficial effect of fiber (3). Some attempts have also been made to identify which types of fiber give the best protection, since this could lead to diets that are more protective than those which rely only on a high intake of fiber-rich foods in general.

In only one study has an attempt been made to look at one type of fiber alone (3). This study concluded that although the total fiber intake did not make a difference, the *pentosan* fraction of fiber, which is found mostly in whole grains, did give protection against colorectal cancer.

In a study that compared the risk of colon cancer among Indians living in northern India with those living in the south, it was found that the disease was absent in the north where the diet contained high levels of vegetable fiber, and quite common in the south where little fiber was eaten (6). Similar results were found when the diet of high-risk Danes was compared to that of low-risk Finns (5). Other studies have not always been as convincing, but this may have been due to other factors.

Experimental evidence from laboratories in different parts of the world has also led to mixed results. But a recent report has revealed that fiber derived from wheat bran and from citrus fruits can protect rats from chemically induced colon cancer (7). If there is a conclusion to be drawn from all the evidence, it is that some components of fiber can protect the colon against certain types of cancer-causing chemicals, but no single type of fiber can protect the bowel against all such chemicals.

However, of the fibers that have been examined, those that are found in whole grains (bran), citrus fruits, and vegetables seem to be the most beneficial, and will therefore be a substantial part of your cancer prevention diet.

FIBER IN YOUR CANCER PREVENTION DIET

If we use accurate methods of measurement, the average American consumes only about 25 grams of dietary fiber daily, and some consume a good deal less. The Kikuyu tribe in Kenya, and the Buganda tribe in Uganda, consume between 130 and 150 grams of fiber each day, perhaps competing for the world record! Most of the poorer peoples in Africa and Asia are a little less ambitious, and consume a modest 40–60 grams a day.

There is little doubt in my mind that these people benefit tremendously from this aspect of their diet, and probably without even knowing it. We in the "advanced" countries of the West should not miss this opportunity to learn from people who live so much closer to nature than we do.

Although there is no precise amount of fiber needed for good health, your dietary fiber intake should be increased to about 50 grams a day: double the present average American intake. This should be derived mainly from an increase in your consumption of unrefined cereals, vegetables, and fruit.

And remember, it is important to increase your daily fiber gradually so that your body has time to make the necessary adjustments to this lifelong commitment.

Although one day we will learn precisely how much of each type of fiber we need for perfect health, that day has not yet arrived. In the meantime, the balance of fiber that you will get on a diet of fruit, cereals, and vegetables will not only include the essential types of fiber, but also many of the vital nutrients that give you cancer protection. This is almost certainly more important anyway, for it is likely that cancer protection does not depend upon the intake or exclusion of any single dietary factor, but rather upon the effect of a number of different factors that work together. The Cancer Prevention Diet is designed to make these factors work for you.

WHERE YOU CAN FIND YOUR FIBER

It's all very well for me to urge you to eat about 50 grams of fiber every day, but you are obviously wondering how on earth this is going to be accomplished. Merely increasing your intake of whole wheat, cereals, fruits, and vegetables will help, although the chances are that most of you would do this without any idea of the amount of fiber that had been added to your diet.

To make this easier, Table 7–1 lists the amount of fiber in typical foods that make up your daily menu. When you discover the structure of your new diet, you will see that your fiber needs will be provided for automatically.

I think that you will easily be convinced from this table that foods which are high in fiber are often low in calories. These figures also suggest that fruit and vegetables are the obvious foods to concentrate on if you wish to eat well and control your weight.

Remember, a gradual increase in your dietary fiber should also be accompanied by an increase in your fluid intake as well as an adequate intake of vitamins and minerals.

Finally, if you have any doubt about whether a high-fiber diet is right for you, or if you have any medical problems that might be influenced adversely, please contact your personal physician for advice.

Table 7–1
SOURCES OF DIETARY FIBER

| | | BREAD AND CEREALS | | |
Food	Amount	Weight (in grams)	Fiber (in grams)	Calories
CEREALS:				
All-Bran	½ cup	35	12.0	105
Bran, Wheat	¼ cup	14	6.0	28
Corn Flakes	1 cup	28	3.4	95
Cracked Wheat	⅓ cup	60	6.0	200
Grape-Nuts	¼ cup	33	3.6	110
Grits	¼ cup	45	4.8	90
Oat Bran	¼ cup	20	5.3	58
Rolled Oats	½ cup	50	5.8	140
Shredded Wheat	1 biscuit	21	2.8	70
Wheaties	1 cup	19	3.5	97
BREADS:				
Cornbread	1 square	30	1.4	58
French bread	1 piece	30	0.8	85
Muffin, bran	1 medium	40	3.3	105
Pumpernickel	1 slice	32	1.9	77
Rye	1 slice	25	0.8	62
White	1 slice	25	0.7	64
Whole meal	1 slice	25	2.1	56
Whole wheat	1 slice	25	1.3	59
Graham crackers	2 squares	15	1.5	53
		FRUIT		
Apple	1 large	166	4.0	84
Applesauce	1 cup	240	3.4	100
Apricots	1 average	36	0.7	16
Banana	1 medium	108	3.0	116
Blackberries	1 cup	144	8.9	53
Blueberries	1 cup	145	3.4	90

Table 7-1 (continued)

FRUIT (continued)

Food	Amount	Weight (in grams)	Fiber (in grams)	Calories
Cantaloupe	½	477	4.8	80
Cherries	10 large	68	1.1	38
Cranberries	1 cup	192	8.0	62
Figs (dried)	1 medium	20	3.7	46
Grapefruit	½	87	0.8	31
Grapes (red)	15	60	0.5	45
Grapes (green)	15	75	0.75	54
Honeydew	⅕	452	4.0	100
Nectarine	1 small	69	1.5	44
Orange	1 small	78	1.6	35
Peach	1 medium	100	2.3	38
Pear	1 medium	164	4.0	88
Pineapple	1 cup	156	1.6	82
Plum	3 small	85	1.8	38
Prunes (dried)	2	15	2.8	38
Raisins (dried)	½ cup	28	2.0	78
Raspberries	1 cup	124	9.2	42
Strawberries	1 cup	143	3.1	45
Tangerine	1 large	101	2.0	39
Watermelon	4 × 8 inch wedge	926	8.1	110

VEGETABLES

Food	Amount	Weight (in grams)	Fiber (in grams)	Calories
Asparagus	1 cup	186	7.0	36
Bean sprouts	1 cup	116	3.0	26
Beans (green)	1 cup	128	4.2	20
Beans (kidney)	1 cup	186	19.4	188
Beans (lima)	1 cup	170	16.6	126
Beans (white)	1 cup	180	15.8	168
Beets	1 cup	170	4.2	66
Broccoli	1 cup	186	7.0	36
Brussels sprouts	1 cup	156	4.6	40
Cabbage	1 cup	170	4.2	20
Carrots	1 cup	110	3.6	30
Cauliflower	1 cup	180	3.2	28
Celery	1 cup	120	2.2	16
Corn (sweet)	1 ear	126	5.2	144
Cornmeal	½ cup	34	3.2	114
Cucumber	½ cup	140	2.2	12
Eggplant	1 cup	200	5.0	32
Lentils	1 cup	200	7.4	194

Table 7-1 (*continued*)

VEGETABLES (*continued*)

Food	Amount	Weight (in grams)	Fiber (in grams)	Calories
Lettuce	1 cup	55	0.8	10
Okra	½ cup	50	1.6	13
Onion	½ cup	58	1.2	14
Peas (canned)	1 cup	170	13.4	126
Pepper (green)	½ cup	58	1.1	10
Potato (baked)	1 medium	150	3.8	144
Radishes (raw)	½ cup	58	1.3	7
Rice (brown)	½ cup	97	2.4	108
Rice (white)	½ cup	102	0.75	114
Spinach	1 cup	55	0.2	8
Squash (summer)	½ cup	90	2.0	16
Squash (winter)	1 cup	240	7.0	82
Tomato	1 small	100	1.5	18

MISCELLANEOUS

Food	Amount	Weight (in grams)	Fiber (in grams)	Calories
FLOUR:				
Dark rye	1 cup	100	12.5	315
Light rye	1 cup	80	2.5	280
Self-raising	1 cup	90	3.5	305
White wheat	1 cup	90	2.5	310
Whole meal	1 cup	95	9.0	300
Whole wheat	1 cup	95	7.0	310
Macaroni	½ cup	70	0.6	77
Spaghetti	½ cup	70	0.8	76
NUTS:				
Almonds	1 tablespoon	8	1.1	46
Chestnuts	3	26	1.8	46
Peanuts	1 tablespoon	9	0.8	52
Pecans	1 tablespoon	7.5	0.5	49

These fiber analyses are derived from the published data of Dr. James W. Anderson, Professor of Medicine and Clinical Nutrition, University of Kentucky Medical Center, Lexington, Kentucky; and from "The Composition of Foods," edited by A. A. Paul and D. A. T. Southgate, published by Her Majesty's Stationery Office, London.

CHAPTER 8

Vital Vitamins

Most of us are fascinated by the almost magical power of vitamins. This isn't surprising. Many scientists share this fascination because these micronutrients are indeed *vital*—to human health. The power of vitamins is so enormous that a chronic deficiency of minute quantities of these chemical substances can cause the body to develop serious and even fatal disease. In fact, the total supply of vitamins that are needed to prevent vitamin deficiency diseases amount to only a teaspoonful per week!

Although many of you already have great faith in vitamins as a source of good health, it is only relatively recently that we have found hard scientific evidence that the presence of some of these vitamins in your daily diet *can reduce your risk of cancer.*

WHAT ARE VITAMINS?

The human body is built of, and sustained by, both the *macronutrients* (fats, proteins, and carbohydrates) and the *micronutrients* (vitamins and minerals). The macronutrients provide us with structural strength and energy, while the micronutrients help critical chemical reactions to occur inside each living cell.

Vitamins are organic substances that are essential for life. This was recognized even in antiquity. However, it was not until the eighteenth century that our modern understanding of vitamins began. The discovery of the value of limes for the prevention of scurvy among British sailors was one of the early triumphs of "modern" medicine, one which ultimately led to the discovery of vitamin C. At about the same time, it was found that cod liver oil could treat rickets; this ultimately led to the understanding of the need for vitamin D for proper bone growth. But it was only in 1912 that F. G. Hopkins, in England, proved that animals required "accessory factors" in addition to protein, carbohydrates and fat, if they were to grow normally. These "factors" turned out to be vitamins.

Dietary vitamins are derived from plants and animals. They can also be synthesized in the laboratory. Altogether thirteen genuine vitamins have been discovered, each having special functions of vital importance to your body. In recent years, some people have tried to add laetrile to the list of vitamins, but rigorous scientific evaluation has proved this substance to be valueless.

Vitamins are either *fat-soluble* or *water-soluble*. This is an important distinction because more fat-soluble vitamins are stored in the body than water-soluble ones.

The fat-soluble vitamins are A, D, E, and K. Their efficient absorption into the body depends in part on dietary fat and bile from the liver. Because these vitamins are stored in the body, their long-term effects are less predictable. And serious toxicity can result from a chronic excess of vitamins A and D.

The water-soluble vitamins are the vitamin B complex (including niacin, riboflavin, folacin, pantothenic acid, pyridoxine, B_{12}, and biotin) and vitamin C, sometimes called ascorbate or ascorbic acid. An excess of these vitamins is normally excreted in the urine or sweat, and so toxicity is not usually a problem.

The health of the body depends upon its ability to perform its vital functions. These vital functions involve chemical reactions which in turn depend upon chemical substances called *enzymes*. Enzymes induce chemical reactions to occur without themselves being used up.

Vitamins are important because they, too, cause important chemical reactions to occur, usually by helping the enzymes. Unlike enzymes, however, they do get used up, which is why we must constantly replace them. Maintaining a balanced intake of vitamins is usually achieved through a sensible diet that includes plenty of fresh fruit, vegetables, and whole grain cereals. Often an appropriate intake is attempted by an almost indiscriminate use of vitamin supplements taken in doses that are based more upon intuition than scientific guidance. Your use of vitamins must be based on a thorough understanding if you hope to benefit fully.

I will now outline the important vitamins to you, with special emphasis on how they might reduce your chances of getting cancer. This chapter will also be a very useful guide to those of you who wish to select vitamin supplements more wisely.

VITAMIN A

As with most vitamins, our first awareness of vitamin A resulted from its deficiency. This produced night blindness, which simply means the inability to see well in the dark. As long ago as 1500 B.C., in Egyptian medical writings, roast ox liver or the liver of black cocks was recommended to cure this disorder. One thousand years later the famous Greek physician and philosopher, Hippocrates, prescribed raw ox liver for night blindness, while the modern medicine men of Ruanda-Urundi in Africa were prescribing chicken liver as recently as 1955. How wise they all were!

It was not until 1915, however, that fat-soluble vitamin A was actually identified, and it was in 1923 that its ability to prevent night blindness and dryness of the eyes was scientifically established.

Research eventually led to the realization that there is more than one form of vitamin A, and that there are other substances such as beta-carotene that can be converted by the body into active vitamin A. Foods that contain these inactive forms of vitamin A will be a very important part of your new diet.

Only two of Vitamin A's basic forms need be considered here because they constitute most of the dietary vitamin A. The first is retinol. It is the active form of vitamin A and is derived from animal sources. The second is *beta-carotene*. This is the inactive form, or *pro*vitamin A, and is derived from plant sources. Inactive beta-carotene is an antioxidant that resists carcinogenesis, and it is converted by the body into active vitamin A, in which form it has other anticancer properties.

While it has been clear for a long time that a certain amount of vitamin A in your diet will prevent you from getting a deficiency disease, it has also been known for some time that huge amounts of vitamin A can actually be very harmful, causing lethargy, fatigue, and malaise. This toxic amount of vitamin A is often associated with abdominal discomfort, and a whole range of other symptoms that include hair loss, dry skin, and emotional problems.

Vitamin A toxicity usually results from a reckless intake of sup-

Table 8-1
THE ACTIONS OF VITAMIN A AND BETA-CAROTENE

- Maintain the integrity of skin, and lining of airways and intestinal tract.
- Necessary for normal color and night vision.
- Necessary for normal growth and development of cells.
- Necessary for normal body defenses (the immune system).
- Vitamin A can inhibit carcinogenesis.
- Beta-carotene is an antioxidant that can also inhibit carcinogenesis.

plements, and is very rarely associated with diet. Only Arctic explorers have been known to get vitamin A toxicity, as a result of subsisting on large amounts of polar bear liver—a very rich source of vitamin A.

The vitamin A in your diet is also affected by your dietary level of protein, fat, vitamin E, and zinc. Proteins are required to carry the vitamin around the body; some fat is needed to stimulate release of the bile necessary for vitamin absorption; vitamin E prevents the destruction of vitamin A in the gut and works with vitamin A to ensure healthy cell membranes; and zinc encourages cell growth, which uses up vitamin A. The level of vitamin A in the bloodstream, on the other hand, is influenced by oral contraceptives (which increase it) and by some diseases (which decrease it).

Can Vitamin A Prevent Cancer?

Vitamin A and beta-carotene are the most exciting of all the vitamins that can protect us from cancer. Tremendous progress has been made in our knowledge of these substances, and especially of their role in preventing carcinogenesis.

In studies involving groups of patients with cancers of the lung, breast, larynx, bladder, esophagus, stomach, colon, rectum, cervix and prostate, it was found that their vitamin A consumption was considerably less than in comparable groups of people without cancer.

In patients with lung cancer, the intake of fresh, green vegetables was found to be low (1); the intake of vitamin supplements was low (2,3); and the intake of liver—a good source of vitamin A—was also low (2). In another study, the low intake of beta-carotene appeared most important (4).

It seems that the commonest cause of cancer deaths in women, breast cancer, may also be reduced by vitamin A (5,6).

Studies of patients with cancer of the larynx found the dietary intake of both vitamin A and C to be lower than in healthy controls (7).

Patients with bladder cancer have also revealed a low intake of vitamin A (8). Of course, other risk factors such as the effects of coffee consumption, smoking, and chemical exposure had to be excluded first before the impact of diet alone could be assessed. A similar approach had to be adopted for other studies too, particularly with respect to the influence of smoking on cancer of the lung and larynx. Even alcohol intake had to be considered when studying the causes of cancer of the larynx.

This illustrates just how careful scientists must be if they are to identify the dietary risk factors in the presence of other risk factors. This certainly was the case in a series of studies that established the importance of fruit and vegetables in lowering the risk of cancer of the esophagus (9,10). It was assumed that since both fruit and vegetables were potent sources of Vitamin A and C, it was the presence of these vitamins that made the crucial difference. This is likely to be correct because laboratory tests have supported this assumption.

In Japan, where stomach cancer is rampant, a convincing study of 265,118 people showed that by simply taking two glasses of milk a day, and by including green and yellow vegetables in the daily diet, the risk of this fatal cancer could be reduced substantially (11). This benefit was ascribed to vitamin A.

And if you need more convincing, comparable benefits of milk, fruit, and vegetables can be implied from studies of patients with both colorectal cancer (12) and prostate cancer (13).

This dramatic evidence of the importance of vitamin A as a cancer-inhibitor is supported by experimental laboratory studies. These experiments showed that tumors occurred more frequently in animals that were deliberately made deficient in vitamin A (14), and less frequently in animals given vitamin A supplements (15,16). Of special interest was a report that vitamin A was protective even after exposure to the carcinogen (17).

Although most experiments have been with vitamin A, some experiments with beta-carotene have also shown a protective effect against ultraviolet light–induced skin tumors (18), and chemically induced gastrointestinal tumors (19).

Certain types of vitamin A may also have a role in cancer treatment. A form of vitamin A, 13-cis retinoic acid, is currently being used in a clinical trial to see whether its direct application to the uterine cervix will reverse cancerous changes. Interestingly, at the University of Arizona a recent case of mycosis fungoides, a skin cancer, responded dramatically to treatment with 13-cis retinoic acid. All visible disease disappeared!

Considering the power of vitamin A and beta-carotene to protect and even reverse cancerous change, these vitamins obviously must be a vital part of the Cancer Prevention Diet.

My Dietary Recommendation for Vitamin A

The evidence clearly indicates that the ideal cancer prevention diet should include a substantial increase in the dietary intake of vitamin A and beta-carotene.

The Recommended Daily Allowance (RDA) published by the National Research Council suggests a modest 1,000 micrograms per day for men, and 800 micrograms per day for women. It is recommended that children should have about half the adult amount. It is very likely, however, that these levels do not give you the maximum protection against cancer.

By the way, you should know that 0.3 micrograms of vitamin A is equivalent to 0.6 micrograms of beta-carotene, and either of these amounts is equivalent to 1 international unit (IU). In case you are wondering, 1 microgram is 1 millionth of a gram, and 1 gram is 1/28 of an ounce. Hardly something you could measure on the kitchen scale!

Toxicity from vitamin A can result from an uncontrolled intake of supplements that provide a regular daily intake of at least 50,000 IU. Toxicity virtually never results from dietary sources of vitamin A. Beta-carotene does not cause toxicity, but can cause the skin to turn yellow if taken in very large amounts. And there have been reports from the National Cancer Institute that the oil carrier of beta-carotene found in typical commercial preparations of that micronutrient may cause some minor side effects in large doses.

However, because of the inherent safety of beta-carotene and the strong evidence of a cancer-prevention effect, you should increase your dietary vitamin A, mainly by increasing your beta-carotene intake, using foods that are naturally rich in these crucial vitamins. This ensures that you will receive any other important cancer-inhibiting substances that may coexist alongside vitamin A or beta-carotene, but which have yet to be identified.

Ideally, the level of vitamin A and beta-carotene in your diet should reach at least 25,000 IU per day. This represents 7,500 micrograms (7.5 milligrams) of vitamin A, or 15,000 micrograms (15 milligrams) of beta-carotene. This is about seven and a half times the amount recommended by the National Research Council. Such a level should be quite safe because even daily doses of 100,000 IU have been given to adults for many months without serious side effects (20):

Remember, the dietary intake for children should be less than half that of an adult.

Where to Find Your Vitamin A

Although vitamin A is fat-soluble and therefore capable of being stored in the body, it is likely that the reduced intake of fat—such an important feature of your new diet—will also tend to reduce your intake of vitamin A, and its absorption. It is therefore particularly important that you deliberately seek out foods that contain vitamin A and beta-carotene, and make them a larger part of your daily diet.

Some of the more popular sources of vitamin A and beta-carotene are listed for you in Table 8–2. Remember, most dietary sources of vitamin A are in the form of beta-carotene.

THE B VITAMINS

The water-soluble B vitamins are an essential part of your diet, although their potential importance in the prevention of cancer is not yet fully established.

The B vitamins are thiamin (B_1), riboflavin (B_2), niacin, pantothenic acid, pyridoxine (B_6), vitamin B_{12}, folacin (folic acid), biotin, and choline; the latter is usually considered part of the vitamin B complex even though it is not actually a B vitamin.

Table 8–2
SOME COMMON SOURCES OF VITAMIN A

Source	Weight (in grams)	Serving	Vitamin A (In IU)	Calories
Bran, wheat (fort.)	35	1 cup	1,650	106
Corn flakes	25	1 cup	1,180	97
Corn meal	118	1 cup	566	427
Corn	117	1 cup	400	431
Pasta (whole wheat)	112	average	200	400
Waffles	75	1 medium	250	210
American cheese	28	average	340	107
Brie	28	average	189	95
Camembert	28	average	262	84
Cheddar	28	average	300	112
Cottage cheese (2% fat)	226	1 cup	158	203
Roquefort	28	average	297	105
Eggs	57	1 large	590	82
Egg yolk	17	1 large	590	59
Milk (2% fat)	244	1 cup	500	121
Pumpkin pie	150	1 piece	3,700	317
Crab	226	½ pound	4,916	211
Halibut	226	½ pound	1,000	227
Mackerel, fresh	226	½ pound	1,020	433
Salmon, fresh	226	½ pound	1,359	482
Whitefish	226	½ pound	5,125	352
Apricot	37	1 average	960	19
Apricot (dried)	65	½ cup	7,085	170
Avocado	200	1 average	580	334
Cantaloupe	100	¼	3,400	30
Elderberries	112	¼ pound	685	83
Mango	300	1	11,090	152
Orange	200	1	290	72
Orange juice	250	1 glass	510	114
Peach	115	1 average	1,330	38
Prune (dried)	185	1 cup	2,580	411
Watermelon	600	1 slice	3,540	156
Liver (beef)	112	¼ pound	49,782	159
Kidney	112	¼ pound	783	147
Butter	14	1 tablespoon	470	102
Margarine	14	1 tablespoon	470	102
Cod liver oil	14	1 tablespoon	11,900	126

Table 8-2 (*continued*)

Source	Weight (in grams)	Serving	Vitamin A (In IU)	Calories
Asparagus (cooked)	75	3 spears	675	15
Black-eyed peas	165	1 cup	580	178
Broccoli (cooked)	155	1 cup	3,800	40
Brussels sprouts	155	1 cup	810	56
Carrots (raw)	100	1 Large	11,000	42
Carrots (cooked)	155	1 cup	15,750	48
Carrots (canned)	155	1 cup	22,500	47
Carrot juice	227	1 cup	24,750	96
Corn (cooked)	165	1 cup	660	137
Endive (raw)	50	1 cup	1,650	10
Lettuce (Boston)	55	1 cup	530	8
(looseleaf)	55	1 cup	1,050	10
Parsley (chopped)	60	1 cup	5,100	26
Peas (cooked)	160	1 cup	860	114
(canned)	170	1 cup	1,170	150
Pimientos	34	1 medium	760	9
Soybeans (raw)	210	1 cup	846	170
(cooked)	180	1 cup	140	234
Spinach (cooked)	180	1 cup	14,580	41
Squash (winter)	205	1 cup	8,610	129
Tomato (raw)	150	1 medium	1,350	33

These data are derived from U.S. Dept of Agriculture reference publications and other scientific sources.

The dietary importance of the B vitamins will now be reviewed briefly, so that those of you who take regular supplements will have a reliable source of information as to their known effects.

THIAMIN (VITAMIN B_1)

A dietary deficiency of thiamin causes beri-beri. This disease, which was common among prisoners of war in Japan, is associated with mental confusion, loss of appetite, muscular weakness and wasting, unsteady walking, paralysis, eye muscle weakness, and heart failure—a fairly dismal state to be in as you can imagine.

Fortunately, a deficiency of thiamin is rare in the United States;

what little there is, is found mainly among alcoholics. In the rest of the world, thiamin deficiency is associated with poverty, the consumption of large amounts of raw fish, heavy tea drinking, and the consumption of white flour and rice (both of which have been stripped of many of their nutrients). In Western countries, flour is deliberately enriched to compensate for some of what is lost through the milling process, and so thiamin is replaced.

Thiamin is needed for the metabolism of carbohydrates and for the normal working of the heart and nervous system. As your carbohydrate intake increases, so does your need for thiamin.

Although there is no direct evidence that thiamin influences your chances of getting cancer, there is evidence that thiamin can influence the immune system, and we know that the immune system is an important part of our defense against cancer. This is illustrated by some experiments which have shown that thiamin-deficient animals have an increased risk of infection when exposed to certain bacteria (21).

The amount of thiamin in your new diet will automatically increase as a result of your greater consumption of whole grains and whole wheat cereals. This increased intake of thiamin will help to release energy from the increased starch in your diet.

The RDA for thiamin is 0.5 milligrams per day for each 1,000 calories in your diet, or approximately 1–1.5 milligrams per day. Although the thiamin requirement for elderly people is less, they tend to use it less efficiently, and so they should not reduce their dietary intake. Women should be aware that the daily intake of thiamin should be increased by another 0.5 milligrams per day during pregnancy and lactation.

Your dietary intake of thiamin need not reach a specific level above the RDA, but a convenient target would be about double that of the RDA, or about 3 milligrams per day. This is appropriate for your new diet because of its high starch content, and because of the potential benefits of thiamin to your immune system.

Where to Find Thiamin (Vitamin B_1)

Thiamin is present in a wide range of foods, which is one reason why a deficiency is seldom found in prosperous Western countries where most people have enough to eat.

Common sources of thiamin are whole grain and enriched cereals, pasta, bread, fish, liver, pork, poultry, oatmeal, lima beans, oysters, and peas. Most of these foods are part of your cancer prevention diet.

Fortunately, there have been no reports of thiamin toxicity even at high doses, but there is no evidence that very high doses of vitamin B_1 confer any benefit either. Given our present state of knowledge, megadoses are best avoided.

RIBOFLAVIN (VITAMIN B_2)

Vitamin B_2 helps to convert proteins, fats, and carbohydrates into energy. It is therefore essential for building and maintaining body tissues such as the skin, blood, and brain.

A deficiency of riboflavin causes certain changes in the skin. Cracks appear around the corners of the mouth and nose, and the tongue can become sore. The eyes become more sensitive to light, and corneal changes and cataracts can occur.

Riboflavin is also vital to the development of *T lymphocytes* (T cells), special white blood cells that are part of our immune system. Lack of riboflavin results in fewer T cells being made, and a consequent increase in our susceptibility to infection—and possibly to cancer. However, no direct evidence exists that links dietary riboflavin levels to the risk of cancer.

The RDA for riboflavin is derived from measurements of urinary excretion of the vitamin. When the daily intake of riboflavin is about 0.5 milligrams per day, the urinary loss is quite low. As the daily intake increases, so does the amount lost in the urine. So you see, any benefit that might arise from a water-soluble vitamin must be produced by a temporary increase in the amount of the vitamin in the body, and supplements would have to be taken frequently to maintain an increased body level.

Because riboflavin requirements used to be thought by some scientists to be influenced by total caloric intake, the RDA is expressed as 0.6 milligrams per day for every 1,000 calories in your diet. In fact, the daily requirement for riboflavin is more closely related to dietary *protein*. This daily allowance of about 1–1.5 milligrams should be increased by 0.5 milligrams per day during pregnancy and lactation, and probably also while using oral contraceptives.

Although there is no evidence that the level of riboflavin intake directly influences your chances of getting cancer, a higher intake could help your immune system. Therefore, aim for a riboflavin intake of about 3 milligrams per day, nearly double the RDA.

Where to Find Your Riboflavin (Vitamin B$_2$)

If your diet did not include any animal protein or dairy products, then you might run the risk of developing riboflavin deficiency. However, as with vitamin B$_1$ (thiamin), your new diet will inevitably increase your intake of riboflavin, so it is nice to know that this will be accomplished effortlessly. It is also nice to know that there have not been any reports of toxicity, even to megadoses of vitamin B$_2$.

Foods that supply most of our riboflavin include liver, milk, meat, whole grain and enriched cereals, dark-green vegetables, pasta, eggs, bread, dried beans, and peas.

NIACIN

Niacin helps thiamin and riboflavin convert food into usable energy. When the diet is deficient in niacin, a disease called pellagra develops.

The first known appearance of pellagra was in Europe around 1720. It seems to have resulted from the introduction of corn into the diet. The name pellagra was first used by Italian peasants to describe the rough skin that is characteristic of the disease. However, it wasn't until 1913 that it was suggested that pellagra was due to a deficiency of the amino acid tryptophan in the corn, and it was another sixteen years before it was realized that tryptophan (which, you may remember, is found in protein) could be converted into niacin within the body.

Early signs of niacin deficiency include weakness and loss of appetite, progressing to dermatitis (skin rashes), diarrhea, and dementia (mental confusion). Fortunately, there has not been an epidemic of pellagra in the United States since 1913, when 200,000 cases per year were being reported in the South. Since then we have all become much more aware of the need for variety in our diets so as to avoid such needless suffering.

Because some of our dietary niacin comes from protein, it is obviously necessary to find some way of standardizing the dietary measurement. This is done by calling 1 milligram of niacin by another name: the *niacin equivalent*. Studies have shown that one niacin equivalent (1 milligram niacin) is produced from 60 milligrams of dietary tryptophan. So now we can estimate our intake of niacin directly, or indirectly from our protein intake.

In practice, however, we need make no lengthy calculations because even the average diet in the United States supplies more than enough niacin to meet the body's needs. In fact, the average diet supplies about 500–1,000 milligrams of tryptophan and 8–17 milligrams of niacin each day. This equals about 16–34 milligrams of niacin equivalents.

I recommend that you follow the RDA for niacin: 6.6 niacin equivalents per 1,000 calories, or about 13 niacin equivalents per day.

Where to Find Your Niacin

As with all the B vitamins, your new diet will more than take care of your niacin needs—especially since there is no evidence that niacin influences your cancer risk.

Apart from the process whereby the body converts protein-derived tryptophan into niacin, this vitamin is also found in liver, poultry, meat, whole grain and enriched cereals, pasta, bread, nuts, dried peas and beans, as well as eggs and tuna fish.

Unlike thiamin and riboflavin, large amounts of niacin are toxic and not in the least beneficial! I therefore urge you to avoid being seduced by wild claims that megadoses contribute to good health. The only situation in which large doses of niacin have been used is in the treatment of heart attacks under close medical supervision. And in this situation niacin was found to cause potentially dangerous changes in heart rhythm, gastrointestinal upsets, and liver damage.

VITAMIN B$_6$ (PYRIDOXINE, PRYIDOXAL, PYRIDOXAMINE)

Vitamin B$_6$ is a collective term for three interrelated vitamins. Pyridoxine is the one that is best known. It helps in the absorption and metabolism of proteins, and in the use of dietary fat. It also plays a role in the chemistry of the central nervous system (the brain), the formation of red blood cells, and in the proper development of the immune system.

The need for pyridoxine was first established in 1939. Patients on poor diets were found to have vague symptoms of weakness, irritability, nervousness, insomnia, and some difficulty in walking. About the same time, infants who were being fed a commercial milk product that was low in pyridoxine developed convulsive seizures. These seizures responded to treatment with pyridoxine—but not the other B vitamins—within twenty-four hours.

Fortunately, the modern American diet is seldom associated with a deficiency of pyridoxine, except in alcoholics and in the elderly. Nevertheless, certain conditions are suspected of increasing the dietary requirement for the vitamin. The most important of these include a high-protein diet, pregnancy, the use of oral contraceptives, and certain drugs that oppose the action of pyridoxine.

Except for its importance in the immune system, there is no direct evidence as yet that vitamin B_6 can influence your chance of getting cancer.

The toxicity of pyridoxine was thought to be quite low, even at doses as high as 1 gram per kilogram of body weight—at least in animals. Recently, there has been a report of severe toxic neuropathy (damage to nerves) that resulted from daily doses of 2–6 grams of pyridoxine for two to forty months in two men and five women (22). In three cases it was medically prescribed, in the rest it was self-imposed in the misguided belief that "more might be better."

The RDA for vitamin B_6 is based upon protein intake, and a diet that includes 50 grams of protein would require 1.0 milligrams per day. (This can be obtained from less than two bananas!)

Although there is no direct evidence of a link with cancer risk, there is evidence that vitamin B_6 can influence the cancer-destroying T cells of the immune system. I therefore recommend that you increase your intake of vitamin B_6 to about 10 milligrams per day. If you wish to take supplements, then keep this supplement to *less than* 10 milligrams per day. Remember, your new diet will provide you with an abundance of pyridoxine at no extra cost!

Where to Find Your Vitamin B$_6$

Typically good sources of vitamin B$_6$ are whole grain cereals, liver, meat, fish, avocados, bread, spinach, poultry, green leafy vegetables, nuts, and potatoes—and of course, bananas.

VITAMIN B$_{12}$

Vitamin B$_{12}$ is required for normal growth of cells, particularly blood cells. It is also needed for maintaining the health of nervous tissue.

When the body is deficient in B$_{12}$, predictable changes occur. You guessed it. Red blood cells are not made properly so anemia develops, later followed by certain degenerative changes in the nervous system. Numbness and tingling in the fingers and toes eventually lead to loss of balance, and pain and weakness in the arms and legs.

The first report of anemia due to a deficiency of vitamin B$_{12}$ was made in Edinburgh to the Royal Medical Society in 1822. Of course, at that time nobody knew the precise cause, and it wasn't until 1948 that the vitamin was actually isolated—almost simultaneously in the United States and in England.

B$_{12}$ dietary deficiency is rare in the United States, except among alcoholics, strict vegetarians, and a few people who are unable to absorb the vitamin due to a missing factor inside the stomach.

The only known relationship of vitamin B$_{12}$ to cancer is the increased risk of stomach cancer among people who have pernicious anemia—the failure to absorb B$_{12}$ due to a missing stomach factor. I remember feeling great pride when, as a medical student, I discovered that a patient who was in hospital for treatment of pernicious anemia had an unsuspected stomach cancer, a cancer that was causing no symptoms, and which had consequently been missed by his physicians. That early diagnosis saved his life.

Where to Find Your Vitamin B$_{12}$

This vitamin is found mainly in animal foods such as liver, kidneys, meat, fish, shellfish, poultry, clams, oysters, yeast, milk, and eggs. Toxicity from large doses of vitamin B$_{12}$ is unknown; so are any benefits. The only indication for supplemental B_{12} is for the treatment of a deficiency, although some physicians do use it as a harmless placebo—after all it is bright red and looks impressive, especially when injected!

It would take about three years to use up your body stores of B_{12} even if your diet completely lacked the vitamin. You will certainly not worry, because your cancer prevention diet will provide you with all the B_{12} you will ever need.

There is, however, one special reason to make sure that you have enough B_{12}. It has been reported that *megadoses* of vitamin C (1 gram *with* each meal) can destroy vitamin B_{12} in your food (23,24), although there is still some controversy about whether this actually causes B_{12} deficiency. This is potentially important because there are very good reasons to increase your intake of vitamin C, as you will soon discover. (My recommendations therefore do *not* include 1 gram of vitamin C with *each* meal.)

The present RDA is 3 micrograms per day, and there is no reason to aim for more. Even the (unsound) typical American diet supplies 5–15 micrograms per day—and, as mentioned above, your new diet will provide even more.

FOLIC ACID

Folic acid is an important vitamin because it is essential for cell growth, blood formation, and immunity, and it may influence your risk of cancer. At this stage the evidence is preliminary, but animal studies have shown that a deficiency of folic acid can lead to impaired immunity, genetic damage, and an increased susceptibility to environmental carcinogens. An interesting report recently appeared in the prestigious journal *Science*. It indicated that folic acid supplementation could prevent the chromosomal (genetic) damage in human cells that was induced either by folic acid deficiency or by caffeine (25). The chromosomal damage observed in these studies was in many respects similar to the genetic damage seen in many human cancers. However, until the proper clinical studies have been done, it is premature to claim that folic acid supplements will prevent the genetic damage produced by all carcinogens. Yet this evidence is compelling enough to encourage moderate supplementation with folic acid.

Body stores of folic acid will last three to six months if the diet is totally deficient in this vitamin. Folic acid deficiency is probably the most common vitamin deficiency in the world. A deficiency of folic acid causes an anemia which is indistinguishable from that caused by vitamin B_{12} deficiency; and it is especially likely during pregnancy. Folic acid deficiency is usually the result of an inadequate diet, and occurs in alcoholics and as a consequence of various diseases.

Where to Find Your Folic Acid

Only about 25–50 percent of dietary folic acid is in a form that can be used by the body, and it has been estimated that 100–200 micrograms are needed each day to maintain tissue reserves. The present RDA is 400 micrograms per day, and this is doubled during pregnancy and lactation.

Good sources of folic acid include liver, kidneys, dark-green leafy vegetables, fruit, wheat germ, and dried peas and beans. These foods will be part of your new diet anyway and so a good intake of folic acid will occur automatically.

Since there is a possibility that folic acid could give you some protection against cancer, and since there is no evidence that an increased intake is harmful in any way, it would seem reasonable to increase *dietary* folic acid. Since this vitamin is stored in the body, dietary supplements should not be necessary. However, for those who wish to take supplements, I would suggest 400 micrograms per day.

A word of warning: I must caution you that folic acid can mask the symptoms of vitamin B_{12} deficiency by curing the anemia but failing to protect the nervous system. This is not a problem in normal, healthy people, but as a general rule, if you have any illness that is under medical supervision, you should discuss any dietary changes with your personal physician.

BIOTIN

Biotin plays an important role in the metabolism of carbohydrates and fat. There is no evidence yet that it influences the cancer risk.

A deficiency of biotin is rare in the United States. When it occurs, it produces loss of appetite, nausea, vomiting, a smooth tongue, mental depression, and a scaly skin rash. It is now thought that the scaly dermatitis sometimes found in infants under six months of age may be due to this vitamin deficiency.

Good sources of biotin include liver, kidney, egg yolk, and some vegetables. Poor sources include meat, cereal grains, and fruit. Quite a lot is also made by intestinal bacteria, which we all have in abundance.

For biotin deficiency to occur in humans, it is necessary to consume the protein avidin, which renders the dietary biotin useless. Avidin is found in raw white of eggs—hardly something to which most of us are addicted!

The RDA for biotin is not yet established, but a dietary intake of 100–300 micrograms per day is considered more than adequate, and it so happens that this is the amount in the average American diet.

Your cancer prevention diet will not significantly influence your biotin intake.

PANTOTHENIC ACID

Pantothenic acid is also involved in the metabolism of carbohydrates and fat. It has no known role in dietary cancer prevention. This vitamin is found in meats, legumes, whole grain cereals, fruit, and vegetables.

A dietary deficiency of pantothenic acid does not occur in man, although it can be artificially induced. When it occurs, it causes widespread failure of many organs.

The RDA is 4–7 milligrams per day for adults, and the present American diet gives us between 5–20 milligrams per day. Your new diet will provide abundant pantothenic acid, so supplementation is pointless.

VITAMIN C (Ascorbic acid)

Vitamin C is one of the most interesting vitamins, and one that will play a very important role in your new diet. Evidence exists that foods rich in vitamin C can reduce the risk of esophageal cancer (26), stomach cancer (27,28), laryngeal cancer (7), and uterine cervical dysplasia (premalignant changes) (29). Possibly other cancers can also be inhibited by vitamin C, but this remains theoretical and may partly depend on the dose of vitamin C ingested.

In 1536, when the French explorer Jacques Cartier found that many of his men were dying (of scurvy) near what is now the city of Quebec, local Indians told him that their affliction could be treated by drinking tea made from the bark of leaves of an arborvitae tree. This tea contained vitamin C. In those days the greatest suffering from scurvy was among sailors; and the Portuguese explorer Vasco da Gama lost 100 of his crew of 160 during a voyage around Africa to India in 1497–98.

Later, on May 20, 1747, the famous experiments of the British naval surgeon Dr. James Lind were performed. Sailors who had scurvy were given either citrus fruit (two oranges and one lemon a day) or other treatments (such as cider or vinegar). Those who received the citrus fruit recovered within a few days; the others showed no improvement. This cure was no small achievement when you realize that the sailors who had scurvy probably had extreme weakness and prostration, swollen bleeding gums, internal bleeding, joint pain, weakness, and diarrhea—and faced imminent death!

It was not until 1928 that L-ascorbic acid was discovered by the Nobel laureate Albert Szent-Gyorgyi, but the world had to wait four years before this substance was shown to be vitamin C. It did not then take long for people to realize that this substance might improve their health, and some began taking vitamin C as a dietary supplement.

Perhaps more than any other vitamin, the amount of vitamin C ingested may influence the range of its effects on the human body. Less than 10 milligrams per day is enough to prevent scurvy—only one five-thousandth of an ounce! If you think of all the horrible manifestations of scurvy, and the fact that it is fatal, then the real power of this small protective dose of vitamin C is evident. Yet, despite this enormous power, large doses of vitamin C are not dangerous, and have never killed anyone.

Massive doses (5–20 grams per day), on the other hand, have been shown in animal studies to cause some side effects, such as infertility, abortion, and a reduced absorption of copper. In humans, massive doses can cause diarrhea, and are suspected of slightly increasing the risk of kidney stone formation. The main caution is that if you use large supplements for prolonged periods you may develop scurvylike symptoms if you stop them abruptly.

In contrast, a medicine like aspirin, which we take for granted, is potentially far more hazardous than vitamin C because it can cause much more serious side effects, such as gastric bleeding (or even death from a suicidal overdose).

Can Vitamin C Prevent Cancer?

Vitamin C has a number of important actions, some of which help to reduce your risk of cancer.

Although much remains to be learned about vitamin C, one effect is particularly well understood—*the antioxidant effect.* For those of you who have forgotten your chemistry, this simply means that vitamin C can react with certain chemicals in the body (including potential carcinogens) and prevent their oxidation into potentially harmful substances.

The kind of chemicals that are neutralized by vitamin C include the very common meat preservatives, nitrates and nitrites. Nitrates and nitrites can react with amines in the body to form *nitrosamines,* which are potent mutagens and carcinogens (30). Much of the increased risk of stomach cancer in Japan is now thought to stem from the traditional Japanese habit of eating nitrate-preserved, smoked sanma fish. Vitamin C has been shown to block the conversion of the nitrate into the carcinogenic nitrosamines, so rendering the fish safe.

The antioxidant action of vitamin C (as well as of beta-carotene, vitamin E, and selenium) is also an effective way to destroy cancer-causing *free radicals,* which are made spontaneously in our bodies. Free radicals are chemical substances that have an odd number of electrons. The odd number is the result of a free, high-energy electron attaching itself to a new atom. The new atom does not like this because the new electron has disturbed its energy balance. So the new atom decides to get rid of the surplus electron at the earliest opportunity. When it does so, there is a sudden transfer of this energy to adjacent body tissue, causing damage, and sometimes leading to cancer.

Free radicals are also formed by the splitting of life-giving oxygen into a dangerous form called singlet oxygen—a free radical that can both cause cancer itself and can activate carcinogens within the body.

Other ways in which free radicals are formed in the body can involve: the interaction of oxygen with polyunsaturated fats (another good reason to limit fat intake); the interaction of oxygen with certain metals; and finally, the effects of sunlight (ultraviolet light), smog (ozone), and radiation.

And remember, it is very fortunate that cancer-causing free radicals can be neutralized not only by vitamin C, but also by vitamin E, beta-carotene (provitamin A), and indirectly by selenium. These antioxidants are naturally a vital part of the Cancer Prevention Diet.

There are a number of other actions of vitamin C which are worth reviewing because they appear to influence the resistance of your body to cancer.

Potentially the most important is the postulated effect of vitamin C on your immune system. Although there is some controversy about this, it appears that vitamin C in large doses can increase your resistance to some infections. Any agent that can increase the general effectiveness of your body's natural defense mechanisms could also increase your defense against cancer. However, this theoretical benefit has yet to be proven scientifically. What is known is that a deficiency of vitamin C leads to a reduction of specialized white blood cells called T cells, which are the defensive killer cells of the immune system.

When cancers form in the body, part of our defense is to try to wall them off with *collagen,* a substance similar to scar tissue. It forms a dense capsule around some tumors that helps to restrict the spread of the deadly cancer cells. Vitamin C is needed for the production of protective collagen.

To help their escape from this restricting capsule, cancer cells produce enzymes (such as hyaluronidase) that dissolve the "cement" that binds cells together. This is one way that cancer cells can facilitate their spread, but it, too, is an action that can be neutralized by vitamin C.

Another controversial action of vitamin C that has attracted much interest is its effect on blood cholesterol and the lipoproteins that carry it around the body. It has been claimed that high doses of vitamin C can increase the level of beneficial high-density lipoproteins (HDLs), and reduce the level of harmful low-density lipoproteins (LDLs) (31). For years, Russian doctors have used vitamin C to try to reduce the risks of heart disease, although it is unclear whether these efforts have paid off.

Vitamin C also protects the body against carcinogenic hydrocarbons, and it has always intrigued me that smokers in fact have a much lower level of vitamin C in their blood as well as in their lung tissue. Possibly, this is because more vitamin C is used up trying to clear away the numerous carcinogens in tobacco smoke.

Well, now you have a very good idea of why vitamin C should protect you—but does it?

There is some epidemiological evidence that diets that are relatively rich in vitamin C do give some protection against some cancers (28), but many other studies have failed to demonstrate any protective effect of vitamin C. Diets that have suggested a protective role for vitamin C have usually been rich in fruit and vegetables. Of course, these diets also contain other important nutrients, but experimental evidence does support the idea that vitamin C may play an important role, particularly in its capacity to neutralize carcinogens (30). This support makes the positive epidemiological evidence somewhat more convincing.

The evidence so far suggests that vitamin C is most influential in reducing the risk of getting esophageal, gastric, and laryngeal cancer, and reducing the chance of developing precancerous changes in the uterine cervix.

A potential anticancer effect of vitamin C was demonstrated in patients who had an inherited condition called familial polyposis of the colon. In this condition, small premalignant growths develop in the colon and rectum, some of which are likely to undergo cancerous change. High doses of vitamin C (3 grams per day) reduced or cleared these growths in five out of eight patients (32), reducing their risk of colon cancer.

Finally, there is evidence that patients with cancer frequently have low blood levels of vitamin C, but it is uncertain whether this is due to the disease itself, or whether a low level of vitamin C contributes to an increased risk of getting cancer in the first place.

How Much Vitamin C Should You Take?

For most of the animal kingdom, this question has been taken care of by the Creator. Except for the whole of mankind, the guinea pig, a fruit-eating bat, some fish, and some species of grasshopper, all animals make the vitamin C they need inside their own bodies!

All vitamins used to be made by primeval animals themselves, but this ability was lost during the long course of evolution—except for vitamin C. Presumably, this is because it was important for the survival of most species. Imagine what it was like for primitive man, struggling to find about 2,500 calories each day from whatever food was available. It is very likely that his intake of vitamin C was much higher than ours is today because much of his diet was vegetation, which is low in calories but relatively high in vitamin C. Yet, despite the inconsistency in the ability of different animal species to synthesize their own vitamin C, our biochemistry is virtually the same as the biochemistry of those animals that make their own vitamin C in large amounts. So would you expect our needs to be any different from the needs of these animals?

Another way of considering this has been espoused with much enthusiasm by Dr. Linus Pauling—the winner of two Nobel prizes—in his book *Cancer and Vitamin C.* Dr. Pauling, who takes 10 grams of vitamin C each day himself, has suggested that if you consider how much vitamin C various animals make in relation to their body weights, and adjust this for the average human body weight, then we all should be taking between 2 and 20 grams of vitamin C each day!

Dr. Pauling also claims that high doses of vitamin C give protection against the common cold, but this has not been convincingly substantiated by independent studies.

The present RDA for vitamin C is a mere 60 milligrams per day, but remember, less than 10 milligrams per day is needed to prevent scurvy. So even the cautious recommendation of the National Research Council is for a dose of vitamin C that is more than six times the minimum needed to prevent deficiency disease.

A diet which is high in vitamin C is already known to be protective against cancers of the esophagus, stomach, larynx, and uterine cervix. Since it is very difficult to achieve levels of vitamin C much above 250–500 milligrams with modern dietary habits, we probably should be taking supplements to achieve the cancer-protecting levels of vitamin C that we need. (These supplements, however, are probably well below the true megadose levels of 5–20 grams a day.)

There are good theoretical reasons why a rich supply of vitamin C could be most effective in eliminating unavoidable carcinogens. Although the National Research Council and the American Cancer Society do not actually recommend vitamin supplements because the evidence that they will *definitely* reduce the cancer risk has yet to be established, some of you will take supplements anyway. Therefore, for those readers who decide to take supplements, I offer the following advice.

After considering all the evidence carefully, I have come to the conclusion that a reasonable vitamin C intake, which might lower your cancer risk and which is completely safe, is 1 gram a day, preferably in divided doses. This should be achieved by combining a 1-gram daily supplement with a diet that is rich in vitamin C.

Although it is better to take your 1 gram daily supplement of vitamin C as 250 milligrams four times a day, I know that you will find 500 milligrams in the morning and 500 milligrams in the evening much more convenient. Alternatively, if you are wealthy, you can choose the new time-release version of vitamin C.

For those of you who already take megadoses of vitamin C, you should know that in our present state of knowledge, taking much more than 1 gram of vitamin C a day is based more upon speculation than science, but will probably do you no harm. After all, as your vitamin C intake increases, your absorption of it decreases.

Where to Find Your Vitamin C

Now you must remember that this is a vitamin that you will find in your diet, but which you may choose to reinforce with a supplement.

As with all postulated dietary cancer-inhibitors there is the possibility that there are substances that coexist with vitamins which have not yet been identified, but whose participation is essential. Therefore, I must emphasize that your prime objective should be to increase your intake of *naturally* rich sources of vitamin C.

Here is a table of some of the better natural sources of vitamin C that will become part of your new diet.

Table 8–3
SOME GOOD SOURCES OF VITAMIN C

Source	Weight (in grams)	Serving Size	Vitamin C (in milligrams)	Calories
FRUIT:				
Acerola (Barbados cherry)	100	10	1,066	23
Acerola juice	242	1 cup	3,872	56
Black currants	100	1 cup	200	54
Grapefruit	200	1 whole	76	82
Grapefruit juice	250	1 cup	95	98
Guava	100	1 whole	242	62
Mango	300	1 average	81	152
Orange	180	1 average	66	64
Orange juice	248	1 6-oz. glass	124	112
Strawberries	150	1 cup	88	56
Watermelon	600	1 slice	42	156
VEGETABLES:				
Asparagus	150	6 spears	39	30
Broccoli	155	1 cup	140	40
Brussels sprouts	155	1 cup	135	56
Cauliflower	125	1 cup	69	28
Loose lettuce	55	1 cup	75	10
Mustard greens	180	1 cup	117	29
Parsley	60	1 cup	103	26
Peppers (green)	80	1 cup	102	18
Spinach	180	1 cup	50	41
Tomato	150	1 average	34	33

These values will be reduced by cooking.

Unlike vitamin A and the vitamin B complex, vitamin C is an unstable vitamin that is easily destroyed during cooking. Care must therefore be taken during food preparation to avoid its loss or destruction.

VITAMIN D (CHOLECALCIFEROL)

Vitamin D is important to human health because it regulates our calcium and phosphate metabolism. This is critical for the growth and maintenance of bones and teeth, particularly during childhood and adolescence. There is no evidence, however, that it directly influences our cancer risk.

There are two types of vitamin D, both equally effective. One is formed naturally by plants, the other by animals. The formation of both require the sun's ultraviolet rays—those rays which give you that beautiful—but dangerous—summer tan. In fact, you are making vitamin D while you tan because this process takes place in the deeper layers of the skin.

Only lack of sunlight or heavily pigmented skin can limit the formation of vitamin D. In the old days, vitamin D deficiency—rickets—did occur. This led to "bowing" of the legs because they were unable to grow in a balanced way during childhood. Rickets, fortunately, is very rare in the United States nowadays.

Vitamin D is found in animal foods such as fish, eggs, liver, and butter. Although milk is a poor natural source, nearly all milk that is sold today is fortified with 10 micrograms of vitamin D per quart.

An excess of vitamin D can cause very serious toxicity. About 2.5 micrograms per day can prevent rickets, while 10 micrograms is the daily dose suggested by the National Research Council to maintain optimum growth during childhood and adolescence.

In adult life, the need for vitamin D actually declines, and the RDA is 7.5 micrograms per day between ages nineteen and twenty-two. The RDA falls even further, to 5.0 micrograms per day, after the age of twenty-two.

Apart from increased requirements during pregnancy, this is a vitamin that you can really ignore because it will be adequate in your new diet.

VITAMIN E

Vitamin E is very important in dietary cancer prevention. Altogether, there are seven types of vitamin E, and all are equally effective. Like vitamin C, vitamin E has antioxidant properties, potentially enabling it to destroy cancer-causing free radicals and to inhibit the formation of carcinogens.

Vitamin E, which was discovered in 1936, is different from other vitamins insofar as there is no evidence of a deficiency disease in man, even when vitamin E deficiency has been deliberately created in volunteers. In animals, however, signs of deficiency do occur when dietary vitamin E is reduced. These signs involve the reproductive system, the blood vessels, the red blood cells, the nervous system, and the muscles. Contrary to the popular myth, vitamin E does not influence human sexuality.

Can Vitamin E Prevent Cancer?

Vitamin E helps to protect the body by reducing the conversion of polyunsaturated fats into dangerous cancer-causing free radicals. The more polyunsaturated fats there are in the diet, the more you need vitamin E. This protection depends upon its antioxidant properties.

The ability to destroy free radicals has led to some interest in the potential of vitamin E to slow down the aging process, but this has never been convincingly established scientifically. However, aging is a very difficult process to study because animals that are used in laboratories do not live very long, and nobody knows whether such research information is relevant to humans. To study humans directly would require about thirty years—and a group of volunteers who would be willing to place themselves on a diet low or high in vitamin E for that long!

Nevertheless, there is evidence that aging is associated with the reaction of tissues with oxygen, and that this process could theoretically be slowed by an antioxidant like vitamin E.

Vitamin E is also used to treat a benign condition called fibrocystic disease of the breast, a condition that affects about half of all women. Fibrocystic disease usually involves both breasts, which become tender and cystic. These cysts are felt as many small lumps or nodules. What is especially important is the fact that women with fibrocystic disease have a two- to eightfold increase in risk of breast cancer (33,34).

Apparently, physicians have successfully treated fibrocystic disease with a program of 600 IU of vitamin E daily for eight weeks, with many women finding pain relief, and some even experiencing complete disappearance of their disease.

Although there is no direct evidence that vitamin E can reduce your risk of cancer, it should be part of your diet. Unlike other vitamins, it is difficult to find populations that have naturally high or low vitamin E consumption for comparison in terms of cancer incidence and mortality. However, in one study that measured the vitamin E level in blood samples taken and stored years before cancer developed, no difference was found between the cancer patients and those who did not develop cancer (35). Although this could be interpreted as negative evidence, it is possible that vitamin E could reduce the risk of certain cancers but not others—information that was unavailable from this study. Another interpretation could be that since vitamin E is stored in body fat, blood levels are not representative of the levels in the tissues that matter. Nevertheless, there is some evidence that vitamin E can inhibit carcinogenesis in the laboratory (36).

The relative lack of evidence does not necessarily mean lack of efficacy. As one often discovers in science, it may simply mean that the right experiments have yet to be done.

The theoretical reasons to which I have alluded in the preceding section form a rational argument, I believe, for readers who wish to take supplements of vitamin E—a substance with no demonstrable toxicity.

In particular, I regard the antioxidant properties as being critically important, especially when it has been shown in animal studies that vitamin E can prevent the formation of carcinogenic nitrosamines.

I should also mention that studies with experimental tumors in animals have yielded inconsistent results. But even if vitamin E does not protect against all carcinogens (and it would be astonishing if any single substance did), it may work with other dietary anticancer agents to give you valuable protection.

Where to Find Your Vitamin E

Vitamin E is present in a variety of foods such as eggs, whole grain cereals, and vegetable oils. Since it is fat-soluble, it is usually found in dietary fat, and can of course be stored in the body.

Since your dietary fat intake is going to be reduced to approximately 20 percent of total calories, your access to vitamin E will naturally fall. Unlike with other vitamins, there is no need to make a special effort to increase your intake from natural sources, for two reasons. Firstly, there is no evidence that dietary vitamin E is better than a simple supplement. Secondly, there is every reason to reduce your fat intake, not increase it.

For those of you who decide to take supplements, I recommend that you take 400 IU of vitamin E daily. This provides you with a daily intake which is two-thirds of the dose that has already proved itself beneficial in fibrocystic breast disease. It is, of course, substantially higher than both the average daily intake of 15 IU of vitamin E in the American diet and the RDA of 10–20 IU (neither dose having ever demonstrated any special value).

VITAMIN K

Vitamin K, which is needed for blood clotting, is obtained from the diet and is also made by bacteria in our intestines. It has no part in dietary cancer prevention.

A deficiency of vitamin K usually occurs because of liver disease, and is consequently more common in alcoholics. There is no RDA for vitamin K, because dietary deficiency does not occur.

Fat soluble vitamin K is found in a wide variety of foods such as dairy products, eggs, meat and liver, fats, some cereals, vegetables, and fruit.

I have summarized the material presented in this chapter in Table 8–4 to provide you with a quick guide to vitamins.

It is essential that you also be aware of how the method of food preparation influences the availability of some vitamins, particularly those that are either water-soluble or heat-sensitive. Consult Chapter 14 for details about the effect of food preparation techniques.

It is also important for you to understand that vitamins help you only when they are taken regularly—for life. Short courses of vitamin supplements are of very little value, except in the treatment of certain medical conditions.

SHOULD YOU TAKE VITAMIN SUPPLEMENTS?

The enormous annual sales of vitamin and mineral supplements in the United States has been estimated in the billions of dollars.

Table 8–4
A SUMMARY OF YOUR VITAL VITAMINS

Function	Cancer Prevention	Some Sources	Recommended Daily Intake
VITAMIN A			
• Needed for normal growth, immune system, healthy skin and hair. • Prevents night blindness.	• Lung, breast, larynx, bladder, esophagus, stomach, colon, rectum, prostate, cervix.	• Liver, broccoli, spinach, cantaloupe, watermelon, fish, endive.	• 25,000 IU in diet. • Beta-carotene supplement optional. • Vitamin A (not beta-carotene) is toxic in excess. • RDA* is 4,000–5,000 IU.
VITAMIN B$_1$ (Thiamin)			
• Needed for normal function of heart, nervous system. • Releases energy from carbohydrates. • Prevents beriberi.	• Not established. • Helps immune system.	• Liver, pasta, whole grain cereals, fish, poultry, peas.	• 3 mg in diet. • Not toxic in excess. • RDA is 1.0–1.4 mg.
VITAMIN B$_2$ (Riboflavin)			
• Releases energy from proteins, carbohydrates, fats. • Needed for normal T cell growth.	• Not established. • Deficiency lowers T cells of immune system, and low T cells can increase cancer risk.	• Liver, milk, meat, whole grains, pasta, dark-green vegetables.	• 3 mg in diet. • Not toxic in excess. • RDA is 1.2–1.7 mg.

NIACIN

- Helps thiamin, riboflavin.
- Prevents pellagra.

- No evidence.

- Liver, meat, eggs, poultry, whole grain cereals, nuts, tuna, pasta.

- 20 mg in diet.
- Toxic in megadoses.
- RDA is 13–19 mg.

VITAMIN B_6 (pyridoxine)

- Helps use of fats, proteins; helps immune and nervous systems.
- Deficient in alcoholics.

- Experimental evidence suggests protection.
- Effects on immune system important.

- Liver, meat, fish, whole grains, poultry, dark-green vegetables.

- 10 mg in diet.
- Toxic in megadoses.
- RDA is 2.0–2.2 mg.

VITAMIN B_{12}

- Required for healthy blood cells, nervous system.

- Not established.
- Absorption defect associated with stomach cancer.

- Liver, kidney, meat, fish, poultry, milk, yeast, eggs.

- 10 mcg in diet.
- Not toxic in excess.
- RDA is 3.0 mcg.

FOLIC ACID

- Deficiency common and can impair immune system, thus increasing cancer risk.

- Some experimental evidence suggests protection at high doses.
- Can reduce chromosome damage

- Liver, kidneys, dark-green vegetables, fruit, wheat germ, peas.

- 1 mg in diet.
- Can mask B_{12} lack.
- Not toxic in excess.
- 400 mcg optional supplement
- RDA is 400 mcg.

Table 8-4 (continued)

Function	Cancer Prevention	Some Sources	Recommended Daily Intake
BIOTIN			
• Metabolizes fats, and carbohydrates.	• No evidence.	• Liver, kidney, egg yolk, vegetables.	• 100–300 mcg in diet. • No RDA exists.
PANTOTHENIC ACID			
• Releases energy from carbohydrates.	• No evidence.	• Meat, fruit, whole grains, vegetables.	• 4–7 mg in diet. • Not toxic in excess. • No RDA exists.
VITAMIN C			
• Needed for formation of bones, teeth, blood vessels. • Antioxidant. • Improves immune system. • Improves formation of collagen and limits cancer spread. • Protects other vitamins. • Increases iron absorption. • Prevents scurvy.	• Esophagus, stomach, larynx, uterine cervix. • Experimental evidence supportive.	• Acerola juice, black currants, oranges, strawberries, broccoli, brussels sprouts, parsley, peppers, spinach, watermelon.	• 1 g if optional supplement taken. Without supplement, eat foods rich in vitamin C. • No serious toxicity. • RDA is 60 mg.

VITAMIN D

- Needed for normal growth of bones and teeth.
- Prevents rickets.

- No evidence.

- Sun-tanning; fish, eggs, liver, butter, milk.

- Diet only: 10 micrograms for children; 5 micrograms for adults.
- Toxic in excess.
- RDA is 5–10 mcg.

VITAMIN E

- Antioxidant, destroys carcinogens.
- Reverses benign breast disease.
- No human deficiency.

- Experimental evidence supportive.

- Eggs, whole grains, vegetable oils.

- 400 IU optional supplement.
- Not toxic in excess.
- RDA is 8–10 mg.

VITAMIN K

- Needed for blood clotting.
- Deficient in alcoholics.

- No evidence.

- Widespread in diet; made by gut bacteria.

- No diet level required.
- No RDA exists.

* The RDA is the recommended daily allowance determined by the National Research Council.

Many people consume large quantities of vitamins impulsively and erratically, and probably with only marginal health benefits.

Against this background, there is now increasing epidemiological and experimental evidence that certain vitamins may have the power to prevent the development of some cancers in man. In consequence, large-scale scientifically controlled studies have recently been initiated by the National Cancer Institute. These ongoing studies are designed to determine whether the regular consumption of certain vitamins could reduce the cancer risk in the general population. The results may turn out to be critically important. As was pointed out in a recent article in the journal *Science* (37), the prevention of cancer should be a top priority in the United States for economic as well as humanitarian reasons, and the success of a cancer prevention program could save the country literally millions of lives and billions of dollars in years to come.

However, these vitamin studies will not produce definitive answers for at least five years, and possibly longer. In the meantime, what should you do? Let us consider the question carefully.

In my opinion, it is medically unethical to recommend that the public should take any drug that has not been proven safe and effective. It is also medically unethical not to discourage smoking. However, there is an important difference between these two examples. The first addresses the issue of taking a drug, while the second addresses the issue of giving one up. In practice, what this means is that withdrawing a drug is much easier to advocate than administering a drug—*when the evidence is incomplete.*

In the case of nutrition the situation becomes rather blurred, since most of us do not think of food as intrinsically harmful. Most public policy dietary recommendations of the past twenty years have been in relation to heart disease. These recommendations have centered on the issue of saturated fat and cholesterol, both of which we were urged to reduce. In general, these recommendations were accepted without too much controversy, probably because they were *negative* actions rather than positive ones. If the public had been asked to *take* something instead, there would have been repeated demands for proof that it worked before the policy would have been widely accepted.

In the case of vitamins we are faced with a form of anarchy. The recommendations of the National Research Council are probably ignored by the majority of the public. If anyone conforms to the recommended levels of vitamins it is more likely to be by chance than by design. In this context, is it appropriate to make interim recommendations for selected vitamin supplementation based upon untested theoretical considerations? In my view the answer is yes, because the vitamins in question are among the safest substances known to man, and because they are presently being consumed in such a haphazard way.

Such provisional guidelines would not be intended to replace proper scientific evaluation. Rather, such guidelines are designed to rationalize the consumption of certain vitamins that are already being purchased and self-administered on a grand scale. Of course, as the results of scientific studies become available, recommendations for vitamin (and mineral) supplementation would have to be updated.

The advantage of such an approach is that the planned intake of dietary vitamin supplements could provide years of valuable cancer protection before the final scientific proof is in. If scientifically controlled studies eventually failed to show convincing protection from a vitamin supplement, what harm would have been done?

For these reasons, I am leaving it to you to decide whether you want to take vitamin or mineral supplements, or not. The details of this optional vitamin and mineral reinforcement program are laid out for you at the end of the Cancer Prevention Diet in Chapter 15.

CHAPTER 9

Minerals—More or Less?

Minerals are intimately involved in the chemistry of the body. Many are part of elaborate enzyme systems which are vital to the life of each cell, while others, like calcium and phosphorus, are the main contributors to the strength and structure of bone. All minerals make up about 4 percent of your body weight, while the trace elements make up only a tiny 0.01 percent.

An increasing number of scientists are now becoming aware of the importance of minerals and trace elements in the nation's daily diet. Not only do these substances in the right amount sustain your general health, but some of them may also make a substantial contribution to reducing your risk of developing cancer.

Scientists refer to *macro*minerals and *micro*minerals, the distinction being based on the different amounts needed for good health. The important macrominerals are calcium, phosphorus, potassium, sulfer, sodium, chloride, and magnesium; the important microminerals, or trace elements, include iron, zinc, iodine, copper, manganese, fluoride, chromium, cadmium, selenium, and molybdenum.

As with vitamins, there is some disagreement between scientists about the exact amount that you need each day, and this need can be complicated by losses during food preparation. Furthermore, the absorption of minerals can be impaired by a high-fiber diet, so it is important that your intake is both adequate and properly balanced; in all events, *megadoses are never necessary*.

I shall now provide you with what you need to know about minerals, with the greater emphasis on those that will influence your cancer risk.

SELENIUM

This is a trace element of fundamental importance to dietary cancer prevention. Scientific evidence has demonstrated that diets that are rich in selenium reduce the chance of developing leukemia and cancers such as those of the colon, rectum, pancreas, breast, ovary, prostate, bladder, lung (in males), and skin (1,2,3,4,5). This evidence was based on information derived from the United States and twenty-two other countries.

The amount of selenium in our diet is influenced to a considerable extent by the amount in the soil. Both internationally and within the United States, geographic areas with low soil concentrations of selenium have higher cancer rates than areas with high soil concentrations. This has been shown most dramatically for breast cancer and colon cancer, two of the commonest cancers in the United States.

In New Zealand for example, there is a very low level of dietary selenium because of local soil conditions. People living there habitually consume less selenium, and their breast cancer rate is one of the highest in the world. Could there be a connection? I think so.

Patients with breast cancer have been found to have lower selenium levels in their blood, but it was uncertain whether a low selenium level predisposed one to the disease or was the result of it. This uncertainty was later resolved by measuring the selenium level in blood samples that had been stored for as long as five years *before* the onset of various types of cancer (6). When compared to healthy people of the same age and sex, the selenium levels were again found to be low, confirming the importance of a low blood selenium level as a predictive cancer risk factor. In fact, the lower selenium levels appeared to be associated with twice the overall cancer risk.

The evidence is not confined to these epidemiological studies. Laboratory experiments have strongly supported the idea that selenium is capable of reducing the cancer risk. For example, there is a strain of mice that have a great tendency to develop breast cancer. After the simple maneuver of adding 2 parts per million of selenite (a form of selenium) to the drinking water, the incidence of spontaneous breast cancers in these mice dropped from 82 percent to 10 percent (7)—impressive evidence of the power of selenium to lower the cancer risk. As with vitamin A, it was also found that selenium could reduce the cancer risk, even when added to the diet a long time after the first exposure to a carcinogen (8). Clearly, this is an important observation if we want to use selenium to reduce our risk of developing cancer due to past exposure to carcinogens.

The beneficial effect of selenium can also be influenced by dietary fat—particularly unsaturated fat. This is important because the diseases that appear to be most strongly inhibited by selenium (breast and colon cancer) are those that are more likely to occur with a high-fat diet.

The precise way that selenium exerts its protective effect is not known with certainty. One important action of selenium may provide a possible explanation. Like vitamin A, beta-carotene, and vitamin E, selenium has antioxidant properties. But unlike these vitamins, selenium does not act directly. Rather, selenium stimulates an enzyme called glutathione peroxidase (and possibly other enzymes) to perform protective antioxidant activity inside all cells. This type of activity is just what is needed to prevent the harmful effects of the free radicals that can be derived from unsaturated fats (9). (Despite this potentially harmful effect of unsaturated fats, however, they remain the safest form of fat from a general health point of view.)

Another action of selenium is its ability to combine with small amounts of potentially toxic dietary metals like cadmium, mercury, and arsenic, making them harmless. This action is probably less important in preventing cancer than the antioxidant effect. It should be remembered, however, that selenium also works in combination with vitamin E, another potential anticancer vitamin.

Finally, there is evidence that selenium may help to destroy carcinogens (10), and improve the body's natural immune defenses (11).

There is one other effect of selenium that is worth mentioning: *it may also reduce your chances of a heart attack!* Countries like New Zealand, Finland, and parts of China all have low levels of dietary selenium and high levels of heart disease (12,13). Although selenium seems to exert its greatest anticancer effect in the presence of unsaturated fat in animal experiments, it is unclear whether this is relevant to the protective actions of selenium in heart disease. In the case of New Zealand and Finland the fat intake is high, and in China the fat intake is low, but the use of selenium supplements apparently has already reduced the heart attack rate in the high-risk areas in China.

How Much Selenium Is Enough?

Selenium can be toxic if it is consumed in excessive amounts. It is therefore very important that you do not indulge in the mistaken belief that the more selenium you take the better. Although selenium toxicity has been recognized for years in animals, there have been few reports of toxicity in humans. Probably the most interesting account of selenium toxicity comes from China. The first description of an animal disease that is now known to be selenium poisoning was made by Marco Polo during his travels in West China in 1295. The next account, which referred to humans, occurred somewhat later.

In 1983, it was reported that between 1961 and 1964 there had been an outbreak of selenium toxicity in Hubei province in the People's Republic of China (14). About half the inhabitants of five villages had been afflicted by strange symptoms that involved the hair, nails, skin, and nervous system. One middle-aged woman had developed paralysis and had subsequently died, and her death had been attributed to selenium poisoning.

The cause of this outbreak was found to be due to weathering of high selenium coal and rock formations that resulted in an increased uptake of selenium by crops that had been fertilized with lime from the region. The concentration of selenium in vegetables was consequently increased by as much as 1,000-fold compared to vegetables sampled in a region associated with selenium deficiency. These unfortunate people from the Hubei villages had consumed about 5 *milli*grams of selenium daily—whereas the average American intake is about 50–160 *micro*grams per day.

Fortunately, minor signs of selenium toxicity are reversible when the dietary intake is reduced. Nevertheless, it would be wise to minimize your risk of toxicity by avoiding excess selenium. What does this mean in practice?

Although certain foods are usually rich in selenium, there is so much regional variation in the selenium content of the soil in the

United States that you can only make rough estimates of your intake. Regions higher in selenium are found mainly in western plains while lower levels are found in all the heavily populated regions of the country. This variation is further complicated by the fact that the foods you buy in your local supermarket come from different parts of the country as well as being grown locally. However, such variation will only risk a relative deficiency, not toxicity.

In areas of the world with naturally high concentrations of selenium in the soil, such as Caracas, Venezuela, there have been no reports of selenium toxicity despite the fact that the selenium content of local milk is ten times higher than in Beltsville, Maryland (7). It has also been shown that certain Japanese populations can tolerate 500 micrograms of selenium daily without side effects (15). Although the National Research Council now recommends a daily selenium intake of 50–200 micrograms, some scientists have recommended a daily intake of 300 micrograms per day for cancer protection. This is far below the level of 2,400–3,000 micrograms of selenium per day that has been shown to cause toxicity when consumed for prolonged periods (16).

If you want to take selenium supplements, I would suggest that you take 200 micrograms per day at a different time of day than your vitamin C supplement. Use an organic selenium supplement such as that found in yeast. This is better than inorganic selenium because it is less toxic and more stable. Of course, your new diet, being rich in whole grain cereals, broccoli, and other sources, will provide some additional selenium, so that in combination with a supplement you should easily reach the suggested anticancer level of 300 micrograms per day.

Where to Find Natural Sources of Selenium

This is not so easy. Most of the "reliable information" on the trace materials that has been widely used is now known to be rather inaccurate, and is being revised by the U.S. Department of Agriculture.

There is also evidence that the selenium in some foods may be less "available" than in others. Unlike vitamins, whose availability in the diet is influenced mostly by cooking, mineral availability is influenced mostly by the particular chemical form that the mineral is in; by the interaction with other minerals (selenium with zinc; and inactivation by large amounts of vitamin C taken concurrently); and by a high level of dietary fiber. Furthermore, the fact that food processing can itself alter the concentration and chemical nature of selenium makes it almost impossible to estimate dietary selenium accurately.

Nonetheless, known rich sources of selenium include seafood, liver, and kidney, followed by meat and whole grains. Fruit and vegetables, a major part of your new diet, are generally not good sources of selenium.

ZINC

Zinc is an essential part of more than 100 enzymes, and is consequently essential for life. This metal is intimately involved in the growth and division of all cells, and therefore it has a great influence on your immune system—part of your defense against cancer. Any deficiency in your dietary zinc will reduce your production of cancer-fighting T cells (17), which could increase your cancer risk. On the other hand, there is evidence that excessive zinc may also be just as harmful.

Few studies associating dietary zinc with cancer have been done. However, it has been convincingly demonstrated that people whose food was rich in zinc had a higher risk of stomach cancer (18); and of leukemia and cancers of the breast, intestine, prostate, ovary, lung, bladder, and skin (4,5). These findings are not just coincidental; they were supported by the fact that the amount of zinc in the blood of healthy blood donors was higher in regions where these cancers more commonly occurred (5). This means that higher levels of zinc in the blood were placing these populations at greater risk. Interestingly, one study even indicated that when zinc was high, selenium was low, suggesting an antagonism between the two (5). No doubt we have a lot to learn about the precise way minerals react with each other.

In contrast to the effects of a high-zinc diet, at least one study has suggested that a diet that is very low in zinc might increase the risk of esophageal cancer (19).

Experimental studies have generally supported these findings, with both high- and low-zinc diets appearing to increase the cancer risk.

What You Should Do About Zinc

Since the evidence is still inconclusive, there is no reason deliberately to increase or reduce the *available* zinc in your diet by specific dietary changes. However, a modest zinc supplement (5 mg) is advisable to ensure that enough zinc is available for absorption in the presence of a high fiber intake.

Zinc deficiency is rare in the United States, being found most often among the children of low-income families. The average mixed American diet provides about 10–15 milligrams of zinc daily, while the present RDA is set at 15 milligrams per day. Some degree of diet planning is required if you intend to maintain an adequate daily intake only by dietary means.

The availability of zinc varies from one food source to another, even if they contain similar amounts of zinc. Vegetarians can easily become zinc-deficient, and a diet that is high in dietary fiber can restrict absorption. This last fact is of special importance to you, since your new diet will be rather high in fiber.

The best natural sources of zinc are seafood (especially oysters), eggs, liver, and meat. Whole grains such as whole wheat, rye, oatmeal, and corn are poor sources because the zinc they contain is in a form that is relatively unusable.

Because you could take ten times the RDA of zinc for years without any discernible general toxicity, and because your anticancer diet is predominantly whole grains, fruit, vegetables and fiber, you may decide to take a zinc supplement. A reasonable supplement is 5 milligrams of zinc per day to maintain the RDA of 15 milligrams. But remember, a zinc supplement is only worthwhile when you have succeeded in following the Cancer Prevention Diet closely. If your fiber intake is still low, or should you break loose one day and have a feast on oysters (or some other meal rich in zinc), you can skip the supplement!

Ideally, once you have established your new diet as a permanent part of your life, you should arrange with your physician to have your zinc level measured to be sure that it is just right. This takes the guesswork out of zinc supplements.

IRON

Do you know anyone who has not been told of the importance of dietary iron? Pick up any magazine, read any newsaper, look at the small print on any packet of enriched cereal, and you are likely to find some words that extoll the virtues of iron.

Iron is needed for the formation of hemoglobin, a vital substance present in red blood cells. It is the hemoglobin that carries oxygen around the body. A deficiency of iron first leads to a depletion of body stores, then to a failure to form hemoglobin. Lack of hemoglobin produces a pale appearance, tiredness, fatigue, and some shortness of breath on exertion—symptoms of anemia that can also be produced by other diseases.

Iron deficiency has also been associated with cancer of the esophagus and stomach, particularly in Sweden (20). In this instance, iron and vitamin supplements have virtually eliminated iron deficiency, and consequently reduced stomach cancer too.

In Colombia, it was found that iron deficiency prevented the stomach from producing acid, so allowing bacteria to grow. As a result, nitrate in the food was converted by the bacteria into cancer-causing nitrosamines, and it is likely that this was the reason for the increased risk of stomach cancer in these people (21).

Although there have been no reports of a greater risk of cancer in people whose intake of iron was high, there is a greater risk of cancer of the lung and larynx among industrial workers who inhale iron dust.

There are only four situations in which iron deficiency is likely to occur. The first is in infancy, because the iron content of milk is low; the second is in childhood and adolescence, because of the need to fill expanding iron stores; the third is in women during the reproductive period, when menstruation causes increased blood (and therefore iron) loss; and the fourth is in pregnancy, when there are increased demands for iron.

The RDA for iron is 10 milligrams per day for men, and 18 milligrams per day for women of child-bearing age. Although only about 10 percent of the iron in food is available for absorption, the absorption of iron is cleverly controlled by the body. The more the body needs, the more it will absorb. When body stores are full, a message is sent to the intestine that reduces—but does not prevent—further absorption. This is the only way that the body can control iron levels because there is no mechanism for surplus iron excretion. Therefore, excessive iron supplements should be avoided.

There is another way that the absorption of iron can be increased, and that is by the simultaneous intake of vitamin C. On the other hand, iron absorption can be reduced by calcium and phosphate salts, tannic acid in tea, and antacids.

Good sources of dietary iron include liver, pork, fish, poultry, dried fruits and beans, and whole grain cereals. Little iron comes from vegetables.

COPPER

There is weak, though direct, evidence that the higher the level of copper in your blood, the greater the risk of cancers of the intestine, breast, lung, and thyroid (5). It is thought that this may be the result of a direct antagonism between the actions of selenium and copper.

Frankly, there is really no epidemiological evidence that dietary copper is a significant risk factor. And this view is strengthened by the lack of any experimental evidence that dietary copper makes any difference. So breathe a sigh of relief, copper can be ignored!

IODINE

Iodine is an essential part of our diet. Lack of iodine produces a marked swelling (a goiter) of the thyroid gland in the neck, followed by thyroid failure.

Thyroid hormone is responsible for a great many chemical reactions in the body, and any failure in its production has very serious consequences. Fortunately, such a thyroid deficiency can easily be treated with thyroid hormone tablets.

A dietary deficiency of iodine is rare in the United States because table salt is usually sold with added iodine. This has reduced the development of cretinism (children with stunted growth and mental retardation), which used to be seen far too frequently. It has also reduced the risk of thyroid cancer, which was found more commonly in people with goiters.

However, care must be taken to have the right amount of iodine. There is evidence that excess amounts and low amounts of iodine can each predispose you to a different type of thyroid cancer (22).

The present RDA is 150 micrograms per day, and there is some concern being expressed that the people of the United States may actually be getting too much iodine. Iodine is found in seafood, dairy products, bread, and iodized table salt. The current recommendation is that you should use iodized table salt *only if you live inland;* in coastal regions, the environmental iodine levels are high enough.

MOLYBDENUM

Molybdenum is a mineral that plays a key role in the function of an important enzyme, xanthine oxidase. Overt signs of human deficiency have not been documented. However, there is some evidence that a dietary deficiency of molybdenum can increase the risk of cancer of the esophagus. In China, recent reports have indicated that esophageal cancer was higher in regions where the level of molybdenum (and other minerals) in the soil was low (23). This observation has led to a fascinating experiment that is being conducted on a grand scale.

Large amounts of molybdenum have been added to the soil in low-molybdenum regions just as fertilizer is added to soil on our farms. Whole grains and vegetables grown under these conditions are now richer in both molybdenum and ascorbic acid (vitamin C), and lower in cancer-causing nitrates and nitrites. Chinese scientists hope that this change in the soil will eventually cause a substantial fall in the number of people who develop esophageal cancer.

China is not the only country that has this problem. In parts of Africa where the molybdenum content of the soil is low, esophageal cancer also occurs with much greater frequency (24). Even in the United States, where it has been assumed that molybdenum deficiency is virtually nonexistent, more people develop esophageal cancer in areas where the molybdenum content of the local water supply is low (25).

The cancer-inhibitor effect of molybdenum has also been demonstrated in animals (26). And the weight of the evidence certainly suggests that good sources of this mineral—liver, kidney, legumes, and certain dark-green vegetables—should be part of your diet.

Although the National Research Council has not defined an RDA for molybdenum, they estimate that a "safe and adequate" intake is 0.15–0.5 milligrams per day for adults. I would advise you to try to maintain your intake just below 0.5 milligrams per day to be sure of benefiting from its anticancer properties while avoiding toxicity. For it appears that molybdenum at high levels can indeed prove toxic. People living in a Russian province where the environmental molybdenum level was high developed toxic symptoms, probably due to the antagonism that molybdenum has for copper (27).

CADMIUM

Although cadmium has been known for years as a toxic substance, there is evidence now that water supplies which are high in cadmium may contribute to an increased risk of a whole range of cancers.

In the United States, there is a greater risk of myeloma, lymphoma, and cancers of the mouth, pharynx, esophagus, colon, larynx, lung, breast, and bladder, due to trace elements in river water (28). Interestingly, although cadmium increases the risk, a similar risk seems to be produced by arsenic, beryllium, nickel, and lead, but not by iron, cobalt, and chromium.

Studies that investigated this risk in twenty-seven countries also showed that cadmium may contribute to cancer of the uterus, the prostate, and the skin (4,5).

The danger of cadmium has also been confirmed in exposed industrial workers, who have an increased risk of kidney and prostate cancer. Not only that, but cigarette smokers have twice the cadmium level of nonsmokers—and also have a higher risk of cancer of the kidney (29).

So, I don't think I need to emphasize that cadmium is a toxic mineral that should be avoided. And of course, don't smoke!

CHROMIUM

Chromium is an essential element that is also a dangerous carcinogen—catch 22! Normal amounts of chromium are needed to help insulin control blood glucose.

There is no direct evidence that dietary chromium has caused cancer, but there is evidence that Russian and Japanese workers who were exposed to chromium dust had more than their share of cancer of the lung, esophagus, stomach, pancreas, and liver.

The present American diet provides about 60 micrograms of chromium each day, and this mostly comes from brewer's yeast, meat products, whole grains, and condiments. Since not all dietary chromium can be used by the body, the RDA has been set at 50–200 micrograms per day.

Since there is no reason to have more chromium than you need, and some excellent reasons to avoid any excess, you can simply let your new diet safely take care of your needs for you.

ARSENIC

If you have seen the film *Arsenic and Old Lace,* or if you enjoy reading murder mysteries, it may be hard to imagine that arsenic is actually a trace mineral that is present in your normal diet—in minute amounts. It is unique in that it can cause cancer in humans, but not in laboratory animals. Most dietary arsenic is found in trace amounts in foods such as seafood, meats, and vegetables.

Arsenic also contaminates fruit, potatoes, and other foods because of its widespread use as an insecticide. This has led to an increased cancer risk among vineyard workers in France, who drank arsenic-contaminated wine, and who were also exposed to insecticide sprays containing arsenic (30). These workers unfortunately went on to get cancer of the skin, lung, or liver. Even if wine is not to your taste, helping yourself to well water in Taiwan could prove dangerous too. In this instance, it was found that drinking arsenic-contaminated well water, and possibly washing with it, produced skin cancer (31).

Although arsenic is considered essential for the normal growth of animals, no dietary level has ever been determined as either desirable or safe in humans.

OTHER MINERALS

Macrominerals such as calcium and phosphorus are also critical components of a healthy diet. Fortunately, there is no evidence that they influence your cancer risk in any way. Only calcium and phosphorus will be mentioned here because they are the most important.

Calcium is the most abundant mineral in the body. It constitutes about 2 percent of the body weight, and often is lacking in the American diet. Nearly all your body's calcium is in your bones and teeth, and the rest is carefully regulated to ensure the proper functioning of most tissues, including the nervous system and muscle cells.

Calcium absorption is increased by vitamin D, but is usually limited to 20–30 percent of dietary calcium. Foods rich in calcium include milk and cheese, sardines, salmon, oysters, spinach, and broccoli.

The need for calcium is greatest during growth and adolescence, and persists throughout life. During pregnancy and lactation, the daily requirement increases by 50 percent.

The RDA for calcium is 800 milligrams per day, though some scientists think that this should be increased to 1,000 milligrams per day. Although still controversial, modest calcium supplements and regular exercise can minimize osteoporosis in postmenopausal women. *Megadose supplements are both unwise and unnecessary.*

Phosphorus is a mineral that works with calcium to provide the strong supporting material for the skeleton. It is involved in many chemical reactions in the body, and is required for the normal functioning of the B group of vitamins.

Since phosphorus is present in nearly all foods, a dietary deficiency hardly ever occurs. Because the ratio of calcium to phosphorus should be 1:1 in adults, the RDA for phosphorus is the same as for calcium—800 milligrams per day.

WHAT YOU SHOULD DO ABOUT MINERALS

Now you should have an excellent idea about the importance of minerals to your health, and particularly to your risk of cancer.

Minerals such as selenium appear to protect you; other minerals, such as iodine, can decrease or increase your cancer risk depending upon the amount. Yet still other minerals, such as zinc, should be maintained at the RDA value, but may require a modest supplement because your new cancer prevention diet tends to limit zinc absorption due to the high fiber content. Finally, some minerals are clearly potent carcinogens, and your exposure to them should be discouraged as far as possible.

So that you can easily review the minerals, Table 9–1 summarizes what you need to know and do.

This has not been a full description of all minerals, for that is beyond the scope of this chapter. Only those that are most critical to your new diet have been discussed. Some very important minerals such as sodium chloride (table salt) have been omitted, but this does not mean that I consider these minerals unimportant. For example, table salt is used much too frequently by most of us, and should be reduced to avoid the dangers of high blood pressure. However, although table salt has no known importance in the dietary prevention of cancer, remember that the high salt content of salt-cured meats has been associated with stomach cancer in Japan.

Obviously, our ability to regulate dietary mineral consumption accurately is rather limited. The same is true of our consumption of the many food additives that are created both by nature and by the food industry—as you will soon find out.

For readers who want to take mineral supplements, Table 15–6 (found in Chapter 15) lists vitamin and mineral supplements that might reduce your cancer risk. Until scientific studies establish whether specific dietary supplements do in fact reduce the cancer risk, you should regard them as theoretically valuable but unproved.

Table 9-1
A SUMMARY OF YOUR IMPORTANT MINERALS

Function	Cancer Risk	Sources	Recommended Daily Intake
SELENIUM			
• Antioxidant. • Neutralizes some toxic metals. • Works with vitamin E.	• Can reduce cancer of colon, rectum, pancreas, breast, ovary, prostate, bladder, lung, skin.	• Milk, chicken, seafood, garlic, whole grains, meat, egg yolk. • Soil level is important.	• 300 mcg daily (200 mcg of this is an optional supplement). • Toxic in large amounts. • RDA is 50–200 mcg. • Do not take at the same time as vitamin C.
ZINC			
• Essential component of enzymes. • Helps immune system. • Interacts with selenium. • Needed for growth, taste.	• High zinc intake increases cancer of stomach, breast colon, prostate, ovary, lung, skin, and bladder. • Low intake also increases risk.	• Liver, meat, eggs, poultry, seafood, milk, whole grains.	• RDA is 15 mg. • Since less is absorbed with high-fiber diet, take 5 mg as optional supplement. • No change in total intake needed.

IRON

• Needed to form hemoglobin, which carries oxygen.	• Deficiency increases cancer of esophagus and stomach. • Iron dust causes cancer of lung and larynx.	• Liver, pork, fish, poultry, dried fruit, whole grains. • Vitamin C increases absorption.	• RDA is 10 mg for men; 18 mg for women. • No change is needed.

COPPER

• Essential component of some enzymes. • Needed for red cells, nervous system, bones, reproduction.	• Very weak evidence.	Oysters, liver, nuts, kidney, dried legumes.	• RDA is 2–3 mg. • No change is needed.

IODINE

• Required for normal thyroid development. • Deficiency leads to goiter.	• Both deficiency and excess can cause thyroid cancer.	• Seafood, dairy products, bread, iodized salt.	• RDA is 150 mcg. • Can be toxic in excess.

MOLYBDENUM

• Part of an enzyme called xanthine oxidase.	• Deficiency may increase risk of cancer of the esophagus.	• Liver, legumes, some dark-green vegetables.	• No RDA exists. • Not more than 0.5 mg. • Toxic in excess.

Table 9-1 (continued)

Function	Cancer Risk	Sources	Recommended Daily Intake
CADMIUM			
• No desirable effects known.	• Considerably increases cancer of mouth, pharynx, colon, lung, larynx, breast, bladder, prostate, uterus, skin.	• Mostly as a contaminant of water.	• No RDA exists. • None if you can help it.
CHROMIUM			
• Helps insulin metabolize glucose.	• Carcinogenic as chrome dust in industry only, where it increases cancer of lung, esophagus, stomach, pancreas, liver. • No evidence of dietary risk.	• Brewer's yeast, meat products, whole grains, condiments.	• RDA is 50–200 mcg.
ARSENIC			
• No desirable effect known.	• Contaminated vineyard workers had more cancer of skin, lung, liver.	• Seafood, meats, vegetables; use of insecticides.	• No need ever established in man.

CALCIUM

- Needed for bones, teeth, muscle, the nervous system, enzymes.
- No risk known.
- Milk, cheese, sardines, salmon, oysters, spinach, broccoli.
- Absorption is increased by vitamin D.
- RDA is 800 mg.
- Megadoses are dangerous.

PHOSPHORUS

- Works with calcium.
- No risk known.
- Most foods.
- RDA is 800 mg.

CHAPTER 10

Food Additives—
Friend or Foe?

On the 23rd of September 1983, the most prestigious scientific journal in the United States, *Science,* had the following dramatically simple message on its cover: EAT—DIE. Inside, was a long article and an editorial that discussed the importance of natural dietary carcinogens and anticarcinogens and the role of diet in the formation of human cancer. Evidently, the general scientific community had become more interested in the potential threat posed to us by a diet that unknowingly places more emphasis on carcinogens than cancer-inhibitors.

Our diet consists of various constituents, not all of which are nutritious. Apart from protein, fat, carbohydrates, vitamins, minerals, and indigestible fiber, there are hundreds of other chemicals that may have important effects. The vast majority of these are created by nature. Some are added by man.

The most important of these nutritionally worthless chemicals in our food function as mutagens, carcinogens, and anticarcinogens. Let me refresh your memory. *Mutagens* are chemicals that can damage the DNA inside cells, thus increasing the chance of a cell becoming cancerous. *Carcinogens* are chemicals that directly cause cancer. *Anticarcinogens* are welcome cancer-inhibitors that can neutralize carcinogens, block the action of carcinogens, or even reverse the changes that have taken place in cancer cells.

The great challenge that scientists now face is to identify all the dietary chemicals that influence our cancer risk, and to determine just how risky or beneficial these chemicals actually are. Eventually, it should be possible to determine with some degree of scientific precision which foods contain a balance of chemicals that favors protection from cancer, and which foods contain a chemical balance that favors carcinogenesis. In the meantime, while this research is in progress, we must plan our dietary defense against cancer with the information that we have already gained from the kind of epidemiological and experimental studies which are by now familiar to you.

To this chemical balance (or imbalance!) of natural carcinogens and anticarcinogens must now be added the effect of the 12,000 contaminants that enter our food supply as a result of the widespread use of insecticides, fertilizers, and packaging materials; and also the effect of nearly 3,000 food additives that are used by food manufacturers to reduce spoilage and to improve the color, taste, or texture of foods.

Although not enough is known yet to be sure, some scientists believe that the greatest threat to our health does not come from all these chemical additives or contaminants, but rather from the even larger number of mutagens and carcinogens that nature has included in our food supply (1).

What is the extent of the problem? Let me give you some idea. About 55 percent of all food eaten in the United States has been processed. This has led to increased concern among thoughtful Americans about possible harmful effects. In fact, the public concern has been far ahead of the concern shown by the Food and Drug Administration, which is supposed to be acting in the public interest (2).

In 1958, Congress passed a law that made it necessary for food additives to be proved safe before they could be used—only to weaken the impact of the law by excluding many established food additives from regulation. The result is that only about 400 of the 2,600–2,700 food additives are regulated! The rest are classified as "Generally Recognized as Safe," saving the food industry the bother and expense of *proving* them so. Not very reassuring! Only the color additives in current use have been thoroughly tested for safety, and then only because some others were found to be potent carcinogens. According to the report of the National Academy of the Sciences (3), only 83 of the 400 regulated food additives have so far been tested, and then not for their potential cancer risk.

Apart from the possible harmful effects of the intentional food additives, how can we know the effects of the 12,000 substances that are *unintentionally* added during food processing? These substances usually are residues of pesticides or drugs given to animals, or accidental contaminants such as polyvinyl chloride or lead. This question is disturbing because *we simply have no idea of the effects of long-term, low-dose exposure to these substances.* We keep our fingers crossed and blindly hope that our bodies will find a way to get rid of these potentially dangerous chemicals before they harm us.

But, before you abandon eating altogether, let us put this information into perspective. All food is made of chemicals, and the vast majority of chemicals found in food are presumably safe. A perfectly good potato is made up of 150 chemicals, including one that is actually poisonous if eaten in large amounts. Milk consists of 95 chemicals, including 6 proteins, 12 fats, 9 salts, 7 acids, 3 pigments, 18 vitamins, and 7 enzymes! Honey is simply sugar in another form—with no nutritional advantages. Natural chemicals have no advantage over their synthetic counterparts, and certainly your body cannot tell the difference.

To the natural mixture of chemicals that make up our food, the food industry has added its own—calling them "additives." The benefits of most additives have actually been considerable and may in the end outweigh the possible risks. For example, over 90 percent of Americans depend upon food that has been grown and processed by less than 10 percent of the population. Processing and refrigeration have enabled food to be transported and stored and made available nearly all year round. Consequently, wastage is greatly reduced and costs are minimized.

Despite these benefits, the power of food processing has created an irresistible temptation for the food industry to make up all sorts of "junk" foods. These foods are dangerous to the degree that they displace really nutritious food from the national diet. Additionally, they often contain high concentrations of fat, sugar, and salt. And, to cap it all, they are invariably bad nutritional value for your money.

INTENTIONAL FOOD ADDITIVES

Intentional food additives are chemicals that are deliberately introduced into food in order to reduce the risk of spoilage, and often to improve the taste, texture, appearance, nutritive value, and sales appeal. Some of these chemicals are derived from natural sources: carrageenin and agar from seaweeds, monosodium glutamate from corn, sugar from sugar cane, and lecithin from soybeans. Sometimes, natural substances are more economically produced in the laboratory; fortunately, the synthesized chemicals are functionally identical. For example, the vitamin C found in fresh orange juice and the organic rose-hip vitamin C from the health-food store are chemically indistinguishable from cheaper, laboratory-made ascorbic acid; and remember, your body cannot tell the difference either.

Chemical additives may also be completely synthetic, having no natural counterpart. Familiar examples of these chemicals include the artifical sweetener saccharin, the antioxidant preservative BHA, and EDTA (which is used in processed food to trap metal impurities). You should not think that these chemicals must be harmful just because they are not found in nature. Many dangerous chemicals occur naturally, so do not be fooled into thinking that all food chemicals must be good simply because they are natural.

As it happens, most intentional food additives are natural foods. The average American consumes food additives each year that add up to about 102 pounds of cane sugar, 15 pounds of salt, 8.4 pounds of corn syrup, and 4.2 pounds of dextrose. These represent approximately 93 percent of all additives. The remaining 7 percent of additives are taken in much smaller quantities. Thirty-three additives make up 6.5 percent of the total—about 9 pounds a year; and 2,600 additives make up the final 0.5 percent—about 1 pound a year. Put another way, additives make up 10 percent of our total food intake, and more than 90 percent of these additives are sugars and salt, which are not linked to cancer.

WHY ARE FOOD ADDITIVES NECESSARY?

Apart from improving taste, texture, and appearance, the most important justification of food additives is their use for food preservation.

Without preservatives, food rapidly deteriorates. This not only limits the storage and availability of food, but it also raises the dreaded specter of food poisoning from deadly bacteria such as *Salmonella* and *Clostridium botulinum.*

Many foods are preserved by antioxidants, which help to prevent fats and oils from becoming rancid—a process that can form carcinogens. BHT, BHA, vitamin C, vitamin E, lecithin, and isopropyl citrate are examples of antioxidants. BHT and BHA have been criticized as possibly dangerous, but these antioxidants can block the action of some carcinogens and are, on balance, desirable. Possibly, their use has contributed to the steady decline in stomach cancer in the United States. Incidentally, I am sure it has not escaped your notice that some of these antioxidants are also valuable nutrients.

Another important group of preservatives act to inhibit the growth of molds, yeasts, and bacteria. Food poisoning has been almost eliminated from processed foods by the use of chemicals like sugar, salt, calcium propionate (which prevents bread from becoming moldy and provides calcium), sodium benzoate, potassium sorbate (in cheese), sodium bisulfite, and sodium nitrite (which prevent deadly botulism in processed meats and fish). We will look more closely at nitrates and nitrites below, because these preservatives can form powerful carcinogens.

CAN INTENTIONAL FOOD ADDITIVES CAUSE CANCER?

Obviously, some food additives are essential because they enable food to be stored and distributed widely, without risk of infection. Because of the consequently lower cost of food production and because of wide distribution, more people now have access to a balanced, nutritious diet than in any other period of human history. Unfortunately, many people are unaware of this. Instead, this abundance of food has led to indulgent, unbalanced diets that have caused an increase in cancer as well as degenerative diseases. Some—but not all—additives may have contributed to this process.

Commonly used preservatives are the *nitrates* and *nitrites.* These chemicals have been used as curing agents for over 2,000 years, and are probably the most important of the suspected carcinogens. These chemicals also are of special interest because they are used not only to preserve, color, and flavor meats and other cured food products, but because they also occur naturally in many plants and vegetables. Even more surprisingly, we produce about four times as much nitrite in our saliva as we ingest each day. And it has been estimated that only 20 percent of our daily nitrite intake comes from additives, while the rest comes from natural sources.

By themselves nitrates and nitrites are not harmful, but they are converted in the stomach to chemicals called N-nitrosamines, which are powerful carcinogens. This reaction can be blocked by antioxidants such as vitamin C *if they are taken at the same time.* The importance of this protection has not been lost on a few food manufacturers who have begun to include vitamin C with the nitrites or nitrates in order to prevent carcinogen formation. This does not necessarily mean that the food manufacturers care about your health, but it does demonstrate what a few sensible government regulations could do!

Another group of additives that we have all heard about is the artificial sweeteners. The most widely used is saccharin, which has had a rather stormy course. Although saccharin has been used since 1902 by diabetics without any evidence of an increased cancer risk, some experiments with rats have demonstrated that high doses of saccharin over a short period of time can cause bladder cancer.

However, so many people depend on saccharin that attempts by Congress to ban it were vigorously resisted. Instead, saccharin is now sold with a label warning that it can cause cancer in animals. This decision was taken after many hours of testimony from expert witnesses, who often failed to agree on how the evidence should be interpreted. The difficulty is understandable. Can one really predict the risk of low-dose exposure to saccharin in humans over many years, using experimental evidence derived from rats that had been given very high doses over a few weeks or months? The current view held by most scientists is that saccharin is, at worst, a weak carcinogen. My advice is to use it as little as possible, unless you are a diabetic.

Of all unnecessary food additives, artificial coloring is probably the one we can do most easily without—and with good reason! During the past fifty years, at least twelve artificial coloring agents have been banned because they were found to cause illness—including cancer—in laboratory animals. Yet, 10 percent of American food still contains artificial coloring.

Although color additives now in use have been tested for carcinogenicity and found to be safe, these chemicals are suspected of causing other problems. Red dye no. 3, for example, interferes with an important chemical that is needed for carrying messages between brain cells. It has been found to change mood and behavior in people, and some parents with hyperactive children have found that behavior problems are diminished if the dye is removed from the children's diet.

If you avoid junk foods, you will substantially reduce your exposure to artificial coloring agents and probably improve your health at the same time. Meanwhile, further testing of food dyes will almost certainly be necessary to understand their long-term effects on human health.

Fortunately, the widely used food preservatives BHT (butylated hydroxytoluene) and BHA (butylated hydroxyanisole) have been extensively tested for cancer risk. So far there have been no reports of any studies linking BHT or BHA with human cancer. However, BHT has been shown to encourage the development of two animal cancers when given in low doses. But actually this story is not as simple as it might appear. In high doses, BHT can *inhibit* the carcinogenic action of a long list of powerful carcinogens. So I consider BHT to be much more likely to work for us than against us. This is important because this preservative is in so much of what we eat. Fortunately, BHA also is a powerful inhibitor of many carcinogens. So now we have two food additives that are both food preservers and cancer-inhibitors.

UNINTENTIONAL FOOD ADDITIVES

Unintentional food additives can be thought of as those chemicals used in food production and packaging that contaminate food and thus enter our food supply.

Hormones

One group of unintentional additives that may be carcinogenic are *hormones,* powerful natural chemicals that have specific actions on various organs or tissues of the body.

They were used to stimulate growth in cattle until the Food and Drug Administration finally succeeded in banning their use in 1979.

Unfortunately, some owners of livestock still defy the ban. The risk is that a hormone like DES (diethylstilbestrol) may occasionally be found in minute quantities in beef or beef liver. The potential danger lies in the fact that DES is a powerful carcinogen that is known to have caused cancer of the vagina and cervix in the children of mothers treated with DES during pregnancy. And furthermore, therapeutic doses of DES given to men with prostate cancer have sometimes caused breast cancer to develop (4). Since this risk of breast cancer also showed up in tests of DES in laboratory animals, the story of DES serves to illustrate the potential value of animal tests in predicting the risk in humans. Although the hormone dose levels that are used in treatment could never result from eating contaminated meat, the effects of chronic low-dose exposure always remain somewhat unpredictable.

Pesticides

One of the most important groups of possible contaminants are *pesticides.* The risk that they pose was well illustrated in late 1983 when the widely used pesticide EDB (ethylene dibromide) was found to be strongly carcinogenic. Evidence was found that EDB persisted in some citrus fruits and much of the nation's grain supplies. Federal regulations were introduced to restrict its use— slowly. Despite the convincing evidence of high risk, economic considerations prevailed sufficiently to prevent an immediate, outright ban. Some states took the initiative and passed very strict controls on its use. Other states, whose economic interests were more vulnerable, appeared relatively indifferent. While the federal regulations gradually take effect, more of us will be exposed to dangerous levels of this pesticide with inevitable consequences. What can we do to protect ourselves when some contaminated foods are still left, unlabeled, on supermarket shelves?

The basic danger of pesticides is that residues remain on vegetable and fruit produce after harvesting. Even food processing fails to remove them. Pesticides also can get into the drinking water to provide us with another unwelcome source. Although many of the pesticides in use today are known to be carcinogenic at high doses over short periods of time, we actually ingest these chemicals at much lower doses over a long period of time.

How can we accurately estimate the risk? Frankly, it is impossible. It is hardly a consolation that no case of human cancer has ever been directly attributed to previous exposure to a food additive or to a contaminating pesticide. This could just reflect our difficulty in understanding a process that takes so long and is so chemically complex.

Probably the most sinister aspect of pesticide contamination is the fact that pesticides are not easily destroyed by the body. Rather, they actually accumulate in our bodies over months and years, with unknown consequences. Just the sort of insidious risk that we should try very hard to minimize.

Other Unintentional Additives

Another example of an unintentional food additive is a carcinogenic substance called acrylonitrile. Don't worry about the name. Think of it as a chemical that can get into some foods from certain wrapping and packaging materials. In practice, the amount that any of us might be exposed to is so small that it is unlikely to be significant. Only certain industrial workers exposed to higher concentrations have so far shown any increased cancer risk.

NATURE'S FOOD ADDITIVES

As if the intentional and unintentional food additives were not enough to contend with, we must now try to understand the subtle influence of all the complex chemicals that nature has included in every source of food we use. Ever since our first exposure to mother's milk, we have taken the benefits of food for granted. As children we are told to eat this or that because it is good for us. In fact, no one who has given such advice has ever understood anything about the reaction of the body to each and every chemical that the food contains. The degree of trust that we all must place in the benefits of food and maternal advice is truly astonishing. Some of that trust is now being challenged by the discovery that eating certain foods once thought beneficial may be harmful, and that eating other foods once thought worthless may be beneficial.

A new science is gradually emerging which is in the process of discovering hidden enemies and hidden friends: nature's own food additives! These are called dietary mutagens, dietary carcinogens, and dietary anticarcinogens.

Dietary mutagens are chemicals that can alter the DNA of a living cell, so increasing the risk that the cell will become malignant (a cancer cell). Since the DNA of all living organisms is basically the same, it is possible to test chemicals for mutagenicity using simple bacterial systems.

A mass of information has been generated about mutagens in food, but interpreting it is another matter. You see, just because a substance is shown to be mutagenic it does not mean that it will necessarily prove to be carcinogenic. But even if tests in animals do prove that a mutagen is carcinogenic, one still has to consider carefully the consequences of removing the mutagen from the diet. You'll see what I mean in a moment.

Mutagens arise in food in all sorts of ways, some of which will really surprise you. Let's consider something as "harmless" and as important as cooking. What would you think if I tell you that cooking destroys germs and makes food much more palatable, and is therefore vital to our health? I have no doubt that you would be in complete agreement with me. Right? But if I also told you that cooking caused mutagens to form you'd probably be astounded! Well they do, and this is how. When you place a juicy, tender steak on your charcoal grill, fat drips down onto the hot coals below. Smoke is formed which rises to penetrate the meat, and this process forms mutagenic chemicals such as benzo[a]pyrene and polynuclear aromatic hydrocarbons (PAH's). Experiments revealed that the more fat there was in meat, the more mutagens were found in the meat after cooking (5). But when meat was cooked in such a way that exposure to smoke was eliminated, these mutagens were hardly formed at all (5,6).

Similar mutagens have been found in smoked foods and, I am sorry to say, in roasted coffee (7). Even vegetables can sometimes become contaminated by PAH's from air, soil, or water. Occasionally, fish and shellfish have become contaminated with these chemicals in their marine environments (7).

During the past few years, it has become apparent that there are many other mutagens beside the PAH's that can be formed by cooking. Most mutagens seem to be formed by an effect of cooking on proteins. This occurs to a greater extent at high temperatures, but can even occur at temperatures below the boiling point of water (8). Broiling hamburgers, beef, fish, chicken, or any other meat, for that matter, will create mutagens, so it appears to be an unavoidable consequence of cooking.

Other mutagens are formed through the action of cooking on carbohydrates. Even an action as innocent as toasting bread has been shown to create mutagenic chemicals through a process known as *the browning reaction* (9). This reaction also occurs when potatoes and beef are fried, or when sugars are heated. Safer methods of cooking will be discussed in more detail in Chapter 13.

There are a number of other chemical mutagens that are found in a great many foods. These have a variety of names, and one of the most common is a group of chemicals called the *flavonoids*. Examples of common foods that contain flavonoids are tea, coffee, Japanese pickles, dill weed, cocoa, fruit jams, beer, red wine, vinegar, raisins, onions, and grape juice. And if you thought your favorite whiskey or brandy was an exception, I'm afraid you're in for a disappointment (10).

Fortunately, extracts of very few fruit and vegetables are mutagenic. In fact, quite the contrary. Laboratory tests have demonstrated that a number of substances in foods can actually inhibit the action of many mutagens. *Anti*mutagenic activity has been shown in extracts of some common vegetables, fruit, and spices, including cabbage, broccoli, green pepper, eggplant, shallots, pineapple, apples, ginger, and mint leaf (11). Other studies have shown similar antimutagenic activity in extracts of wheat sprouts, parsley, lettuce, brussels sprouts, spinach, mustard greens, and other vegetables (12). Although chlorophyll has been touted as the principal antimutagen, there are many others yet to be identified.

Other protective antimutagens include unsaturated fatty acids, folic acid, sodium nitrite (which can also be converted into a carcinogen unless an antioxidant is present), and a variety of antioxidants such as BHA and BHT (preservatives) (13), vitamin A, vitamin C, vitamin E, and selenium (14).

Since cooking is essential to eliminate the very serious illnesses that result from bacterial infection of food, we must continue to eat mutagens if we are to avoid food poisoning. In any case, who among us can even contemplate a raw diet? A much better approach is to make sure we include plenty of the fruit and vegetables in our diet that supply antimutagens and protective antioxidants.

As if natural mutagens are not enough for us to contend with, we now have to contemplate the existence of the many *natural carcinogens* that are found in our traditional diet. Incidentally, most of these carcinogens are also mutagenic, so the distinction becomes a little blurred in practice.

For over a hundred years, scientists have been uncovering an enormous variety of chemicals in plants, and recent tests reveal that many of them are toxic. It appears that plants make many of these toxic chemicals to defend themselves against attacking hordes of insects, bacteria, and fungi. Familiar food items that contain carcinogens include root beer, black pepper, mushrooms, celery, parsnips, figs, parsley, rhubarb, coffee, tea, cocoa, herbal teas, broad beans, cottonseed oil, trout, alfalfa sprouts, and alcoholic drinks; not to mention rancid fat, nitrate preservatives, nitrosamines and foods with mold contamination. The list seems endless!

The influence of mold contamination has also been very important. Certain common molds produce a potent carcinogenic toxin called *aflatoxin B_1*. This kind of contamination often results from storage of food in tropical climates. In the United States, mold contamination is usually found only in crops that are infected before harvesting. Typically, peanuts, corn, and cottonseed are infected, but occasionally tree nuts such as almonds, walnuts, pecans, and pistachios are involved.

Our main exposure to this toxin is from peanuts and corn, and although efforts are made to minimize this exposure, the Food and Drug Administration has classified some aflatoxin contamination as unavoidable. This is not very reassuring because aflatoxin is one of the most potent liver carcinogens known. Studies of people in many countries have associated aflatoxin exposure with an increased risk of cancer. In Mozambique, where aflatoxin contamination of food is thought to be the highest in the world, liver cancer is very common (15). Contaminated groundnuts have increased the incidence of liver cancer in parts of Africa, while similar aflatoxin contamination has been associated with liver cancer in Thailand, Taiwan, and parts of China (16). The effects of aflatoxin are not limited to liver cancer, however. In Henan province in northern China, esophageal cancer has been linked to pickled vegetables and other fermented and moldy food (17). It is a relief to know that there is no evidence linking aflatoxin contamination in the United States with human cancer—yet! So you can continue to eat peanut butter in moderation, provided you remember that it is a rich source of fat.

Now consider this question: since hydrazines are chemicals found in ordinary mushrooms, and since these chemicals cause cancer in mice, should we eat mushrooms? This problem symbolizes the dilemma which we face each day—if we care to think about it. The answer is not simple because the risk is not known with certainty. My own view is that if mushrooms are very important to you, then continue to eat them—in moderation. If they are unimportant, then leave them out of your diet. If you do eat mushrooms, or any other foods containing carcinogens for that matter, then your diet must provide anticarcinogens to protect you. Until we know more, I think that this is a rational approach to this kind of problem.

Coffee is one of the most popular drinks in America. Without it, some of us feel we would not make it through the day. Yet, although there is some evidence which suggests that coffee may cause us to develop pancreatic cancer (18), subsequent studies have failed to substantiate this observation. Despite the fact that coffee has also been shown to have mutagenic activity in experimental studies, I consider that the direct evidence against coffee still remains slight.

Another group of dietary carcinogens that are of unusual interest are the nitrites, nitrates, and nitrosamines. As you no doubt remember, nitrites and nitrates are used to preserve meats and other processed foods. These same preservatives are also used by nature. Beets, celery, spinach, lettuce, radishes, and rhubarb each contain substantial amounts of nitrate. The amount varies to some extent with the composition of the soil, but equally important is the fact that nitrates often coexist with inhibitors or with catalysts that influence their conversion into toxic nitrosamines.

As so often appears to be the case in nature, a balance exists between the good guys and the bad guys. If nature supplies unwanted carcinogens, it also supplies anticarcinogens. The goal of your new diet is to shift this balance very definitely in your favor.

Dietary anticarcinogens are being increasingly recognized as an important part of our defense against cancer. To help you to understand the significance of this, I would like to share a few observations with you.

The majority of cancers arise in parts of the body that are exposed to the environment. For example, the gastrointestinal tract is constantly exposed to an amazing array of chemicals; the lungs are exposed to polluted air (tobacco being by far the worst pollutant); the skin is exposed to sunlight; the urinary tract is exposed to internally produced "pollutants"; the liver is exposed to ingested carcinogens which it concentrates and destroys; and the lymphatic system defends us against infections, including infection by carcinogenic viruses.

For the body to shield itself against this onslaught, sophisticated defense mechanisms have evolved that come to the rescue. Firstly, in most of the tissues that have a high risk of becoming cancerous, cells die and are replaced quite rapidly. As cells divide rapidly, they have a much greater chance of making a genetic mistake during cell division. When this happens, the inherited genetic instructions may be so abnormal that the daughter cells divide uncontrollably—becoming cancer cells. However, sometimes this rapid cell turnover can actually be protective. For example, the lining of the small intestine is completely replaced every two to three days. This means that any cell which is damaged (by mutagens or carcinogens) has a very high chance of dying spontaneously, and it is thought that this is the reason that cancers so rarely occur in the small intestine. In contrast, the cell turnover is slower in the large intestine (colon), which is exposed longer to bacterial and chemical carcinogens, and in which cancer occurs so frequently. Secondly, it is thought that the body's immune system possesses cells which can recognize and eliminate cancer cells and that cancer may arise in the body when this process fails.

In addition to these mechanisms, certain enzymes (chemical regulators) exist within cells that both help to protect cells from damaging carcinogens, and help to repair any damage that might occur. They form part of a really remarkable defense organization!

How then can we relate dietary anticarcinogens to these processes? Unfortunately, nobody really knows the answer to this question. What scientists do know is that there are many chemicals in food that can protect us from cancer. We are far from knowing all of them, however, and are far from fully understanding how they work.

Fortunately, what is becoming clear is that increasing your intake of vegetables can reduce the cancer risk. For example, studies have revealed that people who eat more raw vegetables, including cole slaw and red cabbage (19), more lettuce and celery, (20), and more green and yellow vegetables (21), all have a reduced risk of stomach cancer. Moreover, an increased intake of brussels sprouts, cabbage, broccoli, and high-fiber foods has been shown to reduce the risk of colon and rectal cancer (22). Many of the epidemiological studies that I have referred to earlier have also revealed the importance of dietary vegetables.

The most obvious anticarcinogenic factors in vegetables are the vitamins and trace elements. However, there are probably many other factors, only some of which have been identified. The list is long, and the names will not mean much to you, but these names should eventually become as familiar as the list on the back of a bottle of multivitamins. Among the most studied are phenols, indoles, flavones, aromatic isothiocyanates, protease inhibitors, and sitosterol.

In studies with laboratory animals that have been purposely exposed to chemical carcinogens, most of these substances have been shown to block the two key processes in carcinogenesis: the initiation and promotion of cancer.

Phenols occur naturally in many vegetables, and artificially as the synthetic preservative, BHA.

Indoles are found in cruciferous vegetables such as brussels sprouts, cabbage, cauliflower, and broccoli.

Flavones are present in most fruit and vegetables.

The *aromatic isothiocyanates* are found in cruciferous vegetables like those mentioned above.

Protease inhibitors are also common in plants, but they occur in the highest concentration in seeds, particularly soybeans and lima beans. One study suggested that protease inhibitors prevent the formation of those infamous free radicals referred to earlier! (23)

The last of these nonnutritive dietary cancer inhibitors is *beta-sitosterol,* which is also found in many vegetables and vegetable oils.

Among the nutritive dietary anticarcinogens, let me remind you of the great value of vitamin A and beta-carotene, folic acid, vitamin C, vitamin E, and selenium. Finally, let me bring your attention to another powerful anticarcinogen called *glutathione.* Glutathione is present inside our cells and also in many of our foods. This is a strong antioxidant that may be an effective defense against many carcinogens, including that notorious liver carcinogen, aflatoxin (24).

Using the knowledge derived from animal experiments, some fascinating studies have been done in human volunteers to prove the value of vegetables in our defense against carcinogens. One group of people had a normal diet, and a second group had a diet that was rich in cabbage and brussels sprouts! It almost seems an absurd experiment, except that the results were dramatic, and they confirmed that the people on the vegetable diet could break down two test carcinogens much faster than the group on a regular diet (25). This represents direct evidence of the influence of diet on our cancer defenses.

FOOD ADDITIVES AND YOUR GENERAL HEALTH

Although I have concentrated on factors that might influence your cancer risk, it is also important not to forget that other food additives can also affect your health, even if they do not cause cancer. Of special interest are a group of additives known as the *sulfiting agents.* These antioxidants are important because they are widely used by restaurants to keep fruit and vegetables looking fresh; and because your new diet will significantly increase your intake of fruit and vegetables. Sulfites are also used in many restaurant foods, particularly seafood and fried potatoes. Often they are included in processed foods such as fruit drinks, wine, beer, baked goods, dried fruit and vegetables. So there is a good chance that most of us are exposed to sulfites.

By July of 1983, the Food and Drug Administration had received reports of ninety cases of allergic reactions, including one death, all attributed to the consumption of sulfites! Most often they occurred after eating restaurant salads or other foods, eating processed foods, or drinking wine or other beverages. More than half of these cases were in people who already suffered from asthma, but a third were in people with no history of illness. I would suggest that you ask about the use of sulfites before ordering food in a restaurant, and avoid them whenever possible, particularly if you are an asthmatic.

The only other additive that you should be particularly aware of is *monosodium glutamate,* commonly known as MSG. MSG is used by most Chinese restaurants to enhance flavor, but it has been associated with adverse reactions in some people. These reactions occur quite soon after eating MSG, and consist of headache, faintness, sweating, and, rarely, collapse. However, there is no evidence that MSG influences your cancer risk.

WHAT YOU SHOULD DO ABOUT ADDITIVES

You should now think of some food additives as being harmless, some as being harmful (carcinogenic), and some as being beneficial (cancer-inhibitors). It is also important to recognize the extraordinary contribution that food preservatives have made to our general nutrition; they must not all be dismissed as dangerous.

Although food additives appear in our food as a result of food processing, natural carcinogens and anticarcinogens are found in our food because they have been important to the evolution and survival of plant life. And since natural carcinogens and anticarcinogens often occur together in many foods in varying proportions, it will take a lot more research before we can both establish the complete chemical profile of each food item and understand the precise balance of protective and risk factors. When we ultimately achieve such knowledge, it will be possible to design the perfect diet.

In the meantime, certain foods are clearly more protective than others, and with the evidence already available, a diet can be constructed that emphasizes protective foods, and minimizes those foods which enhance your cancer risk. This approach forms the basis of the Cancer Prevention Diet.

At a practical level, it is much better to eat fresh, unprocessed foods whenever possible. But if you can only find processed foods, then at least you should be aware of the ingredients that are listed on the label of any processed or packaged food items. Although it is impossible to eliminate only dangerous additives, it is still worth trying to reduce your exposure to them. I always try to avoid artificial coloring, nitrates and nitrites, and foods that contain a lot of saturated fat and cholesterol. I also avoid foods that contain large amounts of sugar and salt, two of the most common "safe" additives that manufacturers put into foods to stimulate sales. Why should we restrict sugar and salt consumption? The answer is simple: because sugar causes obesity and salt can cause high blood pressure—and both these conditions reduce life expectancy!

All fresh fruit and vegetables should be thoroughly washed to remove any pesticide residues. Peeling fruit or vegetables will remove superficial contamination and nutrients. When you cannot find the fresh fruits and vegetables of your choice, then choose frozen rather than canned; the latter tend to have many more intentional additives lurking within them. Also, don't be fooled when you see the word "natural" in big letters on the label. This is no guarantee that there are no undesirable additives, since many additives are in fact "natural" substances. Of course, I do not mean to imply that such products are necessarily harmful, but often you will be paying much more for them for no good reason!

Finally, what these simple guidelines boil down to is this: *know what you're eating and learn how to control it.*

CHAPTER 11

Alcohol—At What Price?

. . . it provokes the desire, but it takes away the performance . . .
SHAKESPEARE

The word "alcohol" originated in the East, where for centuries it described a fine powder used for painting the eyebrows! The effects of alcohol were discovered thousands of years before Christ turned water into wine. Early man discovered that when he left some mashed fruit around in a warm corner of the cave, fermentation would produce a crude form of wine. And then he discovered that when he drank this concoction, he experienced certain pleasant effects that went well beyond simply quenching his thirst. The history of ancient civilizations is littered with anecdotes about wine, and it is clear that it did not take long for mankind to see the merits of the deliberate production of alcohol.

Until about 500 years ago, such efforts at production were confined to beer and wine. Then, in the fifteenth century, distillation techniques were developed to produce spirits, and the alcohol content of drinks rose from about 14 percent to 50 percent or more. Needless to say, this "progress" was enthusiastically welcomed by many people. This is not surprising, for alcohol must have been one of the first drugs ever found to induce dramatic effects on mood and behavior.

The discovery of the power of alcohol led to its use as a sacred drink, and this "respectability" has led to its traditional use at a great variety of festive occasions. Yet, despite this acceptance, warnings about the harmful effects of excessive drinking have been found in ancient Egyptian writings as long as 3,000 years ago.

In the United States, after the failure of Prohibition, drinking continued to cause major problems, and is now estimated to cause industrial losses of nearly $50 billion each year. If you then add to this staggering total the social cost of about half of all traffic deaths and about two thirds of violent crime, you can see that alcohol is probably the most socially destructive of all drugs.

In 1976, the average American consumed the alcohol equivalent of two glasses of wine each day. This is the same as two beers or 2.5 ounces of whiskey. Since about 10 million Americans are either alcoholics or very heavy drinkers, the rest of us drink somewhat less than the national average of 2.68 gallons of pure alcohol every year!

THE GENERAL HEALTH EFFECTS OF ALCOHOL

What does all this alcohol do to you? Apart from the immediate effects, which few of us have escaped at some time or another, there are the lasting effects. Among heavy drinkers, the most serious consequences are due to nutritional deficiencies, and to cirrhosis of the liver. Other well-known effects involve the heart and blood vessels. Less well known is the fact that alcohol can accelerate the conversion of chemical procarcinogens into active carcinogens, thereby increasing the cancer risk.

The nutritional deficiencies commonly found in heavy drinkers arise mainly because alcohol is substituted for a proper diet. Various vitamin deficiencies can occur, sometimes with dramatic effect. One example is a brain disease called Wernicke-Korsakoff syndrome. This syndrome, which leads to memory loss and confabulation, is found almost exclusively in alcoholics and is caused by a deficiency of vitamin B_1 (thiamin). Fortunately, this can usually be treated successfully.

The poor diet of the alcoholic, which typically lacks fresh fruit and vegetables, often leads to other deficiencies too, such as a lack of B vitamins, vitamin C, iron, and other minerals. The result is a multitude of physical problems, including peripheral nerve defects, liver disease, eye disease, infertility, impotence, and cancer. Now do you still feel like "one for the road"?

Although alcohol has never been shown to cause cancer directly in any experiment, there is a good deal of epidemiological evidence that strongly links alcohol consumption to the development of many cancers. In Japan, cancer of the esophagus has been associated with the drinking of whiskey and *shochu,* cancer of the rectum with wine, and cancer of the prostate with *shochu* (1). In Africa, a popular alcoholic drink is made from corn, and its consumption increases the risk of cancer of the esophagus (2). In France, home-distilled apple brandy also increases the risk of esophageal cancer (3), and this risk is definitely made worse by smoking (4). As early as 1910, one study found that absinthe drinkers had an increased risk of esophageal cancer (5), so the potential danger of alcohol should have been known by physicians for some time.

In the French city of Lyons, a study of patients with stomach cancer found that they drank about twice as much red wine as a similar group of people without cancer (6). (I'm tempted to suggest that the solution is to drink less wine, but of a better vintage!)

Another recent study, which was done in Denmark, was most revealing (7). As you may know, Danish beer is famous for its strong, rich taste. And the brewery workers are rewarded for their labors with four free pints of beer each day! As it happens, this generosity is misguided. These workers, who consequently drink far more beer than other men in Denmark, have a much greater chance of getting cancer of the esophagus, larynx, lung, and liver, even when the effects of tobacco are allowed for. In contrast, workers in soft-drink factories have the same risk as the general population.

Another way of studying this question is to look at the cancer risk among groups of people who are known to abstain from alcoholic drinks for religious reasons. The most famous are the Mormons and the Seventh-Day Adventists. Predictably, these people have a significantly lower risk of these cancers (8,9).

In other countries, too, there have been many studies that have demonstrated the association of alcohol consumption with cancer. In England, Ireland, and Norway, beer increases the risk of colorectal cancer (10,11,12); in China, a strong alcoholic drink called *pai-kan* increases cancer of the esophagus (13); and in another study, of twenty countries, it was also shown that heavy drinkers had an increased risk of cancer (14).

Well, if you think that the evidence against alcohol is bad, you should know that it is made much worse by combining alcohol with smoking.

I am sure that you have noticed that people who drink heavily often smoke heavily too. Most studies have shown that it is the smoking that really makes the greatest contribution to the danger of alcohol. This is especially true for cancers of the mouth and larynx, but it is also true for cancer of the esophagus. When scientists have studied groups of nonsmokers for the effect of alcohol on cancer risk, the results have been rather vague and unconvincing.

Some investigators have suggested that it is the accompanying malnutrition that increases the cancer risk among alcoholics, and this may indeed be an important factor. Certainly, the same nutrient deficiencies that are commonly found in alcoholics produce an increased susceptibility to experimental cancers in laboratory animals.

Furthermore, since alcohol can stimulate the liver enzymes that convert procarcinogens into dangerous carcinogens, and since tobacco smoke is full of procarcinogens, it does not require a major leap of the imagination to suspect that alcohol could make smoking substantially more dangerous. If you then add to this time bomb the carcinogens that are often found in alcoholic drinks—nitrosamines, polycyclic hydrocarbons, and asbestos fibers in wine and gin—then the combined pleasures of smoking and drinking begin to look suicidal!

WHAT YOU SHOULD DO ABOUT ALCOHOL

Before you totally give up alcohol, there is one vital point that might save the day—or perhaps part of the day. Cancer is not the only disease to fear in life. Heart disease is, after all, the number-one killer and although very heavy drinking can cause damage to the heart, drinking in moderation can actually reduce your risk of a heart attack! This is thought to be due to protective *phyto-estrogens* (female hormones) present in some alcoholic drinks. What then is "moderation"? This is arguable, but we might agree on less than two glasses of wine each day. For reasons that remain obscure, wine seems to be more protective than other drinks, and is therefore the preferred savior. Well, that's not so bad, is it?

So, on balance, I think that it is reasonable to enjoy alcohol in moderation if you are a nonsmoker. If you must persist in smoking, restrict your alcohol intake to less than one glass of wine per day.

Best of all, smokers should use all these reasons to give up smoking, and thereby reduce their risk of cancer and heart disease, while really tasting the pure pleasure of a glass or two from a great bottle of Cabernet-Sauvignon. After all, life is also for living, and this was beautifully expressed in 1600 by the Frenchman Olivier de Serres in his book *Theatre d'Agriculture,* where he wrote "After bread comes wine, the second element given by the Creator for the preservation of life and the first celebration of His excellence."

In the final analysis, alcohol is thought to be the direct cause of about 3 percent of all cancer deaths in men and women (15). And since smoking already causes about a third of all cancer deaths, alcohol clearly makes a bad situation even worse.

So if you want to live dangerously, smoke. If you want to live very dangerously, smoke a lot. If that is still too boring, smoke and drink a lot at the same time. Only remember, you may find that the price you pay is your life!

CHAPTER 12

Obesity, Calories, and Girth Control

. . . a little more than a little is by much too much . . .

SHAKESPEARE

Weight control is a subject that is close to the hearts and minds of all women and most men. Controlling weight has become a private battle that many Americans wage with themselves, day after day, year after year. Vanity and a desire to remain young and attractive even into old age provide tremendous motivation to make great sacrifices. Agonizing efforts at jogging and heroic deprivation at the dinner table have improved the physique and strengthened the character of many Americans of all ages. We have bought millions of copies of hundreds of books espousing the virtues of one diet or another.

Eat more protein; eat less protein; eat less carbohydrate; eat less fat; eat grapefruit; eat pineapple; avoid sugar; eat more fiber. You feel completely confused! Each book has a battle cry that is supposed to distinguish it from the others. In most cases there is little scientific evidence to justify the proposed diet, and the success of these books is a measure of the desperation that many people feel in their search for health and success.

Obesity is America's most serious nutrition problem. The average weight of both men and women is between 15 and 30 pounds *above* the level considered healthy by scientists and the life insurance companies. Government figures indicate that 25 percent of males and 42 percent of females are overweight. This is a serious matter because statistics reveal that being overweight increases the risk of developing such serious diseases as high blood pressure, heart disease, stroke, and cancer. What is more, obesity is associated with an increase in diabetes, respiratory diseases, kidney disease, gastrointestinal problems, gallbladder disease, liver disease, and arthritis of weight-bearing joints. To this grim list can be added the fact that fat people have a higher accident rate and suffer many more complications following surgery.

How did this deplorable state of affairs come about? To understand this, it is necessary to understand how the body regulates its energy balance.

First of all, to maintain a constant weight, the energy provided by your diet should equal the energy required for the body to function. Every person burns up calories just maintaining the blood circulation, breathing, digesting food, contracting muscles, producing chemicals, and so on. This is called the *basal metabolic rate*. To this baseline calorie requirement are added those calories that are needed for any additional activity, whether it be strolling down a quiet country lane or climbing Mount Everest.

Any excess calories in the diet are either stored as fat or burned off as surplus. When we are young, we usually manage to burn off excess calories fairly effectively, but as we get older and are less physically active, this ability to burn off the excess calories insidiously declines. We thus tend to gain weight even if our total calorie intake remains the same.

Secondly, the total number of fat cells in the body influences our tendency to gain weight. Fat cells are created mainly in infancy and early childhood, and infants who are fed high-calorie diets develop more fat cells—cells that remain with them for the rest of their lives. The more fat cells you have, the greater your capacity to store fat. And we all know what that means! Obviously, all parents have a responsibility to protect their defenseless children from the disastrous consequences of an indulgent diet.

As you age, the deliberate pursuit of exercise does more than improve your muscle tone and improve your heart and circulation. It makes you feel better. It also can restore to some extent the ability of your body to burn off those excess calories that we all fear— rather like resetting the thermostat. So, regular exercise is clearly vital to your physical and mental well-being.

The way you exercise is really up to you. Some forms of exercise are naturally much more strenuous than others, but even the most active exercise, such as squash or jogging, does not burn up much more than an extra 600 calories per hour. Since a pound of fat provides nearly 4,000 calories, it would take more than six hours of squash or jogging to lose a pound of fat. There has got to be a better way to lose weight! Actually, there is a better way, and that involves eating less of the "wrong" foods and more of the "right" foods. Fortunately, the National Cancer Prevention Diet provides a natural balance that will also make weight control much easier.

But, unlike fad weight-reducing diets, which last only a few weeks, your new diet will be for life.

Clearly, the only successful weight-reducing diet plan must be one that makes you develop new dietary habits that are permanent. And these new habits should be the right ones for you in every way, both minimizing your cancer risk and helping you with your weight control. For each person with a weight problem, there is an optimum amount of food energy that can be processed each day without gaining weight. Once you have established this amount, then you know that any deviation from this amount will eventually cause your weight to change.

If you are fortunate enough not to have a weight problem, these words of advice are still important because they could prevent you from developing a weight problem later. Why, you may ask, am I so concerned with your weight anyway? How important is your weight when it comes to assessing your cancer risk?

Although it is very difficult to identify the effect of total calorie intake on the risk of developing cancer in humans, there is evidence that being obese does increase the cancer risk. The reasons for this inconsistency are not too difficult to understand.

Calories are the fuel which the body needs twenty-four hours a day in order to function properly. And as you know, calories can be derived from fat, protein, and carbohydrates. Fat provides about 9 calories per gram, while protein and carbohydrate each provide only 4 calories per gram. Fortunately, fiber provides no calories.

The calorie content of a meal can therefore be modified by changing the proportions of fat, carbohydrate, and protein, and by changing the amount of nonnutritive fiber. And since both dietary fat and fiber can influence carcinogenesis, their effects must be distinguished from the effects of calories alone. In practice, this is very hard to do.

Although there have not been very many epidemiological studies

that have tried to relate calorie intake to cancer risk, those that have
been done have been quite provocative. Some studies have looked
at the cancer risk in various economic groups and have found that
hormone-dependent cancers like breast cancer and prostate cancer
are related to affluence (1). In Hong Kong, colorectal cancer causes
twice the mortality among the rich as among the poor (2). In this
case, the calorie intake of the rich averaged 3,900 calories per day,
while the poor averaged 2,700 calories per day.

A major study of thirty-two countries has also revealed a correlation of total calorie intake with colorectal cancer in males, leukemia
in males, and breast cancer in females (3).

A different approach was used in Holland and Japan, where evidence was found that postmenopausal women who were both taller
and heavier had a higher incidence of breast cancer (4).

In the United States, the American Cancer Society carried out a
long-term study of 750,000 men and women between 1959 and 1972
to assess the relationship between weight and various diseases, including cancer (5). Deaths from cancer were found to be significantly increased among those men and women who were more than
40 percent overweight. In men, there was an increased risk of cancer
of the colon and rectum; in women there was an increased risk of
cancer of the gall bladder and biliary system, breast, cervix, lining
of the uterus, and ovary. However, this large study was unable to
distinguish between the effect of nutrients such as fat, and the effect
of total calorie intake per se.

In animals, the results of several experiments have indicated that
animals fed restricted diets live longer than those that are allowed to
eat as much as they want. Similarly, animals that have been exposed to carcinogens, and then placed on a restricted diet, have developed fewer tumors than those given a free diet (6).

WHAT YOU SHOULD DO ABOUT CALORIES

Although the evidence is still rather limited, it would seem that
excessive calories and obesity may well contribute to an increased
cancer risk. There is little doubt, however, that obesity shortens life
expectancy due to cardiovascular and other diseases—ask any insurance agent! So we should all make strenuous efforts to maintain

our ideal weight through greater food consciousness and sensible exercise.

Your new diet should make this relatively easy for you because the increase in fruit and vegetables will provide you with larger volumes of low-calorie foods and filling fiber.

If you are overweight, the adoption of this new diet will greatly assist you to reduce your weight, and to control it more effectively. But don't look for rapid, dramatic changes in your weight. Diets which claim to reduce large amounts of weight rapidly are grossly misleading. The early weight loss that these diets produce is mostly due to water loss, and because they are usually short-term solutions to long-term problems, they never actually solve anything. Instead, they are often dangerous, and can really put the health of the dieter at risk. Far better to adopt a lifetime diet that will gradually normalize your weight while reducing your chance of developing life-threatening diseases. Nevertheless, a 1200-calorie version of the Cancer Prevention Diet that is designed for weight control is included in Chapter 15 for your convenience.

In an ideal world, eating would be for necessity and pleasure, not for the relief of stress or depression. You must therefore develop control over how much and how often you eat, and not allow your mood to dictate your eating habits. This may not be very easy for some people. Researchers at Duke University have studied the relationship of obesity to taste perception. Interestingly, obese people were found to be more aware of taste and to have a greater ability than normal-weight people to identify foods by taste alone. This means that obese people may require more taste stimulation before they feel satisfied by a meal. Between meals, the craving for taste stimulation is also greater in obese people. If you think of the effect that the smell of good cooking has on your appetite, imagine if you felt the same hunger most of the time even without that stimulation.

Such flavor-craving probably results from childhood feeding patterns. Parents are often tempted to give their infants and children sweets or sugary drinks when they are unhappy or as a way to keep them quiet. After a while, anything less sweet becomes tasteless to the child and the problem is established—often permanently.

The body reacts to foods physiologically as well as psychologically. For example, carbohydrates increase the level of serotonin, the brain hormone that provides a feeling of relaxation and well-being. And carbonation of drinks or the use of spices stimulates the nerve receptors in the tongue, which in turn stimulate the production of more adrenaline—and a natural high. Needless to say, these responses encourage one to eat, sometimes too much.

The most practical way to deal with this problem is to try to introduce as much variety into your daily diet as possible. And when you eat, select foods individually rather than mixing them together on your fork. Choose a little of one food, then another, rather than eating all of one item first and then moving on to the next. In this way you can savor different tastes and increase the sense of variety. This should be more satisfying.

HOW DO YOU KNOW IF YOU ARE OVERWEIGHT?

In order to do the right thing, you must first know whether you are in fact overweight, and then you must decide what your daily calorie intake ought be to achieve or maintain your ideal weight.

To know your needs is not always easy. Some people are normal but think that they're overweight, while others are overweight but think they're normal! The glamorous woman of the nineteenth century would be considered fat by today's standards. Modern fashion magazines and the advertising industry influence us in subtle—and not so subtle—ways to be slim, often too slim. This sometimes produces an almost hysterical obsession with dieting that erodes the quality of life. Such a response is never appropriate and should be resisted.

A better way for you to understand your own needs is to refer to the latest table of ideal weights for adult men and women (Table 12–1). This is based upon the Metropolitan Life Insurance Company statistics, which have shown that people of these weights live the longest—and they should know!

HOW TO ESTIMATE YOUR CALORIE NEEDS

Although your new diet will be balanced in a way that will minimize your risk of cancer, it is obvious that the total amount of food that you will need to meet your calorie requirements must be care-

Table 12-1
IDEAL WEIGHT

		MEN					WOMEN		
Height Feet	Inches	Small Frame	Medium Frame	Large Frame	Height Feet	Inches	Small Frame	Medium Frame	Large Frame
5	2	128–134	131–141	138–150	4	10	102–111	109–121	118–131
5	3	130–136	133–143	140–153	4	11	103–113	111–123	120–134
5	4	132–138	135–145	142–156	5	0	104–115	113–126	122–137
5	5	134–140	137–148	144–160	5	1	106–118	115–129	125–140
5	6	136–142	139–151	146–164	5	2	108–121	118–132	128–143
5	7	138–145	142–154	149–168	5	3	111–124	121–135	131–147
5	8	140–148	145–157	152–172	5	4	114–127	124–138	134–151
5	9	142–151	148–160	155–176	5	5	117–130	127–141	137–155
5	10	144–154	151–163	158–180	5	6	120–133	130–144	140–159
5	11	146–157	154–166	161–184	5	7	123–136	133–147	143–163
6	0	149–160	157–170	164–188	5	8	126–139	136–150	146–167
6	1	152–164	160–174	168–192	5	9	129–142	139–153	149–170
6	2	155–168	164–178	172–197	5	10	132–145	142–156	152–173
6	3	158–172	167–182	176–202	5	11	135–148	145–159	155–176
6	4	162–176	171–187	181–207	6	0	138–151	148–162	158–179

Note: These tables reflect the desirable weight for average adults. The optional weights for young adults may be slightly less, and the optional weights for the elderly may be slightly more.
Source of basic data: 1979 Build Study, Society of Actuaries and Association of Life Insurance Medical Directors of America, 1980.
Table courtesy of Metropolitan Life Insurance Company.

fully estimated. If you are presently overweight, you should calculate the calorie needs for your ideal weight and then reduce them by 25 percent.

Calorie requirements can be considered in two parts. The first part is the number of calories that are needed to maintain your basal metabolic rate (BMR). This is simply the energy that you use up just staying alive. The calories that maintain your BMR are like the gas that keeps your car engine idling. To help you to decide how many calories you need, the National Research Council has published (Table 12–2) the range of calories required to sustain the BMR and do some light work (about 100–200 calories per hour). Remember, as your level of activity increases, so do your energy needs; but as you get older, your energy needs decline. The wide range of calories indicates how much people can differ in their energy requirements.

The second part of your calorie requirements can be thought of

Table 12-2
AVERAGE DAILY ENERGY NEEDS BASED ON HEIGHT AND WEIGHT

Age	Weight (in pounds)	Average Height	Energy Needs (in calories)
		MEN	
11–14	99	5'2"	2,700 (2,000–3,700)
15–18	145	5'9"	2,800 (2,100–3,900)
19–22	154	5'10"	2,900 (2,500–3,300)
23–50	154	5'10"	2,700 (2,300–3,100)
51–75	154	5'10"	2,400 (2,000–2,800)
76+	154	5'10"	2,050 (1,650–2,450)
		WOMEN	
11–14	101	5'2"	2,200 (1,500–3,000)
15–18	120	5'4"	2,100 (1,200–3,000)
19–22	120	5'4"	2,100 (1,700–2,500)
23–50	120	5'4"	2,000 (1,600–2,400)
51–75	120	5'4"	1,800 (1,400–2,200)
76+	120	5'4"	1,600 (1,200–2,000)

(For pregnancy, add 300 calories; for lactation, add 500 calories.)
Source: The National Research Council.

as those calories that provide you with the energy that you use up during exercise. The moment you stop doing absolutely nothing, your calorie requirement goes up. The more you do, the more calories you need. Unfortunately, most of us are only too happy to provide our bodies with many more calories than we need—with less than glamorous results.

Now you must consider what your energy requirements are likely to be each day. To do this properly, you should also consider how much exercise is usually part of your daily routine. Table 12-3 provides some examples of the calories used per hour during different types of activity.

These extra calories must be added to those that are needed to maintain your BMR. Thus, by estimating your ideal weight (Table 12-1), your daily energy needs at a light work level (Table 12-2), and factoring in activity above that level (Table 12-3), you should be able to establish the number of calories that you need each day to stay in energy balance and maintain your ideal weight.

Table 12–3
THE EFFECT OF ACTIVITY ON ENERGY REQUIREMENTS

CALORIES	ACTIVITIES
Women: 440 calories	Sleeping 8 hours
Men: 540 calories	
Extra calories used per hour	Various Activities
100+	Slow walking, manual typing, light housework.
200+	Heavy housework, average walking, bicycling about 5 mph, golf.
300+	Walking about 4 mph, tennis doubles, scrubbing floors, bicycling about 8 mph.
400+	Tennis singles, jogging 5 mph, basketball, horseback riding, mountain climbing.
600+	Running 6 mph, squash, handball.

Source: The National Research Council.

To help you understand this in a practical way, let us consider a day in the life of a thirty-five-year-old woman of average height (5′4″) and average weight (128 pounds). According to Table 12–2, her energy needs amount to an average of 2,000 calories daily, doing only light work. If 8 hours' sleep requires about 440 calories, the remaining 16 hours will require nearly 1,600 calories (or 100 calories per hour). However, on the day in question, this woman decides to spend 1 hour jogging (400 extra calories) and 2 hours playing tennis doubles (600 extra calories). This then adds about 1,000 calories to her daily requirements, which now amount to 3,000 calories. Of course, because of variation in basic energy requirements, some women may need more or less than this. The bathroom scale is still your best guide.

If you need to lose weight, then you should maintain the balance of your diet while reducing the total number of calories by about 25 percent below the number of calories required for you to attain your ideal weight. Only when you have achieved your ideal weight can you bring your total calorie intake back to normal—or preferably less than normal.

Table 12–4 summarizes the steps you should take to calculate your caloric needs.

Table 12–4
HOW TO CALCULATE YOUR CALORIE NEEDS

1. Determine your ideal weight based upon your height using Table 12–1. (_____ pounds)

2. Determine your basic daily calorie requirement for someone of your height using Table 12–2. (_____ basic calories)

3. Assess your level of physical activity, and how many calories are required for it, from Table 12–3. (_____ exercise calories)

4. Combine your basic calorie requirement with the number of calories estimated for your level of physical activity. (_____ total daily calories)

5. If you are overweight, reduce the total calorie allowance by 25 percent or more while maintaining the right nutritional balance. (_____ modified daily calorie needs)

6. Record your weight each week and adjust your calorie allowance accordingly. It's a good idea to plot your weight as a graph if you want to have a good idea of the trend.

Now I am sure you would welcome a few words of encouragement. Most readers will tend to maintain their ideal weight much more easily by following the Cancer Prevention Diet than their regular diet. This is because this diet emphasizes foods that are high in fiber, low in fat, and lower in calories. Furthermore, you will inevitably learn more about the nutritional structure of your diet, where the hidden calories are, and how you can restrict them every day.

PART TWO

CHAPTER 13

The Principles of Dietary Cancer Prevention

One must eat to live, and not live to eat . . .
MOLIÈRE, 1668

Diet provides the human body with the most complex mixture of chemicals to which it is exposed. Enormous changes in daily food intake have occurred in Western societies during the past two hundred years, let alone during the past few thousand years. These changes represent a drastic shift in the human diet when compared to the previous millions of years of evolution, during which the diet was relatively stable. From an historical perspective, therefore, our modern diet is one to which we have been only recently exposed and to which we are poorly adapted. The potential effects of this diet are now being further influenced by the "advances" in food technology, which expose us, either deliberately or inadvertently, to an increasing number of chemicals that might affect our health.

It is no secret that the modern American diet is mostly bad, and getting worse. Since the turn of the century, the consumption of meats, dairy products, refined sugars, and processed foods has increased tremendously, while the consumption of fresh fruit, fresh vegetables, milk, and grain products has steadily declined. This high-fat, high-sugar, high-calorie, low-fiber diet has resulted in an epidemic of degenerative diseases and cancer that have already affected or will eventually affect most of us in one way or another. These diseases are almost unknown in societies where the diet is low in fat and high in fiber, and they are increasing in countries like

Japan as some Western dietary habits are adopted. The lessons are obvious.

Most of what we choose to eat is the result of tastes acquired through prosperity, parental example, laziness, advertising, and convention. The great majority of the world's population does not eat the American way. Even in countries where enough food is available, most people have diets that are structured quite differently—fortunately for them! They are spared to a considerable extent the scourge of cancer, heart disease, and hypertension—diseases that cause so much premature illness in Western countries like the United States. Instead, they have to face the diseases of the tropics and the diseases of poverty, which have been mostly controlled in the United States.

During the past few years there has been an increasing awareness that something ought to be done to improve the American diet. Since the turn of the century, there has been a steady increase in the total fat consumption of the average American, so that fat now constitutes about 42–45 percent of his total calories. Then, more than twenty-five years ago, the American medical profession began to learn of the importance of fat in the causation of heart disease. A widespread public awareness campaign was initiated, supported by scientific data. This campaign urged Americans to cut down their dietary fat, particularly saturated fat—the kind that clogs up arteries and kills you!

The food industry reacted positively to this challenge, and began to produce high-quality margarines that helped to replace saturated fats in the diet with unsaturated ones. Many other low-fat products followed, and the public also became aware of the dangers of dietary cholesterol. With the help of sensible food labeling, shoppers were able to buy foods that were low in saturated fats and cholesterol. Probably as a result of this policy, there has been a steady decline in heart disease during the 1970s and early 1980s,. This impressive achievement in preventive medicine must now find its counterpart in reducing the incidence of cancer.

The increasing public interest in diet and nutrition is both welcome and long overdue. Hitherto, nutritional advice has frequently been the domain of self-appointed nutritionists, many of whom managed successfully to exploit the anxieties, ignorance, superstitions, and prejudices of an ill-informed public. Then, in the early

1970s, it became apparent that farm produce was contaminated with pesticides, and that meat was contaminated with hormones and antibiotics. People began to feel concerned. Could these substances be harmful, especially when consumed over a long period of time? Could the farmers or the government be trusted to give an informed or honest answer? This uncertainty and fear led to the birth of the "natural food" movement. This movement attracted a varied collection of followers from the well-informed to the neurotic. It also attracted the exploiters who quickly seized the opportunity to charge more for foods that could often be found for less at the local supermarket!

At last, in 1977, after years of government indifference, the Senate Select Committee on Nutrition and Human Needs, with George McGovern as chairman, challenged the food industry and, in effect, the medical profession. After spending much time collecting evidence, McGovern's committee concluded its investigation with the publication of new nutritional guidelines for the American people. The guidelines were designed to reduce the incidence of many fatal diseases such as cardiovascular disease, diabetes, obesity, cirrhosis of the liver, and cancers of the breast and colon. A start had been made!

Of special significance was the fact that McGovern's committee also encouraged the National Cancer Institute to initiate a thorough review of the interrelationship of diet, nutrition, and cancer. This review culminated in the publication in 1982 of the classic report of the National Academy of Sciences.

Now that you have become familiar with the evidence, you surely will not dispute the fact that we should try to prevent dietary diseases. This offers far more hope for the future than investing more and more money in the treatment of disease. This point is underscored by the fact that despite the huge increase in the cost and the technological expertise of modern medicine, the life expectancy of fifty-year-old American males has apparently increased by only nine months since 1920!

Nevertheless, the accumulation of scientific knowledge is not enough. Knowledge must be put to use, otherwise it is valueless. The philosopher Kant once said, "It is often necessary to make a decision on the basis of knowledge sufficient for action but insufficient to satisfy the intellect." This is the situation that confronts scientists today when trying to decide whether enough is known to justify a radical change in the American diet.

Probably the two most important examples of environmentally induced diseases are lung cancer [smoking] and coronary heart disease [smoking and dietary fat]. Both examples illustrate why it is difficult to make recommendations about diet and cancer with *certainty*. Let me explain why.

Firstly, although the more you smoke the more likely you are to get lung cancer, a substantial number of people who smoke heavily do not get lung cancer. The obvious question is, why not?

Secondly, although people who eat a lot of fat have an increased risk of premature heart disease, many of these people do not get it. Again, the obvious question is, why not?

Presumably the answer is a complex interplay of genetic factors (how well you were made!) and other environmental factors that remain to be identified. But in both these examples the important point to consider is the degree of risk. Think of the problem this way. If you travel at 100 miles per hour down the freeway, your chance of meeting with a fatal accident is much greater than if you travel at 55 miles per hour. Just because you manage to survive one journey at 100 miles per hour does not mean that it is a safe way to travel. It also matters little whether your risk of death at 100 miles per hour is due to a tire blowout, ice on the road, or falling asleep at the wheel. The answer is to slow down! So, without being able to predict the precise cause of any future accident, it is quite reasonable to advocate a policy of driving more slowly to minimize your risks.

It is important that any safety or health recommendation should not introduce new risks. Clearly, no one has been put at risk by being asked to drive more slowly or to give up smoking, and no one appears to have been put at risk by being urged to reduce saturated fat and cholesterol intake. On the contrary, the result of these public health policies has been a reduction in traffic fatalities, a reduction in lung cancer risk among those who stopped smoking, and a progressive reduction in heart disease during the past decade.

The relationship between diet and cancer is not quite as straightforward as between speed and traffic fatalities. Cancer can take many years to develop and can be caused by many different factors.

The association of dietary constituents with an individual's cancer risk will probably never be clear-cut. But harmless changes in our diet, based upon the knowledge we have, can be introduced with considerable benefit. Remember, as much as 60 percent of cancers in women and 40 percent of cancers in men have been attributed to dietary causes (1), and it is thought that as much as one third of cancer in the United States could be prevented by prudent changes in the nation's diet (2).

HOW TO APPROACH DIETARY CANCER PREVENTION

The first thing to do is to understand certain guiding principles that are fundamental to any cancer prevention diet.

1. You must *reduce* the consumption of foods that contain *natural carcinogens* because they may increase your cancer risk. This includes some foods that are smoked, pickled, and barbecued. Even American salt-cured foods and foods cured with liquid smoke, although safer, still contain harmful nitrates and other carcinogens.
2. You must *increase* your consumption of foods that contain *anticarcinogens* because they will reduce your cancer risk.
3. You must *avoid* foods that contain *added carcinogens or procarcinogens.* (Procarcinogens can be converted into dangerous carcinogens in the body.)
4. You must *reduce* your intake of *fat.*
5. You must learn to *restrict* your intake of *calories* so that you achieve and maintain your ideal body weight.
6. You must *increase* your intake of *fiber.*
7. You must *prepare* food in ways that help to *preserve* their vitamin and mineral content.

It must be stressed that all the changes I propose are based predominantly upon changes in diet, not the use of supplements. The evidence that the consumption of certain vegetables, for example, is associated with a lower risk of cancer is probably due to their rich vitamin or mineral content. However, this benefit could also be due to some other accompanying chemical ingredients that remain to be identified. Therefore, it is important not to *rely* on vitamin or mineral supplements. Instead, the judicious use of supplements can *reinforce* the benefits of dietary changes.

To help you to understand the fundamental changes that are needed in your diet, you can see them listed in Table 13–1.

As you can see from the table, the basic objectives are not complicated and can be met easily. After all, the basic dietary constituents are few, and the dietary goals are not designed to be met with absolute precision. A diet of this type, which must be followed for many years to be effective, cannot be too rigid—otherwise it would be ignored.

Although Table 13–1 illustrates the shift in *balance* that should be aimed at on a daily basis, the real objective is to approximate that balance over months and years. You are allowed to deviate from this diet from time to time without guilt or fear, as long as you return to the diet for your regular food guidance. Perhaps you can use one of the oldest ideas of all, and take Sunday off. At least, I think that one day each week could be allowed for social or gastronomic emergencies!

Table 13–1

CURRENT AMERICAN DIET			CANCER PREVENTION DIET	
MACRONUTRIENTS				
Amount	% Calories		% Calories	Amount
About 90 grams	12%	PROTEIN	12%	60–80 grams
		FAT		
Variable, about	16%	Saturated	7%	(65 grams
90–160 grams	19%	Mono-unsaturated	7%	is daily maximum)
	7%	Polyunsaturated	7%	
Variable	28%	CARBOHYDRATES Complex and "naturally occur-ring" sugars	57%	Increase (No gram limit)
	18%	Refined and pro-cessed sugars	10%	Reduce
10–25 grams	None	FIBER	None	40–60 grams
Too high	Too many	ALCOHOL	Reduce	Moderate

Table 13-1 (continued)

MICRONUTRIENTS

RDA		SUGGESTED
	VITAMINS	
4,000–5,000 IU	A	Dietary increase / optional supplement — 25,000 IU
60 mg	C	Dietary increase / optional supplement — 1,000 mg
10.4–13.4 IU	E	Dietary increase / optional supplement — 400 IU
	B complex	
1–1.4 mg	Thiamin	Dietary increase
1.2–1.4 mg	Riboflavin	Dietary increase
1.2–1.4 mg	Niacin	Dietary increase
2–2.2 mg	B_6	Dietary increase
400 mcg	Folacin	Dietary increase / optional supplement — 800 mcg.
3.0 mcg	B_{12}	Dietary increase
500–900 mg	Choline	No change
10 mcg	D	No change
	MINERALS	
50–200 mcg	Selenium	Dietary increase / optional supplement — 200 mcg.
18 mg	Iron	No change
0.15–0.5 mg	Molybdenum	0.5 mg
150 mcg	Iodine	No change
15 mg	Zinc	No change / optional supplement — 5 mcg.
1 mg (RDA = 2–3 mg)	Copper	3 mg
800 mg	Calcium	No change
800 mg	Phosphorus	No change
25–60 mg	Cadmium	Minimize
350 mg	Magnesium	No change
2–5 mg	Manganese	No change
10–60 mcg	Arsenic	Minimize
19–60 mcg	Lead	Minimize

NOTE: High-fiber diets may require vitamin and mineral supplements because of reduced absorption. If you are uncertain about your needs, consult your physician.

With that loophole in mind, let us now review your new "Ten Commandments."

1. *Maintain* your protein intake at 12–18 percent of total calories, or about 60–80 grams daily.
2. *Reduce* your fat intake by half so that it constitutes about 20 percent of your total calorie intake. (Total fat intake should not exceed 65 grams.)
3. *Balance* your fat intake more or less equally between saturated, monounsaturated, and polyunsaturated fats. (Avoid butter; use soft margarine or corn oil.)
4. *Increase* your consumption of complex carbohydrates and naturally occurring sugars to about 60 percent of total calories (about 70 percent by weight).
5. *Reduce* your consumption of refined and processed sugars to about 10 percent of total calories (about 10 percent by weight).
6. *Increase* your dietary intake of vitamin A (beta-carotene), vitamin B complex, vitamin C, and vitamin E, with optional reinforcement of your diet with supplements of beta-carotene, folic acid, vitamin C, and vitamin E.
7. *Increase* your selenium intake through your diet and an optional daily supplement of 200 micrograms.
8. *Increase* your fiber intake gradually to about 40–60 grams daily.
9. *Moderate* your alcohol intake to the equivalent of one glass of wine per day. Do not save up one month's allowance for one evening!
10. *Limit* your calorie intake so that you achieve and maintain your ideal weight.

These "commandments" are deliberately expressed in fairly general terms so that you are not dismayed at the thought of trying to follow them. In practice, the process of food selection, menu planning, and dietary analysis involves few important decisions and should prove quite easy.

Your new diet will develop in the way outlined in Table 13–2.

These dietary guidelines are basically consistent with those recommended by the Senate Select Subcommittee on Nutrition and Human Needs in 1977 in their report entitled "Dietary Goals for the United States" (3), those of the National Cancer Institute issued in 1979 (4), those of the American Cancer Society issued in 1984, and those of the National Academy of Sciences issued in 1982 (5). What is more, following these guidelines will automatically adjust

Table 13-2
ON THE CANCER PREVENTION DIET

- You will eat less fat.
- You will eat more fruit, especially citrus fruit.
- You will eat more vegetables, especially carotene-rich and dark-green vegetables such as carrots, cabbage, broccoli, spinach, collard greens, cauliflower, and brussels sprouts.
- You will eat more whole-grain cereals.
- You will eat less salt-cured, smoked, and pickled foods.
- You will drink alcohol in moderation or not at all.

your dietary intake of most vitamins, minerals, and fiber. All you basically need to do is to select your foods carefully, and monitor your intake of proteins, fats, carbohydrates, and calories.

The basis for reducing fat intake has been described in some detail in Chapter 4. Briefly, there is compelling evidence that several common cancers, including cancers of the breast, colon, and prostate, are all more likely to occur when the diet is high in fat. Both saturated fat and unsaturated fat appear to be responsible. Predictably, the farmers and meat industry feel threatened by such conclusions and recommendations, and sometimes try to discredit them. But since they are hardly impartial, you need not take their statements too seriously. Instead, you should know that the National Cancer Institute is about to undertake a large study to find out whether a low-fat (20 percent of calories) diet will reduce the occurrence of breast cancer in women who are at an unusually high risk. But why wait ten or fifteen years for the result? Surely, it makes more sense to act now while you have time.

It has been shown that cancer of the lung, larynx, bladder, esophagus, stomach, colon, rectum, and prostate are more common among people who eat only small amounts of fruit and vegetables, and less common among those who eat above average quantities of fruit and vegetables. Much of this benefit is attributed to the higher intake of vitamins A and C, as well as a number of specific anticarcinogens found in fruit and vegetables. Needless to say, the fruit and vegetable growers never protested when the National Academy of Sciences published dietary recommendations that extolled the virtues of increased dietary fruit and vegetables!

Increasing your intake of whole grain cereals will provide a wide variety of nutrients, including vitamin B complex, selenium, and fiber. Furthermore, by increasing your intake of whole grain cereals, you will help to exclude other foods from your diet that have a much higher fat content.

The risks of eating nitrate-containing salt-cured, smoked, and pickled foods have become apparent from studies in Japan, China, the Soviet Union, Norway, Iceland, Hungary, and the United States. These studies, like the others, were supported by extensive laboratory evidence. As someone who has been addicted to smoked salmon for years, I find this one of the most difficult temptations to overcome.

Finally, there is no escape from the evidence against alcohol, particularly when it is combined with smoking. Cancers of the mouth, larynx, esophagus, and lung have all been linked to alcohol. More specifically, heavy beer drinkers have a greater risk of colorectal cancer, and wine drinkers have a greater risk of esophageal cancer. Are you beginning to have the feeling that everything that's good is bad? If so, don't despair!

By now you should have a good understanding of the extraordinary role played by diet in the development of cancer and other diseases. And you should already have begun to develop some ideas about how your own diet will have to change. At first you will wonder how you will ever be able to know the amount of protein, carbohydrate, or fat there is in your diet—let alone all the other important ingredients. It seems impossible.

The solution is to ask yourself the nutrient value of everything you eat, and if you don't know it, look it up in the Food Tables in the Appendix. This takes time, but it is time well spent. You will gradually learn the nutrient content of all your favorite foods, and you will also learn what effect cooking has on nutrient content. Once you learn just how much extra fat there is in a fried potato compared to a boiled one, you'll never forget it!

In the cancer-prevention diet I present here, the nutrient content of all the menus and recipes is provided; later you can create your own recipes and menus. You will be able to do this with the help of the specific guidelines and the use of the Food Tables in the Appendix, which provide you with a nutritional analysis of several hundred common food items.

CHAPTER 14

Safer Food Selection and Preparation

The success of dietary cancer prevention depends to a considerable extent upon the ease with which the guiding principles are put into practice. Since food is chemically complex and our knowledge not yet complete, there is no need to be too obsessional about small deviations from the basic dietary recommendations.

If you succeed in shifting the *long-term balance* of your diet so that it *approximates* the goals of your new cancer prevention diet, then you can congratulate yourself and claim this achievement as a personal triumph. And, especially if you are a nonsmoker, you can look forward to greatly reduced chances of getting cancer and other degenerative diseases.

Let us now consider how to change your diet in a practical way. I will assume that you have decided to make a determined effort to turn over a new leaf, to make a fresh start, and to give up past sins!

Since we are now working together, there are several points which you should understand before we can proceed.

1. The most important part of your new diet is the *reduction of fat to about 20 percent of total calories.* The way that this is accomplished should provide you with the right balance of protein, carbohydrates, fiber, vitamins, and minerals. The first step is to learn which foods will give you most benefit, and which may be harmful. Common foods will therefore be listed in groups based upon their predominant characteristics.

2. Within each group there may be foods that are either high or low in some critical nutrient. By combining foods in ways that complement one another, the final dietary balance can be improved.

229

3. When foods contain both good and bad constituents, they can still be used in moderation provided that they are accompanied by other foods that contribute to the desired balance. The exception to this would be foods that are contaminated by carcinogens such as mold. Fortunately, this is so rare in the United States that we can ignore the problem.

4. When creating menus, foods should first be selected to provide you with the essential macronutrient balance (the right amount of proteins, fats, and carbohydrates). Then you should estimate the vitamin and fiber contribution. If you do this properly, the mineral intake should take care of itself.

5. When creating menus, think also in terms of doubling the amount of fruit and vegetables that you traditionally think appropriate, while increasing their variety. This will ensure that your full nutritional needs are met, while providing you with invaluable anticarcinogens.

6. A similar process is involved in creating and selecting individual recipes. For example, if some of your favorite recipes happen to include rather a lot of oil or butter or cream, you may still be able to salvage them by simply cutting down on the fat component and substituting soft corn oil margarine for butter, so that the complete meal provides only about 20 percent of calories from fat.

7. Since fruit and vegetables will contribute much more to your new diet, they should be fresh rather than processed whenever possible. This will help to minimize your exposure to preservatives and food additives such as nitrates and nitrites. However, you should remember that some other preservatives, such as BHA and BHT, may inhibit carcinogenesis, and so need not be avoided.

8. Some awareness of the consequences of food preparation is important, because cooking can influence both the availability of nutrients and the formation of mutagens or carcinogens.

THE BEST FOODS

Before preparing your meals you must know how to plan them. And this means knowing which foods to concentrate on, and which foods to avoid. Your new diet will concentrate mostly on the following foods.

1. *WHITE MEATS:* You will mostly use low-fat meats such as chicken and turkey to supply your protein needs. You see the early pilgrims had the right idea! *Always remove the fat-laden skin before you eat.*

2. *FISH:* Most fish are excellent sources of the right nutrients. Exceptions are herring, mackerel, salmon, and shellfish, which have a high fat or cholesterol content, and should consequently be eaten less frequently. Also remember that freshwater fish in many parts of the United States are polluted with high concentrations of carcinogens and should be avoided.

3. *VEGETABLES:* It is vital that you dramatically increase the variety and quantity of vegetables in your daily diet. Concentrate on dark-green and deep-yellow vegetables, which will provide you with large amounts of vitamin A, vitamin C, vitamin E, and many minerals.

   For example, you can use potatoes to provide carbohydrates, vitamin B complex, and minerals. Soybeans are also an excellent source of protein, vitamin A, vitamin B complex, and minerals such as calcium. They also contain the anticancer chemicals known as *protease inhibitors.* Carrots are of special interest because they are one of the best sources of beta-carotene, the precursor to vitamin A. As you may remember, beta-carotene is an antioxidant and one of the most powerful means for destroying those dangerous cancer-causing substances, the free radicals. Vegetables are also an excellent source of dietary fiber. It doesn't matter if you eat them raw or cooked—just eat them!

4. *FRUIT:* You must also increase the amount and variety of fruit in your diet each day. Like vegetables, fruit represents superb value both nutritionally and economically. Both fruit and vegetables are high in nutrients, low in calories, high in fiber, and low in cost.

   Fruit and vegetable juices provide most of the same nutrients but lack the fiber found in whole fruits and vegetables.

5. *CEREALS:* You will find yourself eating large amounts of whole grain cereals. These will provide you with a wonderful source of micronutrients as well as the B vitamins, vitamin E, and fiber. This is part of your switch from the refined carbohydrates to the complex carbohydrates. Typical examples of whole grain cereals are whole wheat and wheat bran, while brown rice is an excellent source of complex carbohydrates.

6. *LIVER—A SPECIAL CASE:* Liver belongs with the good foods as well as with the restricted foods. As one of the richest sources of vitamin A and the B vitamins, liver clearly has potential cancer-inhibiting properties. But there is a problem with liver. It contains far too much cholesterol and must therefore be restricted in your new diet. I suggest restricting liver to once a month. If tender calf's liver is something you dream about, you will find this advice particularly disappointing. Preparations such as pâté de foie gras are also very high in fat, so don't be deceived by a delightful disguise!

Although only a few foods should be totally banned from your diet, there are some that must be restricted because they are rich in fat, or contain carcinogens, or have been shown to increase your cancer risk in some other way.

Let's now consider what these restricted foods are, even though farmers and food producers will no doubt insist otherwise.

THE RESTRICTED FOODS

1. *HIGH-FAT FOODS:* The use of these foods should be controlled carefully. For example, both eggs and dairy products are a rich source of dangerous fat, and the yolk of one egg contains more than a full day's allowance of cholesterol, as well as other fats. Whole milk, cream, and cheese contain a lot of fat, although some low-fat varieties of cheese as well as low-fat milk and skim milk are available. However, low-fat products often still contain a lot of fat, so it is important to get used to the idea of noting the weight of fat in any product whenever possible and relating this to your daily allowance.

What this short speech implies is that you should reduce your intake of products that contain hidden fat as part of your plan to restrict your fat intake. Choose low-fat milk and cheese whenever possible, and avoid butter because of its high cholesterol and saturated fat content. Instead, try to develop a taste for soft margarine. Recently, some margarines have appeared that contain 25 percent less fat than regular margarines. These represent an obvious choice for daily use.

Whole eggs should also play a modest role in your diet. Use egg whites and discard yolks whenever possible. Remember, your objective is to limit your total fat intake to about 20 percent of total calories. One small consolation—your high-fiber diet may actually help to reduce your fat absorption.

Even "lean" meat can contain more than 60 percent "fat" calories—unfortunately! Red meats are the worst offenders, and of course the best cuts contain the most fat. You must therefore limit your intake of beef, pork, veal, lamb, and processed meats.

Foods like bacon, ham, sausages (hot dogs), and salami, for example, usually contain a high proportion of fat. Hot dogs cannot be sold under that name unless they contain a certain percentage of fat, but this should not exceed 30 percent by weight, or almost 80 percent of total calories! Interestingly, many of the meat producers, while rejecting the evidence that dietary fat is harmful, have been very busy producing low-fat ham and other meat products. Presumably, and understandably, when they have enough of these products available to sustain their profits, they will agree that low-fat foods are definitely better!

2. *SMOKED, PICKLED AND BARBECUED FOODS:* Countries like Japan, where smoked and pickled foods are popular, have a higher incidence of several types of cancer, particularly cancer of the esophagus and stomach. All the evidence suggests that traditional methods of smoking and pickling food creates some of the carcinogens responsible for these cancers. Burning wood and charcoal causes potent carcinogens, the benzopyrenes, to form on the surface of barbecued meat and fish. This process, by the way, is greatly reduced if fat is not allowed to drip onto the coals. Regrettably, exposure to smoked and pickled foods should be minimized because these foods are rich sources of carcinogens, particularly the notorious nitrites and nitrates, and the polycyclic aromatic hydrocarbons and N-nitroso-compounds.

3. *FOODS CONTAINING MUTAGENS AND CARCINOGENS:* Asking you to avoid these foods is like asking you to approve a resolution in favor of motherhood. Obviously you would vote for it. Unfortunately, given our present state of knowledge, it is not easy to avoid these foods. We are only just beginning to learn which foods actually contain mutagens, carcinogens, and anticarcinogens, and our knowledge is far from complete. Nevertheless, certain foods should be eaten infrequently. Mostly, these are processed foods containing chemical additives whose long-term effects are unknown. But a specific reason to avoid the processed meats is the fact that they are a prime source of nitrites and nitrates. These chemicals are usually present in pickled (salt-cured) and smoked foods. Some of the better, more socially responsible manufacturers now produce processed foods that contain added ascorbic acid (vitamin C) alongside the nitrates and nitrites. This simple step can help to prevent the conversion of nitrates and nitrites to cancer-causing nitrosamines. However, the danger list can also include natural foods like mushrooms, which contain potentially dangerous mutagens.

4. *ALCOHOL:* You should limit your consumption of alcohol, particularly if you are a smoker. Of course, if you are already a committed smoker, you may not be the sort of person who cares about taking steps to reduce your cancer risk. Nonetheless, I'd like to encourage you anyway.

Now that you have an idea of where your new diet is leading you, the next step is to learn about the most common foods that are available, and which nutrients these foods will provide. These tables, however, do not constitute an endorsement of all foods listed.

Now that you have familiarized yourself with Tables 14–1 and 14–2, you know the types of foods that can provide you with ex-

Table 14–1
SOME RICH SOURCES OF MACRONUTRIENTS

Proteins	Fats	Carbohydrates
Fish	Butter	Whole grains
Poultry	Margarine	Whole wheat
Vegetables	Oils	Cereals
Red meats	Whole milk	Fruit
Pork	Nuts	Vegetables
Veal	Seeds	Nuts
Cheese	Red meats	Honey
Whole grains	Bacon/ham	Sugar
Soybeans	Cheese	Rice

Table 14–2
SOME RICH SOURCES OF VITAMINS

Vitamin A	Vitamin B Complex	Vitamin C
Liver	Whole grains	Oranges
Fish	Fish	Lemons
Broccoli	Liver	Broccoli
Brussels sprouts	Brown rice	Tomatoes
Spinach	Peas	Green peppers
Lettuce	Yeast	Acerola cherries
Apricots	Legumes	Grapefruit
Peaches		Strawberries
Carrots	**Vitamin E**	Liver
Asparagus	Fish	Asparagus
Soybeans	Peanuts	Spinach
Turnips	Almonds	Turnips
Hot red chilies	Wheat germ	Hot red chilies
Dandelion greens	Walnuts	Currants
Kale	Olive oil	Parsley
Parsley	Margarine	Collard greens
Sweet potato	Soybean oil	Brussels sprouts
Pumpkin	Raw cabbage	Cauliflower
Greens		

cessive fat, necessary protein, an abundance of carbohydrates, and good sources of critical vitamins.

The next step is to learn which foods provide you with minerals and fiber. In order to keep your diet program as simple as possible, only the more important minerals will be considered in Table 14–3.

Fortunately, most of your mineral requirements will be met easily by your new diet because of the relatively high amount of fruit, vegetables, and cereals.

But foods provide more than nutrients; some provide fiber too. Although there is an excellent guide to dietary fiber in Chapter 7, Table 14–4 will remind you of some of the best sources of fiber. You can then relate these foods to those that supply macronutrients and micronutrients.

Don't try to memorize these tables all at once! After you have

Table 14–3
SOME RICH SOURCES OF SELECTED MINERALS

Selenium	Zinc	Iron	Calcium	Copper	Molybdenum
Wheat germ	Wheat germ	Liver	Milk	Liver	Liver
Rice	Liver	Poultry	Cheese	Nuts	Milk
Eggs	Soybeans	Meat	Legumes	Raisins	Whole grains
Shellfish	Seeds	Fish	Shellfish	Legumes	Spinach
Flounder	Eggs	Soybeans	Spinach	Applesauce	
Sole	Shellfish	Spinach	Broccoli	Tea	

Table 14–4
SOME SOURCES OF DIETARY FIBER

Cereals	Fruit	Vegetables	Nuts
All-Bran	Apples	Beans	Almonds
Wheat bran	Blackberries	Broccoli	Brazil nuts
Whole wheat	Black currants	Brussels sprouts	Peanuts
Oat bran	Cranberries	Cabbage	Walnuts
Graham crackers	Pears	Carrots	Pecans
Corn bran	Peaches	Potatoes	
Rye	Raspberries	Peas	
Cracked wheat	Raisins	Eggplant	
Rolled oats	Apricots	Lentils	
Pumpernickel	Prunes	Spinach	
Grapenuts		Brown rice	

completed your three-week introductory course, you will learn what components of your cancer prevention diet are provided by each different food without having to tax your memory even a little. It will have become second nature to you.

Learning about the desirable and restricted food groups is not all that I want you to know. I want you automatically to ask yourself certain specific questions before you buy food, plan menus and recipes, or eat out. The specific questions that you should train yourself to ask are:

1. Does the food primarily belong to the cereal, fruit, vegetable, fish, meat, dairy, fat, or sugar group?
2. How much fat does this food contain? (Multiply weight of fat in grams by 9 to determine "fat" calories.)
3. How much fat is saturated? How much is unsaturated? (Ideally, the ratio of saturated to unsaturated fat should be 1:2.)
4. How much cholesterol is present?
5. How much protein and carbohydrate are present? (Multiply weight in grams of protein and carbohydrate by 4 to determine protein and carbohydrate calories, respectively.)
6. What are the main vitamins that this food will provide?
7. What is the approximate total calorie content?
8. Does this food contain additives such as nitrates or nitrites?
9. How has the food been prepared? Has it been barbecued, fried, pickled, or smoked?
10. Approximately how much fiber will this food provide?

Food labels may be very helpful, but they seldom provide all the answers. If you are in doubt, write to the manufacturer and request a detailed analysis of the food product. This is particularly useful if it happens to be something that you eat frequently.

The need to restrict your fat intake and to increase your dietary fiber will inevitably dictate the kind of foods that you must choose. Relatively large amounts of fruit, vegetables, and whole grain cereals are essential to meet your fiber requirements; simultaneously, they will provide you with fewer calories and most of your vitamins and minerals. Furthermore, the more you use these low-fat food groups, the easier it will be for you to control your weight and your fat intake—the key to your new diet.

Nevertheless, fat does creep insidiously into your diet. It is found hidden in all sorts of places. Most of the sauces used with vegetables tend to contain cream or oil, and fruit is often served with whipped cream, cakes, or pastry. Breakfast cereals are served with milk, and bread inevitably is spread with butter or margarine. Cooking methods such as frying can make a real difference, contributing "fat" calories in abundance. So the best thing to do first is to examine your own dietary habits for evidence of excessive fat intake. This will greatly help you when you start to plan your cancer prevention diet. Some of the commonest sources of dietary fat are listed in Table 14–5. *The fat content of each food item is expressed as the percentage of total calorie content, not as percentage by weight.*

Although you may be astonished at the percentage of "fat" calories that exist in some of your favorite foods, it is also evident that there is considerable variation, even within food groups such as fish. Low-fat fish and chicken provide you with two of the easiest ways to eat animal protein without boosting your fat intake. This does not mean that you cannot eat other meats that contain more fat, it is just that you will have to eat much less of them if you are to keep within the planned daily fat intake of about 20 percent of total calories.

In practice, you can expect your typical dinner plate to contain less meat, more pasta, and more vegetables, because pasta and vegetables contain very little fat. In this way you can compensate for small amounts of high-fat meat with large amounts of low-fat vegetables. Furthermore, this move away from fat can be greatly reinforced by ending lunch and dinner with fresh fruit instead of cream cakes or chocolate mousse!

To achieve a balanced low-fat diet you should therefore substantially increase your consumption of vegetables, fruit, cereals, and selected meats and fish, using those listed in Table 14–6 as a guide.

Apart from desirable foods that are either low in fat or high in fiber, there are also a variety of foods that contain natural carcinogens. Although only some have been identified, the short list of foods in Table 14–7 below will give you some idea of how common foods may expose us to small amounts of powerful carcinogens. No doubt many more natural carcinogens will be identified in the future, and so it is really premature to contemplate banning such foods from your diet. However, it is probably reasonable to reduce the frequency of these foods in your menu planning.

When making food choices you will need to develop a quick way

Table 14-5
SOME COMMON SOURCES OF DIETARY FAT

Meats	Fat (% Calories)	Fish	Fat (% Calories)
Pâté de fois gras	85	Fishcakes (fried)	60
Bologna	81	Mackerel	57
Frankfurters	80	Salmon (Atlantic)	55
Bacon strips	76	Trout	53
Liverwurst	75	Caviar	51
Ground beef	64	Sardines	49
Bacon (Canadian)	57	Bluefish (fried)	43
Pork (lean)	52	Halibut (broiled)	37
Veal	51	Tuna	37
Lean ground beef	46	Flounder	36
Liver (fried)	45	Salmon (baked)	36
Duck	44	Haddock (fried)	35
T-bone steak	42	Swordfish	31
Chuck (lean)	40	Bluefish (baked)	29
Chicken leg (fried)	39	Cod (broiled)	28
Pheasant	37	Salmon (pink)	28
Lamb leg (roasted)	36	Rockfish (steamed)	21
Sirloin	33	Perch	12
Chicken (dark meat)	32	Lobster	11
Liver	30	Northern pike	11
Chicken breast (fried)	37	Halibut	10
		Red snapper	9
Turkey (light meat)	20	Pollock	8
Chicken (light meat)	18	Shrimp	8
		Haddock	1

DAIRY PRODUCTS		MISCELLANEOUS	
Camembert	74	Butter/margarine	100
Roquefort	74	Avocado	88
Cheddar cheese	73	Almonds	82
Egg (fried)	71	Peanuts	76
Omlette (1 egg)	67	Peanut butter	76
Egg (boiled or poached)	63	Ice cream	49
		French Fries	43
Parmesan	59	Apple pie	39
Whole milk (3.5% fat)	48	Soybeans	39
		Popcorn	10
Cottage cheese	36	Spaghetti	1
Yogurt (whole milk)	35	Baked potato	1
Low-fat milk (2% fat)	30		
Yogurt (low-fat)	17		

Data derived from "Composition of Foods," *USDA Agricultural Handbook, No. 8.*

Table 14-6

A SELECTION OF FOODS CONTAINING LESS THAN 10% "FAT" CALORIES

VEGETABLES

Asparagus	Califlower	Lentils	Pumpkin
Beans (green)	Celery	Lettuce	Radishes
Beans	Collard greens	Okra	Rhubarb
(lima, navy, pinto)	Corn (sweet)	Onions	Sauerkraut
Beets	Corn grits	Papaws	Spinach
Broad beans	Cornmeal	Peas	Squash
Broccoli	Cowpeas	Peppers	Tomatoes
Brussels sprouts	Cucumbers	Pimientos	Turnips
Cabbage	Kale	Potatoes	Vegetable
Carrots			juice

FRUIT

Acerola cherries	Cherries	Honeydew	Pineapple
Apples	Cranberries	Lemons	Plums
Apricots	Currants	Limes	Prunes
Bananas	Figs	Loganberries	Raisins
Blackberries	Fruit salad	Oranges	Raspberries
Blueberries	Grapefruit	Peaches	Strawberries
Boysenberries	Grapes	Pears	Tangerines
Cantaloupe	Guavas	Persimmons	Water-
			melon

CEREALS

Barley	Bread	Oats	Rye
Bran	Bulgur	Popcorn (plain)	Pasta
Bran flakes	Egg noodles	Rice	Whole
			wheat

FISH AND MEAT (LESS THAN 20% "FAT" CALORIES)

Bass	Haddock	Perch	Rockfish
Cod	Halibut	Pike	Shrimp
Crab	Lobster	Pollock	Skate
Chicken	Octopus	Red snapper	Turkey

of categorizing each food item. This must also include a quick way of judging the size of an average serving. Many food labels give the weights of protein, fat, and carbohydrate in grams, which is helpful when estimating calorie content but which is of little use to most of us when judging standard portions.

Nevertheless, certain weights and measures are familiar to you and it might help to remind you of how they relate to each other.

Table 14–8 provides you with an accurate weight exchange, and an aproximate guide to volume exchanges. In the kitchen, you can use accurate scales and measuring flasks. The dietary analyses of recipes and menus that you use regularly can be recorded so that you do not have to repeat the calculations each time. Other rough equivalents which may also be helpful to you are presented in Table 14–9.

FOOD PREPARATION

Although the judicious use of these tables should help you to make sensible food choices, buying the right food and planning the right menus is not everything. Food preparation can have profound effects on the nutrient density (the ratio of calories to nutrients). This is well illustrated by some examples that I slipped surreptitiously into Table 14–5. You may have wondered why I included a baked potato, which has only 1 percent "fat" calories, in a table designed to show you which foods are high in fat. Well, it was to highlight the dramatic difference that frying can make to calorie content. In this case, frying increases the percentage of "fat" calories from 1 percent to 43 percent!

This principle applies to all sorts of food preparation in which fats might be added to the final result. Rich gourmet sauces are notorious for their high fat content, and there is little virtue in choosing a low-fat food only to convert it into a high-fat one through the addition of a wickedly delicious sauce! Pasta is particularly susceptible to this dietary decadence.

Apart from adding fat to your food on the sly, there is also the need to preserve the vitamins and minerals that can sometimes be lost in cooking and storage. When purchasing foods such as fruit and vegetables, try to obtain fresh produce. Whenever possible try

Table 14-7
SOME FOODS CONTAINING NATURAL CARCINOGENS

Black pepper	Mushrooms	Celery	Parsnips
Figs	Parsley	Sassafras oil	Bergamot oil
Moldy food	Trout	Lettuce	Herb teas
Coffee	Tea	Cocoa powder	Mustard seed
Fava beans	Mustard oil	Horseradish	Alfalfa sprouts
Cottonseed oil	Kapok oil	Okra oil	Honey

Table 14-8
WEIGHTS AND MEASURES

Weights	Volume Measurements
1,000 milligrams [mg] = 1 gram (g)	1 cup = ½ pint
1 ounce = 28.35 grams	2 cups = 1 pint
3.57 ounces = 100 grams	4 cups = 1 quart
¼ pound = 113 grams	1 cup = 8 fluid ounces
½ pound = 227 grams	1 fluid ounce = 2 tablespoons
1 pound = 453 grams	1 tablespoon = 3 teaspoons
1 pound = 16 ounces	1 tablespoon = ½ fluid ounce
	1 glass = about 6 ounces

Table 14-9
ROUGH EQUIVALENTS

1 fluid ounce	=	28 grams
1 cup — cooking oil	=	200 grams
— water	=	220 grams
— milk	=	240 grams
— cereal	=	50 grams
— flour	=	100 grams
— sugar	=	200 grams
1 tablespoon — oil	=	14 grams
— milk	=	14 grams
— honey	=	20 grams
— flour	=	8 grams
— sugar	=	12 grams
½ tablespoon	=	1 pat butter
1 teaspoonful (oil)	=	5 grams

to select naturally ripened fruit and vegetables. Storage of fresh fruit and vegetables in a refrigerator for more than a few days can lead to significant losses of vitamins, so be careful not to store food for long periods.

Since vitamins such as the B complex and C are water-soluble and sensitive to high temperatures, canned foods have usually lost most of these vitamins. Frozen foods are better preserved and are much preferred if you cannot find the fresh variety. During the freezing process, foods are partially cooked first, which causes some loss of vitamin C and thiamin (vitamin B_1). But this process prevents further losses of many other vitamins that would otherwise occur.

Prolonged storage, even of frozen foods, eventually leads to losses of vitamins. But then there is often a delay between the picking of fresh produce and its subsequent arrival in your kitchen, and this also results in vitamin losses. So unless your vegetables are really fresh, you may in fact find more vitamins in frozen vegetables. Frozen orange juice, however, does retain its vitamin C even when reconstituted, and can be stored for several days. This is good to know because it is such an excellent natural source of vitamin C, and a perfect supplement to the whole citrus fruits that are an essential part of your diet.

COOKING

Cooking food brings with it two important problems that cannot be ignored, although they are not easily solved. The first problem has to do with the *preservation of vitamins* during cooking. The second problem—the formation of mutagens during the *browning reaction* resulting from the effect of heat on proteins and sugars—has already been alluded to in Chapter 9. Since the benefits of cooking far outweigh the known risks of these mutagens, these problems should not be exaggerated.

Vegetables

There is a widespread belief that raw vegetables are more nutritious than cooked ones. Intuitively, raw vegetables appeal to many people because they seem closer to nature. Although cooking undoubtedly can alter the chemical and structural nature of food, our information is mostly limited to the effect of cooking on vitamin content. But, in the context of cancer prevention, very little is known about the effect of cooking on other natural anticarcinogens. In our present state of knowledge, the important point is that you should eat more vegetables—either cooked or uncooked.

The storage and preparation of vegetables can greatly influence their vitamin content. Here are some tips for saving your vital vitamins:

1. Do not soak vegetables in water. This is one way to encourage the loss of water-soluble vitamins such as the B complex and C.
2. Cooking pots should be made of aluminum or stainless steel rather than copper or iron. An improperly lined copper pot can destroy vitamins C, E, and folacin. Iron pots can also destroy vitamin C, and they increase the iron content of your food too.
3. Pressure cooking, though not widely used, actually preserves vitamins best. But this method of cooking must be done with care to avoid any risk of injury.
4. Steaming is almost as good as pressure cooking, and is definitely safer. But steaming can cause the loss of some vitamins such as B_1, B_2, C, and folacin. When steaming vegetables, undercook them slightly.
5. Boiling causes greater vitamin losses, particularly of vitamin C. Nevertheless, you can limit vitamin destruction by boiling vegetables in small amounts of water until only just done. In the case of rice, avoid washing the rice before boiling if you want to limit the loss of B vitamins. In the case of potatoes, baking in the skin is by far the best method. Finally, all these methods are superior to frying because they avoid the addition of fat.
6. Storing cooked food in the refrigerator for subsequent reheating should be avoided if possible, because both storage and reheating encourage further vitamin loss.

Meats, Fish, and Poultry

Meat, and to a much lesser extent fish and poultry, are major sources of fat in your diet. This is not only because some meats tend to have a naturally high fat content, but also because the way they are cooked can really influence the final amount of fat that they contribute. After all, what's the use of choosing a low-fat food if you cook it in a way that greatly increases its fat content? And if you've recklessly chosen a high-fat food, why make matters worse? Therefore choose the way you cook carefully, and think about the effect that cooking has on your diet.

1. *Frying:* Avoid frying whenever there is an alternative. Some mutagens and carcinogens are formed by frying, particularly at higher temperatures. As you are now well aware, frying, especially deep frying, also adds calories. Whenever possible, frying should be done with as little fat as possible, and at lower temperatures (below 300° Fahrenheit).

   Avoid cooking with oils that are rich in saturated fats. Olive oil contains mostly monounsaturated fats, and is rather less good than vegetable oils such as corn, cottonseed, sunflower, safflower, and soybean oil that are rich in polyunsaturated fats. Polyunsaturated fats are the type that lower blood cholesterol and so reduce the risk of coronary heart disease.

2. *Roasting:* This method is better than frying, but roasting usually means that you baste the meat with fat, which makes this method less desirable. It is a good idea to make sure that as much fat as possible drains away, so place the roast on a rack that allows fat to collect in a pan beneath.

3. *Baking:* This method of cooking is better than roasting or frying because it does not contribute any fat to your meal. Nor is it as likely to contribute carcinogens produced directly by the cooking process itself. This method is particularly suitable for poultry and fish dishes.

4. *Broiling:* To a greater extent than either roasting or baking, this cooking technique has the disadvantage of exposing food surfaces to intense heat that usually produces the browning reaction. It does not matter whether the heat source is above or below, the result is just the same. If you wish to broil food, keep the temperature setting below 300° Fahrenheit.

5. *Barbecuing* As you now know, the smoke and flames from the barbecue pit are an excellent way to make your own carcinogens. If you must barbecue, one way to limit this effect is to reduce the exposure of the meat or fish to the smoke and flames. This is easily done by increasing the distance of the food from the coals, and by wrapping the food in aluminum foil or by placing it in a pan. In the case of chicken or fish, it is a good idea to remove the skin on which the carcinogens form when cooking is completed. Lean meats are also preferred because there is less fat to drip onto the fire. Burning fat always produces more smoke and flames, which in turn produce more carcinogens.

6. *Microwave Cooking:* Well, it is nice to know that some things have no relationship to cancer—at least not yet! So far, there is no evidence that microwave cooking leads to the formation of carcinogens. The only caution should be in the use of the browning plate, which of course could cause the formation of carcinogens and mutagens.

By now you should have an excellent understanding of the basic principles of the Cancer Prevention Diet. This will help you to proceed to the detailed structure of the diet which is presented in the next chapter. Planned menus are provided that form the basis of a three-week introductory training program. This training program will provide you with the understanding of nutrition that is essential for a healthy life.

Later, for the more adventurous, or for those with more time, there are easy instructions for planning your own individualized diet program.

CHAPTER 15

The Cancer Prevention Diet: A National Goal

- Reduce fat to 20% of calories
- Increase fruit
- Increase fiber
- Increase vegetables
- Increase whole grain cereals
- Maintain ideal weight
  - Avoid barbecued, salt-cured, and smoked foods

You have now reached the stage when you are ready to begin your diet program. Think of it primarily as a nutrition education program. For it to succeed, you must find your diet easy to understand and easy to follow. Every effort will therefore be made to help you make the transition from your present diet to your new one.

The most fundamental change in your diet will be *fat reduction.* Although a low-fat diet can still be a real pleasure, it may take a while before you feel accustomed to it. Probably your greatest difficulty will be to resist delectable high-fat foods, lovingly prepared by friends who remain ignorant. The only solution to this problem is to educate them—tactfully! Eating out in restaurants will also present some problems until you learn how to choose from a menu sensibly (and until restaurant owners learn that they have a responsibility for the nation's health).

In practice, your new diet program will develop in two stages. The first stage will introduce you to the *ten food groups,* and will explain how they are used to develop menus of the right dietary balance.

The second stage will introduce you to a three-week course of introductory menus that will lower your fat intake to 20 percent o calories. These menus will show you the style of diet that will be yours for life! The five introductory menus are designed to be very simple and completely flexible. Any breakfast can be combined with any lunch, and any lunch can be combined with any dinner. Using this system, you have the power to create 125 different daily meal combinations! Each one of these meal combinations will provide you with the right daily dietary balance and about 2,000 calories. If you need to modify the calorie intake, you will be shown how to do this without significantly changing the vital dietary balance. The impact on the introductory menus of the addition or subtraction of one or two servings from each food group is shown later in this chapter in Tables 15–5 and 15–6.

THE TEN FOOD GROUPS

These food groups are designed to make it easier for you to understand and control the nutrients in your diet. Each of the ten groups supply certain vital nutrients. This means that each group will contribute a different balance of protein, fat, carbohydrate, fiber, vitamins, and minerals to your diet. However *within each group,* foods can be exchanged or traded, using the standardized amounts.

These standardized amounts of food within each group can be thought of as *servings*. Personalized menus can then be created using a certain number of servings from some, or all, of the ten food groups.

Although the most important foods that you need are listed in these food groups in **boldface** type, there may be some that you would like to add yourself. These can be added after you have analyzed them for nutrient content, using the food nutrition tables in the Appendix. The nutrient analysis will enable you to decide not only the group to which the food belongs, but also the amount that is equivalent to one serving within the selected food group.

If variety is the spice of life, it is also a nutritional virtue! However, there are some obligations. *Your daily menus should contain at least three food servings from the vegetable group (Group 7); two from the fruit group (Group 3); two from the cereal group (Group 1); and one from the bread group (Group 2).* These are the food groups that provide the least fat, the most fiber, and the most cancer protection. One more daily obligation remains, and that is to select at least *one serving of meat, fish, or poultry from either Group 5 or 6.* This will provide you with the complete protein that you need for proper general nutrition.

Before you see the introductory menus, you must take a good look at the ten food groups. This will help you to make sense of the introductory menus because it will help you to understand how the menus were created from the food groups.

You will notice that within each food group, the serving size of the selected foods has been adjusted so that it *approximates the average nutrient value* of the group. This means that you can choose any food within a food group and know the calorie content and nutrient value without having to calculate it.

Once you have familiarized yourself with the way the food groups work, I'll introduce you to an easy way to plan and record your new diet.

THE TEN FOOD GROUPS

GROUP 1   CEREALS, RICE, AND PASTA
One serving averages: 200 calories

6 grams of protein
44 grams of carbohydrate
1 gram of fat
6 grams of fiber
10 grams of fiber (cereals only)

vitamin A   900 IU
vitamin C   6 mg
cholesterol   0 mg

CEREALS, RICE, AND PASTA GROUP (Cereals only)

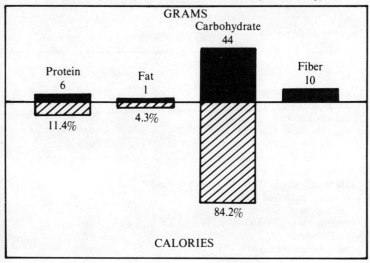

CEREALS, RICE, AND PASTA GROUP

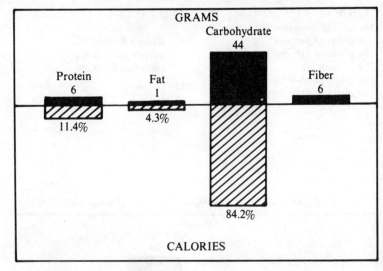

FOOD	SERVING
1. **All-Bran,* Kelloggs**	1 cup
2. **Barley,** pearled, light (uncooked)	⅓ cup
3. **Bran Flakes, 40%**	2 cups
4. **Bran Flakes, 40%, with Raisins**	1½ cups
5. Corn Flakes, plain	2 cups
6. Cornmeal, degermed, dry	½ cup
7. Grape-Nuts, Post's	1½ cups
8. **Macaroni, spaghetti, other pasta (cooked)****	1½ cups
9. **Oatmeal or Rolled Oats**	1½ cups
10. **Oats, puffed**	2 cups
11. **Popcorn (plain), popped**	7 cups
12. **Puffed wheat**	3 cups
13. **Rice, brown (cooked)****	1 cup
14. Rice, long grain (cooked)***	1 cup
15. Rice, puffed	3 cups
16. **Weetabix**	3 bars
17. **Wheat, Shredded**	2 cups
18.	
19.	
20.	

* Contains 25 grams of fiber.
** 2.5 grams of fiber.
*** 1½ grams of fiber.

GROUP 2	BREAD

One serving averages: 180 calories

6 grams of protein	vitamin A	0 IU
1.5 grams of fat	vitamin C	0 mg
35 grams of carbohydrate	cholesterol	0 mg
3.5 grams of fiber		

BREAD GROUP

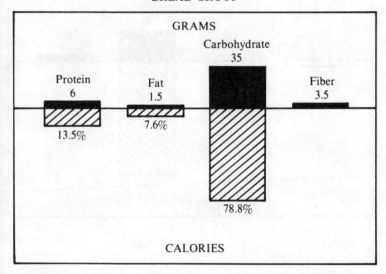

FOOD	SERVING
1. **Bagel, 3", whole wheat**	1
2. **Cracked wheat**	3 slices
3. French bread	2 slices
4. Italian bread	2 slices
5. Raisin bread	3 slices
6. **Rye bread, pumpernickel**	2 slices
7. **Whole wheat, home-baked (recipe #1)**	2 slices
8.	

GROUP 3   **FRUIT**

One serving averages: 100 calories
1 gram of protein	vitamin A 1,000 IU
0 fat	vitamin C 30 mg
25 grams of carbohydrate	cholesterol 0 mg
3.5 grams of fiber	

FRUIT GROUP

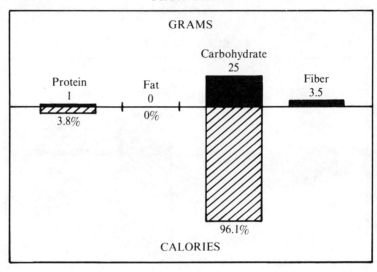

	FOOD	SERVING
1.	**Apples,** unpeeled	1
2.	Applesauce, unsweetened	1 cup
3.	**Apricots**	3
4.	Banana	1
5.	Blackberries	1 cup
6.	Blueberries	1 cup
7.	**Cantaloupe**	½
8.	Cherries	10
9.	**Grapefruit**	1
10.	Grapes, Thompson seedless	30
11.	Honeydew melon	⅕
12.	**Oranges**	2 small
13.	**Peaches**	2
14.	Pears, raw, Bartlett	1
15.	Plums, Japan	3

FOOD	*SERVING*
16. **Prunes**	½ cup
17. **Raisins,** seedless	⅓ cup
18. **Raspberries,** red	1 cup
19. Strawberries	1 cup
20. **Tangerines**	2
21. Watermelon (4″ by 8″ wedge)	1 wedge
22.	
23.	
24.	
25.	

GROUP 4   **VEGETABLES**

One serving averages: 70 calories

5 grams of protein	vitamin A 5,000 IU
0 grams of fat	vitamin C 70 mg
13 grams of carbohydrate	cholesterol 0 mg
7 grams of fiber	

VEGETABLE GROUP

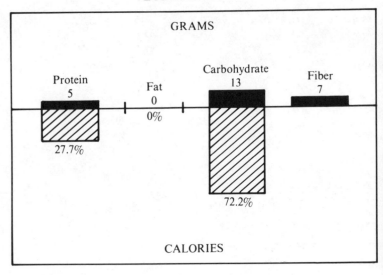

FOOD	SERVING
1. Asparagus spears	20 spears
2. **Beans, great northern**	⅓ cup
3. **Beans, green**	2 cups
4. **Beans, kidney**	⅓ cup
5. **Beans, Lima**	½ cup
6. **Beans, Navy**	⅓ cup
7. **Beans, white**	½ cup
8. **Broccoli, cooked**	1½ stalks
9. **Brussels sprouts, cooked**	1½ cups
10. **Cabbage, cooked**	2½ cups
11. **Cabbage, raw, shredded**	4 cups
12. **Carrots, whole (8" by 1")**	2
13. **Carrots, grated**	1½ cups
14. **Cauliflower, raw, chopped**	2 cups
15. **Cauliflower, cooked**	2 cups

FOOD	SERVING
16. **Collard greens, cooked**	1 cup
17. Corn, sweet, cooked	1 ear
18. **Chard, Swiss**	2 cups
19. Cucumber, with peel	84 slices
20. Endive, curly	7 cups
21. **Kale, cooked**	2 cups
22. **Lentils**	⅓ cup
23. Lettuce, Looseleaf	6 cups
24. Okra pods, 3" by ⅝"	25 pods
25. **Peas, black-eyed**	⅓ cup
26. **Peas, green**	½ cup
27. **Peas, split**	⅓ cup
28. **Potatoes, baked**	½
29. Potatoes, mashed	½ cup
30. **Soybeans, cooked**	⅓ cup
31. **Spinach, cooked**	2 cups
32. **Squash (zucchini), cooked**	2½ cups
33. **Squash, winter, baked**	1 cup
34. Tomatoes	3 small
35. Mixed salad (from your own recipe) ......?	
36.	
37.	
38.	
39.	
40.	

GROUP 5   MEAT AND FISH (High-Fat)
One serving averages: 165 calories

22 grams of protein	vitamin A 3,000 IU
7 grams of fat	vitamin C 0 mg
1 gram of carbohydrate	cholesterol 100 mg
0 fiber	

MEAT AND FISH GROUP
(high-fat)

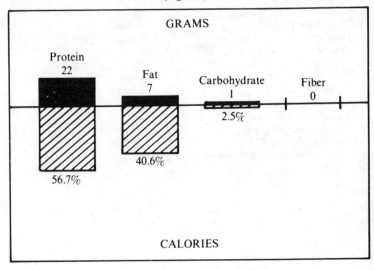

FOOD	SERVING
1. Beef, lean only	4 ounces
2. Beef, ground, broiled (10% fat)	2 ounces
3. Beef, roast, relatively lean only	4 ounces
4. Fish sticks, breaded, cooked	2 sticks
5. Haddock, breaded, fried	4 ounces
6. Ham, lightly cured	1 ounce
7. Lamb, lean only	3 ounces
8. **Liver,* calf**	3 ounces
9. Pork chop, lean	2 ounces
10. Salmon, fresh	3 ounces
11. Salmon, pink, canned	4 ounces
12. Steak, relatively fat, lean only	4 ounces
13. Steak, relatively lean, lean only	5 ounces
14.	

* Not more than once a month.

GROUP 6   POULTRY, FISH (Low-Fat)
One serving averages: 110 calories

21 grams of protein	vitamin A 10 IU
2 grams of fat	vitamin C 0 mg
0 grams of carbohydrate	cholesterol 80 mg
0 grams of fiber	

MEATS, POULTRY, AND FISH GROUP
(low-fat)

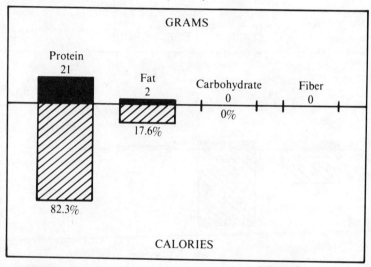

FOOD	SERVING
1. **Bass, broiled**	4 ounces
2. **Chicken, baked (without skin)**	3 ounces
3. **Cod, broiled**	4 ounces
4. **Cottage cheese (1% fat)***	¾ cup
5. Crab meat (white or king)	1 cup
6. Egg, whites only*	7 egg whites
7. **Flounder, broiled**	4 ounces
8. **Haddock, broiled**	4 ounces
9. **Halibut, broiled**	4 ounces
10. **Ocean perch, broiled**	4 ounces
11. **Red snapper, broiled**	4 ounces
12. **Shrimp**	3 ounces
13. **Sole, broiled**	4 ounces
14. **Turkey, light meat, roasted (without skin)**	3 ounces
15. Ham (low-fat)	2 slices
16.	

* Included here because of low fat content.

GROUP 7   EGGS AND CHEESE

One serving averages: 90 calories

6.5 grams of protein	vitamin A 225 IU
6.5 grams of fat	vitamin C 0 mg
1.5 grams of carbohydrate	cholesterol 100 mg
0 grams of fiber	(egg 274 mg)

EGGS AND CHEESE GROUP

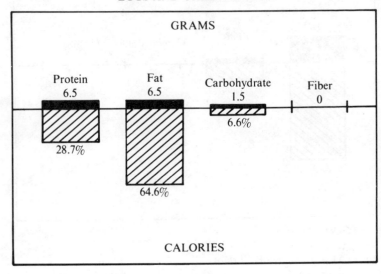

FOOD	SERVING
1. Blue cheese	1 ounce
2. Camembert	1 ounce
3. Cheddar cheese	1-inch cube
4. Egg (boiled, poached, scrambled)	1
5. Mozarella	1 ounce
6. Parmesan cheese, grated	3 tablespoons
7. Pasteurized American cheese	1 ounce
8. Swiss cheese	1 ounce
9.	

GROUP 8   **MILK**

One serving of 1% milk: 100 calories
   8 grams of protein
   3 grams of fat
   12 grams of carbohydrate
   0 grams of fiber

vitamin A   500 IU
vitamin C   0 mg
cholesterol 10 mg

MILK GROUP

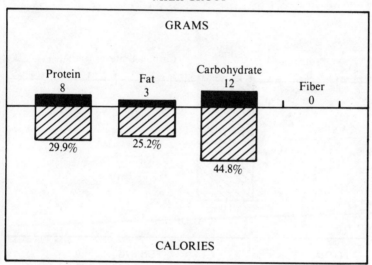

FOOD	SERVING
1. **Milk (1% fat)**	1 cup
2. Milk (2% fat)	See below
3. Milk, non-fat skim	See below
4. **Yogurt, plain (from low-fat milk)**	1 cup
5.	

Please note that the use of 1 cup of 2% low-fat milk instead of 1% low-fat milk provides your diet with an extra half of a Group 9 fat serving (2 grams of fat). If you are obliged to use 1 cup of whole milk instead of skim milk, you will add another 4.8 grams of fat—a little more than one Group 9 fat serving—to your dietary intake. In contrast, the use of one cup of non-fat skim milk saves one Group 9 fat serving.

GROUP 9   FATS AND OILS
One serving averages: 35 calories

0 grams of protein	vitamin A 45 IU
4 grams of fat	vitamin C 0 mg
0 grams of carbohydrate	cholesterol: high in butter and cream
0 grams of fiber	none in vegetable oils

FATS AND OILS GROUP

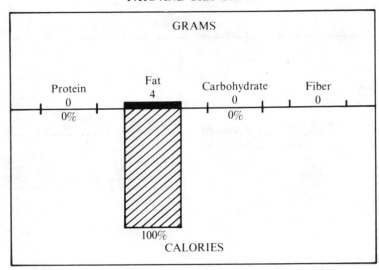

FOOD	SERVING
1. Butter	1 teaspoon
2. **Corn oil**	1 teaspoon
3. **Margarine**	1 teaspoon
4. **Margarine, soft**	1½ teaspoons
5. Mayonnaise, regular	2 teaspoons
6. **Olive oil**	1 teaspoon
7. Peanut oil	1 teaspoon
8. Safflower oil	1 teaspoon
9. Salad dressing, blue cheese	1½ teaspoons
10. Salad dressing, French	1 teaspoon
11. Salad dressing, Italian	1 teaspoon
12. Salad dressing, Thousand Islands	1½ teaspoons
13. Whipped cream topping	4 tablespoons
14. Sour cream	4 teaspoons
15. Vinaigrette (recipe #14)	1½ teaspoons
16. Heavy cream	2 teaspoons
17.	

GROUP 10   **SUGAR, PRESERVES, AND FRUIT JUICES**
One serving averages: 120 calories   cholesterol 0 mg.
  0 grams of protein   (orange juice:
  0 grams of fat   vitamin A 500 IU
  30 grams of carbohydrate   vitamin C 120 mg.)
  0 grams of fiber

SUGAR, PRESERVES, AND FRUIT JUICES GROUP

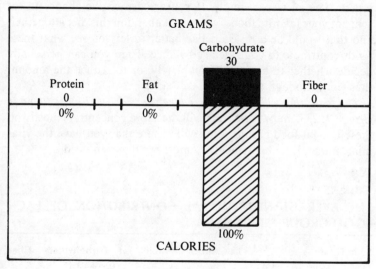

FOOD	SERVING
1. **Apple juice**	1 cup
2. **Grapefruit juice**	1 cup
3. Honey	2 tablespoons
4. Jams and preserves	2 tablespoons
5. **Lemon juice**	2 cups
6. **Orange juice**	1 cup
7. White sugar	2 tablespoons
8. Maple syrup	2 tablespoons
9.	

Now that you have read through the ten food groups, you may feel the need for a short refresher course! Table 15–1 summarizes the information in the previous charts and will make it much easier for you to compare the nutritional contribution made by each food group.

The selection of foods within these ten groups should satisfy the tastes of most people. Nonetheless, you may be puzzled by the inclusion of a high-fat meat group [Group 5] and a high-fat dairy group [Group 7] in a diet plan that is designed to restrict your fat intake. The answer is simple. If you are denied the chance to eat some of your favorite foods, you might abandon this diet altogether, and that would be a disaster. Far better to let you see what these foods contribute to your dietary balance. Then you can personally decide whether to ban them completely, or to reduce the amount that you include in your diet.

The foods that will do most to reduce your cancer risk are found in Groups 1, 2, 3, and 4. Your diet will therefore concentrate mostly on these low-fat food groups. This will ensure that you have the vitamins, minerals, anticarcinogens, and fiber that you need.

Table 15–1
THE AVERAGE NUTRITIONAL CONTRIBUTION OF EACH FOOD GROUP SERVING

Food Group	Calories	Protein	Fat	Carbohydrate	Fiber
				(IN GRAMS)	
1. Cereals, rice, pasta	200	6	1	45	6 (10)
2. Bread	180	6	1.5	35	3.5
3. Fruit	100	1	0	25	5
4. Vegetables	70	5	0	13	7
5. Meat, fish (high-fat)	165	22	7	1	0
6. Poultry, fish (low-fat)	110	21	2	0	0
7. Eggs, cheese	90	6.5	6.5	1.5	0
8. Milk (1% fat)	100	8	3	12	0
9. Fats, oils	35	0	4	0	0
10. Sugar, fruit juices	120	0	0	30	0

HOW TO PLAN A MENU USING FOOD GROUPS

Using the concept of the food groups, it is possible to plan a day's menu by combining various food groups in different proportions.

For example, if you combine food groups as shown in Table 15–2, using the number of servings listed, it is easy to find out their nutrient value from the summary in Table 15–1. You can then add up the nutrients that determine the final dietary balance.

This example of a basic menu plan must now be translated into typical meals by choosing foods from the different groups. This is easier if you make a simple list of your selections from the different groups. This is illustrated in Table 15–3. Of course, each day's menu does not have to contain precisely these choices. However, *you should include a minimum of three vegetable servings and two fruit servings in your daily menu.*

In this particular menu, the fat servings are mostly used to "lubricate" the vegetables, bread, and spaghetti. This makes these foods much more palatable. In another menu, the fat could be used in a salad dressing, a sauce, or for cooking instead.

Table 15–2
A COMBINATION OF FOOD GROUPS THAT PROVIDES ABOUT 2,000 CALORIES AND 20% OF CALORIES FROM FAT
Total fat restricted to 45 grams per day

Food Group	Servings	Calories	Protein	Fat	Carbohydrate	Fiber
			(IN GRAMS)			
1. Cereals	2	400	12	2	90	12
2. Bread	1	180	6	1.5	35	3.5
3. Fruit	3	300	1	0	75	15
4. Vegetables	3	210	15	0	39	21
5. Meat, fish	—	—	—	—	—	—
6. Poultry, fish	1	110	21	2	0	0
7. Eggs, cheese	1	90	6.5	6.5	1.5	0
8. Milk (2% fat)	1	100	8	5	12	0
9. Fats, oils	7	245	0	28	0	0
10. Sugar, juices	3	360	0	0	90	0
TOTAL:		2,030	69.5	45	342.5	51.5
Percent calories:			14%	20%	66%	

Table 15–3
A TYPICAL DAY'S FOOD GROUP SELECTION

Group	Selected Foods	Servings
1. Cereals	Spaghetti	2
2. Bread	Whole wheat bread	1
3. Fruit	Orange, cantaloupe, blueberries	3
4. Vegetables	Carrots, green beans, baked potato	3
5. Meat		
6. Poultry, fish	Chicken	1
7. Eggs, cheese	Parmesan	1
8. Milk	Milk (2% fat, for coffee)	1
9. Fats, oils	Margarine, sour cream	7
10. Sugar, juices	Orange juice, sugar, jam	3

These selected foods can now be arranged into a typical menu such as that shown below:

BREAKFAST	AMOUNT	FOOD GROUP	SERVINGS USED
Orange juice	1 cup	Sugar, juice (10)	1
Whole wheat bread	2 slices	Bread (2)	1
Soft margarine	3 teaspoons	Fats (9)	2
Preserves	2 tablespoons	Sugar (10)	1
Tea or coffee (+ milk)			

SNACK			
Orange	1	Fruit (3)	1

LUNCH			
Cantaloupe	½	Fruit (3)	1
Spaghetti	2 cups	Cereals (2)	2
Parmesan	3 tablespoons	Eggs, cheese (7)	1
Soft margarine	3 teaspoons	Fats (9)	2
Tea or coffee (+ milk)			

Table 15-3 (*continued*)

DINNER	AMOUNT	FOOD GROUP	SERVINGS USED
Chicken breast (baked, no skin)	3 ounces	Poultry, fish (6)	1
Green beans	2 cups	Vegetables (4)	1
Baked potato	½	Vegetables (4)	1
Carrots	2 large	Vegetables (4)	1
Blueberries	1 cup	Fruit (3)	1
Sugar	2 tablespoons	Sugar, juice (10)	1
Soft margarine	3 teaspoons	Fats (9)	2
Sour cream	4 teaspoons	Fats (9)	1

INTRODUCTORY MENUS

Now that you have understood how food groups are used for meal and menu planning, you are ready to begin the introductory course. This lasts for three weeks, and will provide you with the training that will enable you to follow the Cancer Prevention Diet for life.

The introductory menus presented in this chapter are designed to give you a correctly balanced, 2,000-calorie diet that is high in whole grain cereals, fruit, and vegetables, and low in fat. No food is smoked or barbecued, and none should contain carcinogenic preservatives.

A diet that is based upon defined amounts of certain food groups can still be both practical and enjoyable—and simple to plan. The nutritional balance of the breakfasts, lunches, and dinners has been designed for maximum flexibility. When any breakfast is combined with any lunch and any dinner, the fat, protein, carbohydrate, calorie, and fiber content will be virtually the same. This means that even during your three-week introductory program, you will enjoy the freedom to choose from 125 different menu combinations!

Now if you happen to love steak and are dismayed at the absence of your favorite steak dinner from the introductory menus, you could substitute steak for fish or poultry, *but the nutritional balance will change.*

Just substituting one serving of steak (or any red meat) from Group 5 (high-fat) instead of using a choice from Group 6 (low-fat), will add 5 grams of fat to your daily intake. But you could compensate for this by leaving out one slightly generous fat serving (Group 9). In the sample menu plan above, for example, you could replace the chicken breast with 5 ounces of lean steak—and forgo the whipped cream topping on your blueberries. So you see, it really is easy to tailor your diet to suit your own tastes.

For anyone who cannot eat lunch at home, following this diet will be more difficult. Probably the easiest solution is to create a rice-based dish (such as a vegetable risotto) that you can bring to work with you. Just make sure that the lunch you design has the right nutritional balance, and is comparable to those that I have suggested.

If you have to eat out at a neighborhood restaurant, life gets more complicated. Yet there is a simple solution. Salads are always popular. Even restaurants have a hard time doing much harm to a salad—as long as it's fresh! Using either the vegetable food group or the nutrition tables in the appendix, you should be able to calculate the nutritional content of your favorite salad combination. Lettuce provides more decoration than nutrients—remember, it takes 6 *cups* of lettuce to equal one vegetable serving—and a very small quantity of lettuce takes up a disproportionate amount of space on your plate. But if you add tomatoes, carrots, broccoli, green peppers, and beans, for example, and a little dressing you have the makings of an excellent light lunch. Apart from salads, select dishes that can be analyzed easily. For example, a fillet of baked fish with lemon juice is much easier to analyze than a combination of shrimps and scallops in a cream sauce. Therefore, avoid selecting dishes from restaurant menus that include heavy sauces or other sources of fat; order small portions of meat, fish, or poultry; and demand a selection of vegetables without adornment.

It is my hope that restaurants will eventually be persuaded to provide their customers with detailed nutritional information alongside each dish on the menu, which would make it much easier to follow a properly balanced diet.

Now let's look at the introductory menus and how they are planned. These menus have been created from the following combination of servings from different food groups:

Table 15-4

INTRODUCTORY MENUS—DAILY FOOD GROUP SELECTIONS

Food Groups	Breakfast	Lunch	Dinner	Total
1. Cereal	1	1		2
2. Bread	1			1
3. Fruit		1	1	2
4. Vegetables		1	3	4
5. Meat				0
6. Poultry, Fish			1	1
7. Eggs, cheese		1		1
8. Milk (1% fat)	1			1
9. Fats, oils	2	2	4	8
10. Sugar, juices	3			3

Daily Intake:	Calories	Protein	Fat	Carbohydrate	Fiber
		(PERCENT OF CALORIES)			(GRAMS)
Diet Analysis:	2,000	15	20	65	57
Dietary Goal:	2,000 +/−	12–18	20	65	50–60

Note: Calorie total is 2,000 based upon food group averages; however, the actual menus average 2,045 calories per day when analyzed using more precise computerized food tables.

If you need 2,000 calories a day, this diet plan will provide you with an excellent balance of cancer-inhibiting nutrients and fiber. Later you will learn how easily you can increase or decrease your calorie intake according to your needs.

As you can see, the introduction to your diet program has been deliberately designed for gastronomic simplicity. More exotic recipes will come later!

Now, let's look at the actual menus so that you can see just what you're in for!

Now that you have seen how straightforward the Cancer Prevention Diet Program can be, you should feel greatly encouraged to make the small investment of time and effort required to learn the dietary habits that could preserve your health. This is equivalent to a small financial investment turning you into a millionaire! And who would turn down that kind of investment opportunity?

As you follow the introductory menus, remember that lunches and dinners can either be prepared as simple meals, or can be given

YOUR FIRST BREAKFAST MENUS

EACH MENU USES:
    1 SERVING.....GROUP 1 (CEREALS)
    1 SERVING.....GROUP 2 (BREAD)
    1 SERVING.....GROUP 8 (MILK, 1% fat)
    2 SERVINGS....GROUP 9 (FATS)
    3 SERVINGS....GROUP 10 (SUGAR)

	Food Selected	Serving Size	Food Group	Servings
BREAKFAST 1	Orange juice	1 cup	Sugar	1
	40% Bran Flakes	2 cups	Cereals	1
	Milk (1% fat)	1 cup	Milk	1
	Sugar	1 tablespoon	Sugar	½
	Whole wheat bread	2 slices	Bread	1
	Soft margaine	3 teaspoons	Fats	2
	Jam or preserves	3 tablespoons	Sugar	1½
	Tea or coffee			
BREAKFAST 2	Orange juice	1 cup	Sugar	1
	Weetabix	3 biscuits	Cereals	1
	Milk (1% fat)	1 cup	Milk	1
	Sugar	2 tablespoons	Sugar	1
	Whole wheat bread	2 slices	Bread	1
	Soft margarine	3 teaspoons	Fats	2
	Jam or preserves	2 tablespoons	Sugar	1
	Tea or Coffee			
BREAKFAST 3	Grapefruit juice	1 cup	Sugar	1
	Shredded Wheat	2 cups	Cereals	1
	Milk (1% fat)	1 cup	Milk	1
	Sugar	1 tablespoon	Sugar	½
	Whole wheat bagel	1	Bread	1
	Soft margarine	3 teaspoons	Fats	2
	Jam or preserves	3 tablespoons	Sugar	1½
	Tea or coffee			
BREAKFAST 4	Orange juice	1 cup	Sugar	1
	Oatmeal	1½ cups	Cereals	1
	Milk (1% fat)	1 cup	Milk	1
	Sugar	1 tablespoon	Sugar	½
	Whole wheat pancakes	2	Cereals	1

	Food Selected	Serving Size	Food Group	Servings
	Soft margarine	3 teaspoons	Fats	2
	Maple Syrup	3 tablespoons	Sugar	1½
	Tea or coffee			
BREAKFAST 5	Grapefruit juice	1 cup	Sugar	1
	Raisin bran	1½ cups	Cereals	1
	Milk (1% fat)	1 cup	Milk	1
	Sugar	1 tablespoon	Sugar	½
	Raisin bread	2 slices	Cereals	1
	Soft margarine	3 teaspoons	Fats	2
	Honey	3 tablespoons	Sugar	1½

(If you wish, you can transfer any breakfast item to lunch or dinner.)

YOUR FIRST LUNCH MENUS

EACH MENU USES:
     1 SERVING....GROUP 1 (CEREALS)
     1 SERVING....GROUP 3 (FRUIT)
     1 SERVING....GROUP 4 (VEGETABLES)
     1 SERVING....GROUP 7 (EGGS, CHEESE)
     2 SERVINGS...GROUP 9 (FATS)

	Food Selected	Serving Size	Food Group	Servings
LUNCH 1	Carrots (grated)	1½ cups	Vegetables	1
	Vinaigrette	2 tablespoons	Fats	1
	Macaroni	1½ cups (cooked)	Cereals	1
	Swiss cheese	1 ounce grated	Egg, cheese	1
	Soft margarine	3 teaspoons	Fats	2
	Orange	1 average	Fruit	1
LUNCH 2	Brown rice	1 cup (cooked)	Cereals	1
	Beans	½ cup	Vegetables	1
	Poached egg (mixed with rice & beans)	1	Egg, cheese	1
	Soft margarine	3 teaspoons	Fats	2
	Apple	1 average	Fruit	1

	Food Selected	Serving Size	Food Group	Servings
LUNCH 3	Spaghetti	1½ cups (cooked)	Cereals	1
	Tomatoes (small)	3	Vegetables	1
	Basil	to taste		
	Garlic	1 clove		
	Olive oil	2 teaspoons	Fats	2
	Swiss cheese	1 ounce grated	Egg, cheese	1
	Orange	1 average	Fruit	1
LUNCH 4	Tomatoes	2 large	Vegetables	1
	Brown rice	1 cup (cooked)	Cereals	1
	Egg, hard boiled	1	Egg, cheese	1
	Corn or olive oil	2 teaspoons	Fats	2
	Choice of fruit	1 serving	Fruit	1
LUNCH 5	Pasta	1 cup (cooked)	Cereals	1
	Egg (beaten and poured over the hot pasta)	1 raw	Egg, cheese	1
	Nutmeg	1 pinch		
	Peas (green)	½ cup	Vegetables	1
	Soft margarine	3 teaspoons	Fats	2
	Orange	1 average	Fruit	1

(If you wish, you can transfer any lunch item to breakfast or dinner.)

YOUR FIRST DINNER MENUS

EACH MENU USES:
      1 SERVING....GROUP 3 (FRUIT)
      3 SERVINGS...GROUP 4 (VEGETABLES)
      1 SERVING....GROUP 6 (POULTRY, FISH)
      4 SERVINGS...GROUP 9 (FATS)

	Food Selected	Serving Size	Food Group	Servings
DINNER 1	Chicken, baked	3 ounces	Poultry, fish	1
	Broccoli	1½ stalks	Vegetables	1

	Food Selected	Serving Size	Food Group	Servings
	Potato, baked	1 whole	Vegetables	2
	Soft margarine	6 teaspoons	Fats	4
	Choice of fruit	1 serving	Fruit	1
	Beverage (watch out for calories!)			
DINNER 2	Corn	1 ear	Vegetables	1
	Sole, broiled	4 ounces	Poultry, fish	1
	Spinach	2 cups	Vegetables	1
	Carrots	2	Vegetables	1
	Soft margarine	6 teaspoons	Fats	4
	Beverage (watch out for calories!)			
DINNER 3	Turkey, baked	3 ounces	Poultry, fish	1
	Zucchini	2½ cups	Vegetables	1
	Brussels sprouts	1½ cups	Vegetables	1
	Potatoes, mashed	½ cup	Vegetables	1
	Soft margarine	6 teaspoons	Fats	4
	Choice of fruit	1 serving	Fruit	1
	Beverage (watch out for calories!)			
DINNER 4	Lentil soup	⅓ cup lentils	Vegetables	1
	Flounder, broiled	4 ounces	Poultry, fish	1
	Green beans	2 cups	Vegetables	1
	Cauliflower	2 cups	Vegetables	1
	Butter	4 teaspoons	Fats	4
	Choice of fruit	1 serving	Fruit	1
	Beverage (watch out for calories!)			
DINNER 5	Asparagus tips	10	Vegetables	½
	Cornish hen, baked	3 ounces	Poultry, fish	1
	Broccoli	1½ stalks	Vegetables	1
	Brussels sprouts	1½ cups	Vegetables	1
	Carrots (sliced)	1 large	Vegetables	½
	Soft margarine	6 teaspoons	Fats	4
	Choice of fruit	1 serving	Fruit	1
	Beverage (watch out for calories!)			

If you substitute a Group 5 serving such as steak for the Group 6 serving of fish or poultry, you will increase your daily fat intake by 5 grams. This simple substitution will increase your calories from 1,990 to 2,035, and your "fat" calories from 20% to 23%. This effect can be eliminated by omitting 5 grams of fat from other sources—if you have the willpower!

more zest with various herbs or spices. There is no reason for your food to be dull. Just think of this diet as a great opportunity for you to show off your cooking skills! After all, there is certainly no evidence that dull meals are the way to better health!

HOW YOU CAN CHANGE THE INTRODUCTORY MENUS

When you understand the way these introductory menus are structured, you can change them to suit your needs. It should be easy for you to replace a selected food group serving with another choice from the same food group. You can increase or reduce your calorie intake by adding or subtracting servings from different food groups, provided that you calculate the impact such a change would have on the final dietary balance. Details of how to plan menus at different calorie levels are discussed later.

If you are in urgent need of a low-calorie diet plan, you can follow the 1,200-calorie Cancer Prevention Diet for Weight Control which you will find later in this chapter.

When you use a recipe, or if you have to eat out, estimate as best you can the impact on your daily food intake. If you have distorted your dietary balance, don't despair. Try to catch up with your schedule later—but don't leave it too late!

Let's now examine what would happen to the percentage of calories derived from fat if you added one or two extra servings from each food group to the introductory menus. This will help you to understand how different types of food influence your diet, and what to expect if you succumb to temptation!

How to Increase Your Total Calories

If you need more than 2,000 calories to remain in calorie balance, then you need to understand the effect of adding servings from each food group. Table 15–5 reveals the impact of different food groups on your total calorie intake and on the percentage of calories derived from fat, protein, and carbohydrate.

Table 15–5 gives you a good idea of the effect of adding one or two servings from each food group to the introductory menus. Some of these effects need a little explanation. It is clear that you can add servings from the first four groups to increase your calorie intake without raising your percentage of "fat" calories, but you should be cautious when you add servings from Groups 5, 7, 8, and 9.

Unfortunately, the impression is given that adding calories from Group 10 is also a good way to reduce the percentage of "fat" calories. It isn't! Apart from the vitamins in fruit juices, the calories provided by sugar (and alcoholic drinks) are valueless from the nutritional standpoint, and should be kept below 15 percent of total calories.

If you are a devout meat-eater, the introductory menus probably leave you with a craving that reaches your very soul. Salvation could come from adding one or more servings from Group 6 (poultry, fish), which will increase your percentage of protein but not of fat; or you could add one serving from Group 5 (high-fat meat), which will raise your fat intake to 22.1 percent of total calories. Two servings from Group 5 would make that figure even worse, pushing up your fat intake to 24.2 percent. You could try to compensate for this by omitting fat from other groups, but this is not very easy.

Cheese lovers will have a tough time controlling Group 7. But you can see that this is essential because a couple of extra portions of cheese could contribute as much fat as a medium-size steak!

Now let's look at ways to reduce your total calorie intake while still preserving the anticancer effect.

How to Reduce Your Total Calories

If you need less than 2,000 calories to remain in calorie balance, and wish to reduce the amount of food in the introductory menus, then you must understand the effect of removing servings from each food group. Table 15–6 shows you the result of removing one serving of each food group. If you remove more than one serving, just subtract the appropriate nutrient value of that food group—and recalulate the effect on the percentage of fat calories. Obviously, food groups that are relatively high in fat (Groups 5, 6, 7, 8, and 9) can be subtracted in confidence because this will lower the percentage of fat calories. In practice, *do not reduce Groups 1, 2, 3, or 4,* because they form the foundation of your diet.

If an emergency weight-loss program is needed from time to time, you can use the carefully balanced 1,200-calorie version of the diet—the Cancer Prevention Diet for Weight Control, which appears later in this chapter.

Table 15-5
THE EFFECT OF ADDING ONE OR TWO SERVINGS TO THE INTRODUCTORY MENUS

	Calories	Protein	Fat	Carbohydrate	Fiber (GRAMS)
			(PERCENT OF CALORIES)		
Dietary Goal	2,000 +/−	12–18	20	62–68	50–60
Current American Diet	Too many!	12	42	46	10–20
Introductory Menus	2,045	14.8	20.7	64.5	57
ADD 1 SERVING OF:					
GROUP 1 Cereals	2,254	14.5	19.1	66.4	63–67
GROUP 2 Bread	2,222	14.7	19.6	65.7	60.5
GROUP 3 Fruit	2,149	14.2	19.7	66.1	60.5
GROUP 4 Vegetables	2,117	15.2	20	64.8	64
GROUP 5 Meat	2,200	17.7	22.1	60.2	57
GROUP 6 Poultry, fish	2,147	18	20.5	61.5	57
GROUP 7 Egg, cheese	2,135	15.5	22.5	62.1	57
GROUP 8 Milk	2,183	15.5	22	62.5	57
GROUP 9 Fats, oils	2,081	14.5	22	63.5	57
GROUP 10 Sugar	2,165	14	19.5	66.5	57

ADD 2 SERVINGS OF:

GROUP 1	Cereals	2,463	14.2	17.9	67.9	69–77
GROUP 2	Bread	2,400	14.6	18.7	66.7	64
GROUP 3	Fruit	2,253	13.7	18.8	67.5	64
GROUP 4	Vegetables	2,189	15.6	19.3	65.1	71
GROUP 5	Meat	2,383	20.1	24.2	55.7	57
GROUP 6	Poultry, fish	2,249	20.9	20.4	58.7	57
GROUP 7	Egg, cheese	2,226	15.9	24.3	59.8	57
GROUP 8	Milk	2,259	16.2	21.1	62.7	57
GROUP 9	Fats, oils	2,117	14.3	23.4	62.3	57
GROUP 10	Sugar	2,285	13.2	18.5	68.3	57

Table 15-6
THE EFFECT OF REMOVING ONE SERVING FROM THE INTRODUCTORY MENUS

	Calories	Protein	Fat	Carbohydrate	Fiber (GRAMS)
			(PERCENT OF CALORIES)		
Dietary Goal	2,000 +/-	12-18	20	62-68	50-60
Current American Diet	Too many!	12	42	46	10-20
Introductory Menus	2,045	14.8	20.7	64.5	57
SUBTRACT 1 SERVING:					
GROUP 1 Cereals	1,832	15.2	22.6	62.2	47-51
GROUP 2 Bread	1,867	14.9	21.9	63.2	53.5
GROUP 3 Fruit	1,941	15.4	21.8	62.8	53.5
GROUP 4 Vegetables	1,981	14.6	21.4	64	50
GROUP 5 Meat	Not used in introductory menus				
GROUP 6 Poultry, fish	1,943	11.2	20.8	68	57
GROUP 7 Eggs, cheese	1,954	14.1	18.6	67.3	57
GROUP 8 Milk	1,938	14	20.5	65.5	57
GROUP 9 Fats, oils	2,009	15	19.3	65.7	57
GROUP 10 Sugar	1,925	15.7	22	62.3	57

Now you have all the information you need to develop the right dietary habits, and to maintain your own cancer prevention diet. It is very reassuring to know that this permanent approach to your diet will provide you with the best nutritional balance for a long and healthy life.

Your greatest danger is the risk of sliding back into old, indulgent habits. Only you can fight this temptation. As the old saying goes, "Although you can lead a horse to water, you cannot make it drink." Nevertheless, there is some comfort in the thought that, with time, you will acquire new habits that will displace the old ones. Therefore, the longer you continue with your new diet, the more likely you are to make it into a permanent virtue. Be determined; never give up!

HOW TO PLAN YOUR OWN MENUS

Now that you have seen how the food groups are used to construct a menu, you are ready to begin to think of how you could construct one for yourself.

To start with, I suggest that you use the foods that I have selected for you in the food groups when planning new menus. Once you have become familiar with the method of menu planning, then some other food items can be substituted, provided that you stick to the basic principles of the diet.

Remember that, whatever your calorie intake, *it is essential that you include the basic food groups in your daily diet.* These are shown in Table 15–7.

Table 15-7
YOUR BASIC DAILY REQUIREMENT

Food Group	Number of Servings
Cereals (Group 1)	2
Bread (Group 2)	1
Fruit (Group 3)	2
Vegetables (Group 4)	3

It is helpful to know that these foods will contribute about 1,000 calories, a lot of fiber, and some important nutrients to your diet. However, the protein provided by these food groups will be insufficient and incomplete. As you no doubt recall, vegetable protein alone is inadequate because it does not provide all the essential amino acids. It must be supplemented by protein derived from eggs, milk, or meat (Groups 5, 6, 7, 8) to make up for this deficiency. It is therefore very important that you include one or more servings from Groups 5, 6, 7, or 8 in your daily diet as you raise your protein intake above 60 grams a day.

The freedom to choose from many different foods within each food group will inevitably influence your daily intake of vitamins and minerals. It will be too difficult for you to keep track of them, but you will be pleased to know that your new diet will probably provide you with more natural vitamins and minerals than you have ever had before!

What basic nutrients then do these important basic food groups supply? For your convenience I have summarized them in Table 15–8. To these essential food groups, you must then add protein, fats, and sugars from the other food groups.

Variety is important too, so do not always choose the same foods within each group. In the vegetable group, those that are yellow or dark-green are the most valuable because they are such good sources of vitamin A and other anticarcinogens. In the fruit group, citrus fruits are the most valuable.

Now what should you do if you want either to reduce your total calorie intake or to increase it? Let's look at Table 15–2 again and then at Table 15–10.

If you want to plan a *low* calorie intake you will have to be prepared to reduce your fat intake, otherwise you will exceed the guiding limit of about 20 percent "fat" calories. Reducing the amount of each serving from Group 5 (high-fat meats), Group 7 (eggs and cheese), and Group 9 (fats and oils) is likely to have the most impact on calories because these groups have the most fat. In any case, do not reduce the amount of foods that are high in fiber (Groups 1, 2, 3, 4).

If you want to plan a *high* calorie intake—and some of us actually do—then I would suggest that you accomplish this by increasing the foods that are high in carbohydrate, particularly complex carbohy-

Table 15-8
BASIC DAILY MENU PLANNING

Group	Servings	Calories	Protein	Fat	Carbohydrate	Fiber
					(IN GRAMS)	
Cereals	2	400	12	2	88	12–20
Bread	1	180	6	1.5	35	3.5
Fruit	2	200	2	0	50	7.0
Vegetables	3	210	15	0	39	21
TOTAL		990	35	3.5	212	43–51
(Percent of calories)			(14%)	(3%)	(83%)	
AVERAGE:		1,000	35	3.5	200	45

Add protein from Groups 5, 6, 7, or 8 to total 60–90 grams per day

Add fat from Groups 5–9 (20% of calories; maximum 65 grams per day)

Add sugar, preserves, fruit juices from Group 10 (10–15% calories)

This gives you the basic diet structure, but it is important that you use every opportunity to increase your cereal, vegetable, and fruit intake rather than to succumb to the temptation to consume refined sugars, fatty meats, or dairy products. Daily diet planning is much easier if you use this table with Chart 15–1 at the end of this chapter.

Table 15-9

HOW YOUR TOTAL FAT ALLOWANCE RELATES TO CALORIE INTAKE ON A 20 PERCENT FAT DIET

Calories	Total Fat (in grams)
1,000	22
1,200	27
1,400	31
1,600	36
1,800	40
2,000	45
2,200	49
2,400	53
2,600	58
2,800	62
3,000	65 maximum
3,200	65

drate. This is the form of carbohydrate that is rich in fiber (Groups 1, 2, 3, and 4); it is definitely *not* the kind of carbohydrate that is found in refined sugars (Group 10).

It would make no sense to increase your calories only by eating fat (Group 9), since reducing fat is one of the main objectives of your new diet. In any case, whatever your calorie intake, you will need to learn how to measure the fat in your diet, and to calculate the percentage of calories derived from fat. This is essential when you plan your diet. After all, I don't expect you to follow the introductory menus forever!

These food group selections all provide 20 percent of calories from fat. Once you have decided upon your total calorie requirements, try to memorize the number of group servings that make up your daily diet, or if you find that too difficult, write them down on a small card that you can keep with you. It would also be helpful to record the average nutritional content of each food group alongside. Then, as you plan your meals, or when you eat out, you'll have a good idea of what effect various foods have on your nutritional balance.

For those of you who might need to lose weight, or whose calorie

Table 15–10

A GUIDE TO FOOD GROUP SERVINGS FOR DIFFERENT CALORIE NEEDS

Food Groups	1500 cals	1750 cals	2000 cals	2500 cals
1. Cereals	2	2	2	2
2. Bread	1	1	1	2
3. Fruit	2	2	3	4
4. Vegetables	3	3	3	4
5. Meat, high-fat	(optional substitution when diets are above 2000 cals)			
6. Fish, poultry	1	1	1	2
7. Eggs, cheese	0	1	1	1
8. Milk	1	1	1	1
9. Fats	5	6	7	9
10. Sugar	1	2	3	3

needs are exceptionally low, I suggest that you use the detailed Cancer Prevention Diet for Weight Control (1,200 calories).

THE CANCER PREVENTION DIET FOR WEIGHT CONTROL (1,200 CALORIES)

The Cancer Prevention Diet can also be used for weight control and weight reduction. To save you the time and bother of creating a 1,200-calorie diet of the right *balance,* here is a carefully constructed weekly diet plan that does it all for you. Although the diet is planned for one week, you can continue it for two to three weeks, or even longer if you wish. Despite the low calorie intake, this diet will increase your vegetable, fruit, and fiber intake, while lowering your fat intake to 20 percent of total calories.

Fat reduction tends to remove some of the lubrication and flavor that makes food palatable, particularly in a low-calorie diet. To avoid this problem, the secret is to *use herbs, spices, and lemon juice freely to enhance flavor.* Bear this in mind as you prepare your meals. As you follow the menus, use your own imagination and cooking skill to make them as interesting as possible. Some dishes can be served hot or cold, depending upon your preference.

Since the goal of the Cancer Prevention Diet is to alter the *balance* of what you eat over a period of time, you can choose to combine each breakfast with any of the lunches or dinners, provided you do *not* repeat any meal during the week. If you did repeat meals and chose *only* the highest calorie breakfast, lunch and dinner every day, you would find yourself on a 1,500-calorie diet, not a 1,200-calorie diet! Therefore the easiest thing to do is to follow the diet plan exactly.

Although this diet plan is highly nutritious, the calcium and iron level is a little below the daily requirement. Calcium, iron, and other mineral supplements will therefore be necessary if you stay on this diet for more than three weeks.

Some people may find 1,200 calories sufficient to meet their energy needs, but it is likely that more calories will be needed to sustain an optimum body weight. Consequently, it is advisable to work out your ideal weight and calorie needs before choosing a diet for long term weight control.

The daily menus and nutrient analyses are based upon careful attention to portion sizes and the way food is prepared. Resist the temptation to add a little extra fat in the hope that it will not be noticed, or that it does not matter: it will and it does!

One week on this diet will provide you with the following daily average nutrient intake:

Calories	1207		Iron	14.2 mg
Protein	56.3 gm		Cholesterol	115.6 mg
Fat (20% cals)	28.7 gm		Vitamin A	13753 IU
Saturated fat	6.6 gm		Thiamin	1.4 mg
Oleic acid	7.8 gm		Riboflavin	2.2 mg
Linoleic acid	.8 gm		Niacin	19.2 mg
Carbohydrate	199.1 gm		Vitamin C	334 mg
Calcium	611.8 mg		Sodium	2772 mg
Phosphorus	1069 mg		Fiber	37 gm

SUNDAY

Breakfast:

Orange juice ....1 cup
Raisin Bran ....1 cup
Milk ....1 cup
Apple, sliced ....1 average size

(Calories 440; protein 14 gm; fat 6 gm; carbohydrate 98 gm; fiber 13 gm)

Lunch:

Spaghetti, cooked ....1 cup
Tomatoes ....1 large (or 2 small)
Corn oil ....2 teaspoons
Salt ....⅓ teaspoon
Basil ....to taste
Garlic ....to taste
Thyme ....to taste

(Calories 319; protein 9 gm; fat 10 gm; carbohydrate 51 gm; fiber 4 gm)

Dinner:

Chicken, white meat, baked, diced ....½ cup (3 ozs)
Potato, baked in skin ....½ average
Broccoli, cooked, without stems ....1 cup
Peas, fresh or frozen ....½ cup
Salt, in cooking ....½ teaspoon
Soft margarine (corn oil) ....2 teaspoons
Orange ....1 average size

(Calories 426; protein 35 gm; fat 11 gm; carbohydrate 49 gm; fiber 15 gm)

Sunday's Food Analysis

Calories 1185
Protein .... 57 grams
Fat .... 28 grams
Saturated Fat .... 6 grams
Carbohydrate .... 198 grams
Calcium .... 636 milligrams
Iron .... 14 milligrams

Vitamin A .... .9868 IU
Thiamin .... 1.6 milligrams
Riboflavin .... 1.8 milligrams
Niacin .... 23.9 milligrams
Vitamin C .... 420 milligrams
Sodium .... .2657 milligrams
Cholesterol .... 90 milligrams
Fiber .... 33 grams

MONDAY

Breakfast:

Orange juice ....1 cup
Whole wheat bread ....2 slices
Soft margarine (corn oil) ....2 teaspoons
Jams or preserves ....1 tablespoon

(Calories 434; protein 9 gm; fat 11 gm; carbohydrate 78 gm; fiber 7 gm)

Lunch:

Salad
Macaroni, enriched, cooked ....1 cup
Broccoli, raw or cooked ....1 cup
Carrots, grated ....½ cup
Corn oil ....2 teaspoons
Herbs ....to taste
Salt ....⅓ teaspoon

(Calories 331; protein 12 gm; fat 10 gm; carbohydrate 51 gm; fiber 10 gm)

Dinner:

Filet of sole, baked ....3 ozs
Potatoes, boiled, peeled ....1 average
Spinach, cooked ....½ cup
Carrots, cooked, cut crosswise ....½ cup
Soft margarine (corn oil) ....1 tablespoon
Lemon juice ....1 teaspoon
Salt ....⅓ teaspoon
Apple ....1 average size

(Calories 444; protein 20 gm; fat 14 gm; carbohydrate 62 gm; fiber 16 gm)

Monday's Food Analysis

Calories 1210
Protein . . . .   42 grams
Fat . . . .   35 grams
Saturated fat . . . .   5 grams
Carbohydrate . . . .   192 grams
Calcium . . . .   352 milligrams
Iron . . . .   9 milligrams
Vitamin A . . . . .26750 IU
Thiamin . . . .   1.2 milligrams
Riboflavin . . . .   0.9 milligrams
Niacin . . . .   9.7 milligrams
Vitamin C . . . .   328 milligrams
Sodium . . . . 2334 milligrams
Cholesterol . . . .   45 milligrams
Fiber . . . .   33 grams

TUESDAY

Breakfast:
  Grapefruit, pink . . . . .½
  All bran . . . . .1 cup
  Milk (2% fat) . . . . .1 cup
(Calories 299; protein 15 gm; fat 6 gm; carbohydrate 65 gm; fiber 26 gm)

Lunch:
  Salad
  Brown rice, cooked . . . . .1 cup
  Tomatoes, raw or cooked . . . . .1 large (or 2 small)
  Egg, hard-boiled . . . . .½
  Corn oil . . . . .2 teaspoons
  Salt . . . . .⅓ teaspoon
  Apple . . . . .1 average size
(Calories 509; protein 10 gm; fat 14 gm; carbohydrate 88 gm; fiber 13 gm)

Dinner:
  Turkey, white meat, baked . . . . .3 ozs
  Beans, green . . . . .1 cup
  Carrots . . . . .½ cup
  Potato, baked . . . . .½

Soft margarine (corn oil) ....2 teaspoons
Salt ....½ teaspoon
Strawberries ....½ cup
Sugar, granulated ....1 teaspoon
(Calories 385; protein 33 gm; fat 11 gm; carbohydrate 39 gm; fiber 10 gm)

Tuesday's Food Analysis

Calories	1194	
Protein	58	grams
Fat	32	grams
Saturated fat	7	grams
Carbohydrate	192	grams
Calcium	561	milligrams
Iron	15	milligrams
Vitamin A	15224	IU
Thiamin	1.4	milligrams
Riboflavin	3.5	milligrams
Niacin	24.5	milligrams
Vitamin C	219	milligrams
Sodium	3539	milligrams
Cholesterol	220	milligrams
Fiber	49	grams

WEDNESDAY

Breakfast:
Orange juice ....1 cup
Fruited Bran ....1 cup
Milk, (2% fat) ....1 cup
Strawberries ....½ cup
(Calories 404; protein 14 gm; fat 5 gm; carbohydrate 80 gm; fiber 11 gm)

Lunch:
Sandwich
Whole wheat bread ....2 slices
Soft margarine (corn oil) ....½ tablespoon
Tomatoes ....(1 large or 2 small)
Chicken, white meat, baked, diced ....½ cup (3 ozs)

(Calories 431; protein 31 gm; fat 12 gm; carbohydrate 50 gm; fiber 10 gm)

Dinner:
    Flounder ....3 ozs
    Brussels sprouts, steamed ....1 cup
    Cauliflower, steamed ....½ cup
    White beans ....½ cup
    Lemon juice ....1 teaspoon
    Herbs ....to taste
    Salt ....½ teaspoon
    Cantaloupe ....¼
(Calories 385; protein 29 gm; fat 15 gm; carbohydrate 44 gm; fiber 16 gm)

Wednesday's Food Analysis
Calories	1220	
Protein	75	grams
Fat	32	grams
Saturated fat	7	grams
Carbohydrate	174	grams
Calcium	558	milligrams
Iron	16	milligrams
Vitamin A	11123	IU
Thiamin	1.5	milligrams
Riboflavin	1.7	milligrams
Niacin	23	milligrams
Vitamin C	451	milligrams
Sodium	2085	milligrams
Cholesterol	149	milligrams
Fiber	37	grams

THURSDAY
Breakfast:
    Orange juice ....1 cup
    Raisin Bran ....1 cup
    Milk (2% fat) ....1 cup
(Calories 360; protein 13.5 gm; fat 5.5 gm; carbohydrate 78 gm; fiber 9 gm)

Lunch:
    Yogurt, plain ....8 ozs
    Bran muffin 1
    Banana 1
(Calories 350; protein 16 gm; fat 8 gm; carbohydrate 59 gm; fiber 6 gm)

Dinner:
    Shrimp ....3 ozs
    Rice, long grain, cooked ....1 cup
    Lettuce, loose ....1 cup
    Broccoli, raw, without stems ....½ cup
    Tomatoes ....1 small
    Lemon juice ....1 teaspoon
    French dressing (low cal) ....1 tablespoon
    Pear..............................1 average size
(Calories 507; protein 31 gm; fat 3 gm; carbohydrate 93 gm; fiber 11 gm)

Thursday's Food Analysis

Calories 1217
Protein .... 60 grams
Fat .... 17 grams
Saturated fat.........................   7 grams
Carbohydrate .... 230 grams
Calcium ....1099 milligrams
Iron .... 16 milligrams
Vitamin A ....6174 IU
Thiamin .... 1.3 milligrams
Riboflavin ....   2 milligrams
Niacin .... 16 milligrams
Vitamin C .... 277 milligrams
Sodium ....3629 milligrams
Cholesterol .... 146 milligrams
Fiber .... 26 grams

FRIDAY

Breakfast:
Orange juice ....1 cup
All bran ....1 cup
Milk (2% fat) ....1 cup
Banana 1
(Calories 459; protein 17 gm; fat 6 gm; carbohydrate 104 gm; fiber 28 gm)

Lunch:
Salad
Brown rice, cooked ....1 cup
Broccoli, raw, without stems ....½ cup
Carrots, grated, raw ....½ cup
Corn oil ....2 teaspoons
Herbs ....to taste
Salt ....⅓ teaspoon
(Calories 336; protein 8 gm; fat 10 gm; carbohydrate 54 gm; fiber 10 gm)

Dinner:
Leg of lamb, lean only ....2.5 ozs
Potato, baked ....½
Peas, fresh or frozen ....½ cup
Cauliflower, cooked ....½ cup
Soft margarine (corn oil) ....2 teaspoons
Salt ....⅔ teaspoon
Raspberries, red ....½ cup
Sugar, granulated ....½ tablespoon
(Calories 396; protein 28 gm; fat 13 gm; carbohydrate 43 gm; fiber 12 gm)

Friday's Food Analysis
Calories 1192
Protein .... 53 grams
Fat .... 29 grams
Saturated fat .... 7 grams
Carbohydrate .... 201 grams
Calcium .... 551 milligrams

Iron	16	milligrams
Vitamin A	12559	IU
Thiamin	1.7	milligrams
Riboflavin	3.7	milligrams
Niacin	21	milligrams
Vitamin C	318	milligrams
Sodium	2959	milligrams
Cholesterol	85	milligrams
Fiber	50	grams

SATURDAY

Breakfast:

Orange juice ....1 cup
Fruited bran ....1 cup
Milk (2% fat) ....1 cup
Cantaloupe ....¼
(Calories 417; protein 15 gm; fat 5 gm; carbohydrate 84 gm; fiber 12 gm)

Lunch:

Macaroni, enriched, cooked ....1 cup
Beans, green ....½ cup
Peas, fresh or frozen ....½ cup
Peppers, green ....¼ cup
Corn oil ....2 teaspoons
Salt ....⅓ teaspoon
(Calories 345; protein 12 gm; fat 10 gm; carbohydrate 53 gm; fiber 8 gm)

Dinner:

Risotto
Brown rice, cooked ....1 cup
Ground round of beef ....3 ozs
Carrots, grated ....½ cup
Peppers, green, diced ....½ cup
Corn oil ....1 teaspoon
Salt ....⅓ teaspoon
Orange ....1 average size
(Calories 469; protein 22 gm; fat 12 gm; carbohydrate 68 gm; fiber 10 gm)

Saturday's Food Analysis

Calories 1231
Protein . . . . 49 grams
Fat . . . . 28 grams
Saturated fat . . . . 7 grams
Carbohydrate . . . . 204 grams
Calcium . . . . 524 milligrams
Iron . . . . 13 milligrams
Vitamin A . . . . .14576 IU
Thiamin . . . . 1.4 milligrams
Riboflavin . . . . 1.6 milligrams
Niacin . . . . 16 milligrams
Vitamin C . . . . 323 milligrams
Sodium . . . . 2201 milligrams
Cholesterol . . . . 74 milligrams
Fiber . . . . 30 grams

YOUR DIET AND OTHER DISEASES

I must take this opportunity to emphasize the importance of limiting your saturated fat, cholesterol, and salt intake to reasonable levels to protect your heart and blood vessels. As an approximate guide, your cholesterol intake should not exceed 300 milligrams per day; your saturated fat intake should ideally be one third of your total fat intake; and your sodium (salt) intake ideally should not exceed 5 grams per day.

In practice, this means limiting your intake of eggs to about three or four per week (one egg has 274 milligrams of cholesterol); eating soft margarine rather than butter; cooking with oils such as safflower, soybean, or corn oil; and finally, adding only a little salt to your food. Having informed you of present medical dogma, it is interesting that some researchers are now questioning the importance of salt as a cause of high blood pressure. Evidence is coming to light which suggests that only a few people are sensitive to salt, and that lack of other minerals such as magnesium, calcium, and potassium may be as important. However, this research is controversial and not yet firmly established.

One of the most gratifying aspects of your decision to follow the

Cancer Prevention Diet is that it will also reduce your risk of heart disease—the number-one killer in the United States. It is very interesting that as evidence accumulates linking diet to the development of cancer, heart disease, diabetes, degenerative vascular disease, diverticulosis, and aging, the dietary changes that appear most beneficial are basically the same.

By the way, if you currently have any medical problems, you should consult your physician before modifying your diet.

VITAMIN AND MINERAL SUPPLEMENTS

Although your new diet will increase your intake of the many crucial nutrients that you need for cancer prevention, some of you may wish to consolidate your dietary vitamins and minerals with the few supplements listed in Table 15–11. The arguments for and against vitamin and mineral supplements have been discussed earlier.

For the present, I do not recommend these supplements for children under six years of age. It is far better that young children acquire good dietary habits that reflect the *balance* of foods described in this chapter. For children between the ages of six and sixteen, I suggest that any vitamin and selenium supplements be reduced to *one quarter* of the dose in Table 15–11, and zinc should be omitted.

Table 15–11
OPTIONAL VITAMIN AND MINERAL REINFORCING SUPPLEMENTS

Vitamins	Supplement	New Daily Requirement
Beta-carotene (Vitamin A)	25,000 IU	25,000 IU +
Folic acid	400 mcg	400 mcg +
Vitamin C	1,000 mg	1,000 mg +
Vitamin E	400 IU	400 IU
Minerals		
Selenium	200 mcg	200–300 mcg
Zinc	5 mg	15 mg

It is very important that you take vitamin A in the form of beta-carotene. Do not take preformed vitamin A. This ensures that you benefit both from the superb antioxidant (cancer-inhibiting) properties of beta-carotene, and from the effects of the vitamin A which is formed from it in your body. Taking beta-carotene also protects you from the risks of vitamin A toxicity that can result from excessive vitamin A supplements.

Folic acid is a very important vitamin that is potentially valuable in cancer prevention because of evidence that it may limit genetic damage of the type that is often seen in cancer cells. It is also important for the normal growth of cells, and a deficiency causes a form of anemia. A daily supplement of 400 micrograms would be reasonable to ensure adequate body stores, but the optimum dose for cancer prevention has not yet been established. Remember that folic acid supplements can mask the development of a serious disease known as pernicious anemia, so higher dose supplements, except during pregnancy or lactation, are probably unwise until the benefits are better understood.

Vitamin C also has strong antioxidant properties, although there is disagreement among scientists about the precise dose necessary. The recommended dose should prove effective, but no harm should come from doubling this dose.

Vitamin E has antioxidant properties too, and works in conjunction with selenium. Since vitamins A and E are both fat-soluble and thus easily stored by the body, it is difficult to predict the long-term effects of a lifetime supplement. The suggested dose of vitamin E is therefore slightly below that used for the treatment of fibrocystic breast disease, and it should be both safe and effective. However, there have been reports of headaches, tiredness, and nausea being associated with high doses of vitamin E. If this ever appears to be a problem, omit vitamin E from your daily supplements for a week or two.

At the present time, there is really too little evidence that the taking of a wide range of vitamin and mineral supplements would be beneficial to anyone who follows this diet, and so they are not recommended. A high intake of cereals, fruit, and vegetables will provide you with what you need, and a greater variety of nutrients than you will ever find in a bottle at your local drugstore. As it is, there are over fifty known nutrients, and only seventeen have been studied in sufficient detail for the National Research Council to actually make any recommendation for a daily allowance.

The supplement of the cancer-inhibiting mineral selenium is designed to boost the action of vitamin E and to provide further antioxidant-like activity. You should also know that the selected dose is at the upper level of that defined by the National Research Council. This supplement, when combined with *dietary* selenium, should bring your selenium level into the range that gives the most cancer protection without the risk of toxicity.

The need for a zinc supplement depends upon your level of fiber intake. If you follow this diet successfully, it is probably wise to take a modest daily supplement (5 milligrams) unless your physician has determined that your absorption of zinc is adequate.

I would like to emphasize that these six supplements are at doses that have not been reported to cause any toxicity in humans. They are designed to *strengthen* the anticancer effect of your dietary vitamins and minerals; they are *not designed to be a substitute for them!* If you decide to take supplements, this decision only makes sense if you take them regularly for the rest of your life—or until carefully controlled clinical studies have established whether or not they do indeed have a significant preventive role in cancer. However, do not exceed the suggested doses in the misguided belief that more is always better. And do not expect that somehow these supplements will take care of any medical problems that you might have. A good diet cannot replace needed medical care.

Although you can find these supplements in some drugstores, it may be more convenient for you to order them from a reputable supplier. One advantage of ordering them directly is that you can obtain vitamin C in powder form, which is much less expensive than tablets. The ideal way to take your vitamin C supplement is to add one quarter of a teaspoonful (1,000 milligrams) to a glass of orange juice. In this way you really don't taste it, and you have the pleasure and benefits of orange juice at the same time. Alternatively, you can use the slow-release form of vitamin C. This form releases the vitamin into your system more gradually, and is available commercially in some stores.

By now you should have a fairly clear idea of why certain supplements may be worthwhile. It is also clear that the precise dose which is needed is not known with certainty. However, I personally feel that it makes no sense to ignore potentially valuable nutrients simply because we do not fully understand them. If that policy had been followed in other areas of human endeavor, and particularly in medicine, very little progress would ever have been made. For these reasons, you must expect the suggested range and dose of dietary supplements to change as new knowledge becomes available.

Interestingly, studies are either under way, or about to be initiated by the National Cancer Institute, to investigate the potential preventive role of beta-carotene among smokers at high risk of lung cancer, and the potential preventive role for a low-fat diet (20 percent of calories) among selected young women at high risk of breast cancer. So with your new diet, you will be at the forefront of current research into cancer prevention!

HOW TO RECORD YOUR DIET

Although recording a diet is a rather daunting prospect, I am about to ask you to attempt to do this for three weeks only. The purpose of this stressful exercise is to train you to eat properly. Without a record, we all have wonderful knack of forgetting our moments of weakness. After three weeks you should have learned a great deal about your new diet and how it works in practice. This may be enough for you almost instinctively to plan your diet correctly. Of course you can continue to record your diet for as long as you wish, but without the assistance of a personal computer this will be too much for most people.

Recording a diet is much easier if you have a standard approach each day. For this reason I have created some simple charts (Chart 15–1 and Chart 15–2) that will not only help you with record keeping, but will also help you with meal planning. These charts are at the end of this chapter.

You may already have some ideas about how you could record your own diet. In case you haven't, you might like some suggestions and step-by-step instructions.

1. You will need a diet diary and a simple pocket calculator—unless you happen to be a mathematical genius!

2. Copy out Table 15–1, which summarizes the nutritional contributions of each food group, onto a convenient card. Keep it either in your kitchen or in your pocket.

3. If you rigorously follow the introductory breakfasts, lunches, and dinners, your record keeping will be greatly simplified. If you change the introductory menus, and particularly if you use your own menus and recipes, you must record the food groups selected each day, and how many servings you have used. Use a copy of the Daily Nutrient Analysis Chart (Chart 15–2) for this purpose.

4. When you plan your own daily menus, use the Basic Daily Menu Planning Table (Table 15–8) and the Daily Diet Plan Chart (Chart 15–1). Choose the foods you prefer, decide on the number of servings, and analyze them with the help of the Nutritional Contribution table (Table 15–1).

   This analysis first involves adding up the total number of calories consumed and the number of grams of protein, fat, carbohydrate, and fiber contributed by each food group.

   If you then multiply the total number of grams of both protein and carbohydrate by 4, you will obtain the approximate number of calories derived from protein and carbohydrate. Similarly, if you multiply the total number of grams of fat by 9, you will obtain the number of calories derived from fat.

   The percentage of calories derived from protein, fat, and carbohydrate can then be calculated by dividing their individual calorie values by the total number of calories consumed and multiplying this number by 100. You are now able to know whether your fat intake is about 20 percent of your total calories.

   Remember, it is more important that your total fat intake average 20 percent of total calories over weeks and months and years, rather than that it be precisely 20 percent each and every day.

5. Once you have mastered menu planning using the food groups, you can create or use recipes that have known nutrient values. Some examples of such recipes are to be found in Chapter 16.

   A recipe can be thought of as having certain nutrient values that are equivalent to one or more food group servings, or even parts of servings. The nutrient value of a recipe can therefore easily be subtracted from the food group servings that you plan to use during the day. In this way recipes can easily be incorporated into your diet.

6. When you eat out, there is no easy answer to your wish to maintain accurate records. You can only estimate what is in most restaurant meals and try to subtract that from your total daily allowance. Only when restaurants publish nutritional information in their menus will

it be possible to eat out with a clear conscience. Unfortunately, George Orwell never predicted that for 1984!

One way to save your conscience may be to follow the biblical idea of taking one day a week off! That certainly won't harm you, and this "safety valve" may help you to stick more closely to your diet for the rest of the week—and the rest of your life!

As a final encouragement, the next chapter provides you with some simple recipes that will train you to adopt the right dietary habits. I do hope that they will also enhance your eating pleasure as they have mine.

Charts for Planning and Recording Your Diet

Chart 15-1
THE DAILY DIET PLAN

Food Groups:	1	2	3	4	5	6	7	8	9	10
SERVINGS ALLOWED:										
BREAKFAST:										
SNACK:										
LUNCH:										
SNACK:										
DINNER:										
TOTAL:										

Selected Food Groups	Selected Foods	Servings Used
1. CEREALS		
2. BREAD		
3. FRUIT		
4. VEGETABLES		
5. MEAT (high-fat)		
6. POULTRY, FISH (low-fat)		
7. EGGS, CHEESE		
8. MILK		
9. FATS, OILS		
10. SUGAR, FRUIT JUICE		

Chart 15-2
DAILY NUTRIENT ANALYSIS   Date _____

Group / Servings	Calories	Protein	Fat	Carbohydrate	Fiber
				(IN GRAMS)	
1 _____ •	_____ •	_____ •	___ •	_____ •	_____
2 _____ •	_____ •	_____ •	___ •	_____ •	_____
3 _____ •	_____ •	_____ •	___ •	_____ •	_____
4 _____ •	_____ •	_____ •	___ •	_____ •	_____
5 _____ •	_____ •	_____ •	___ •	_____ •	_____
6 _____ •	_____ •	_____ •	___ •	_____ •	_____
7 _____ •	_____ •	_____ •	___ •	_____ •	_____
8 _____ •	_____ •	_____ •	___ •	_____ •	_____
9 _____ •	_____ •	_____ •	___ •	_____ •	_____
10 _____ •	_____ •	_____ •	___ •	_____ •	_____
TOTAL _____ •	_____ •	_____ •	___ •	_____ •	_____

Percent calories: • _____ • ___ • _____

(Goal: • 2,000 +/− • 12–18% • 20% •   62–68%   • 50–60 g)

HOW TO CALCULATE THE PERCENTAGE OF CALORIES DERIVED FROM FAT

1. Estimate your total intake of protein, fat, and carbohydrate in grams.
2. Combine the number of grams of protein and carbohydrate, and multiply this number by 4 (calories from protein and carbohydrate).
3. Multiply the number of grams of fat by 9 (calories from fat).
4. Divide the number of "fat" calories by the total number of calories derived from protein, fat, and carbohydrate.
5. Multiply this number by 100 to discover the *percentage* of "fat" calories.

CHAPTER **16**

Selected Recipes

All of us are naturally gifted when it comes to knowing what we like to eat. Usually this means giving in to all those reckless impulses that should be curbed. Some of us, on the other hand, think that the only way to a healthy diet is one that denies all the sensual pleasure of eating. Fortunately, this is not so. The more pleasure you can get from your new cancer prevention diet program the better. To show you that this really is possible, here are a few delicious recipes that will encourage you to increase your intake of fresh vegetables, fresh fruit, whole grain cereals, and low-fat foods.

Each recipe will be accompanied by a nutrient analysis that includes the protein, fat, carbohydrate, fiber, and calorie content. This will enable you to assess its impact on your daily diet plan. For example, if a recipe for four people uses 4 servings of Group 4, 6 servings of Group 5, and 8 servings of Group 9, then it is easy to divide these servings by four to get the average. In this instance it would produce an *average intake per person* of 1 serving of Group 4, 1½ servings of Group 5, and 2 servings of Group 9. These values can then be subtracted from your daily allowance. If you use more than one recipe, just repeat the process. If you create a recipe or a menu that happens to be a family favorite, then you can record the diet analysis for future use. When a recipe contains more than 20 percent "fat" calories, you will have to reduce other sources of fat during the day if you want to follow your diet program closely.

Each recipe is also accompanied by an analysis of the vitamin A, vitamin B_1, vitamin B_2, niacin, cholesterol, sodium, and fiber content. If you need further dietary information you can use the reference tables in the Appendix or another reliable reference source.

However, information about other important vitamins such as vitamin E, and minerals such as selenium and molybdenum is omitted from the analysis because it is either unavailable or unreliable.

The cholesterol and sodium content are included in the nutritional analysis because your intake of cholesterol should be limited to 300 milligrams per day, and your sodium intake should be limited to about 5 grams per day. This is not because of any effect that these substances might have on your cancer risk (for which there is little evidence in the United States), but because they can make a very real difference to your risk of heart disease and high blood pressure. Finally, I have not included the saturated and unsaturated fat content because this will make the calculations of your dietary food balance far too complicated. Instead, by limiting your total fat intake to about 20% of total calories, and by using fats and oils that are high in unsaturated fatty acids, you will automatically control your fat balance.

Remember, these recipes do not possess magical powers! My purpose is to suggest simple, delicious recipes that emphasize some of the foods that form the basis of your new diet program. The accompanying nutrient analysis will enable you to monitor your intake of some of the major nutrients and fiber, and to calculate the impact of each recipe on your daily diet plan.

BREADS

1.   WHOLE WHEAT BROWN BREAD WITH BRAN

Baking bread is one of the great cooking pleasures! The smell of baking bread is unrivaled, even by that of freshly ground coffee! And since most commercial breads are disappointing in taste and texture—and usually lack fiber—why not discover the delight of cooking your own. This whole wheat bread recipe, which makes two loaves, is guaranteed to delight even the most ardent white bread fanatic!

What you need:

Whole wheat flour	1	pound (450 grams)
Wheat bran	¼	pound (100 grams)
Bread flour (unbleached flour)	1	pound (450 grams)
Warm water	20	fluid ounces
Sugar	1	tablespoon
Yeast	2	cubes*
Coarse salt	1	tablespoon
(or table salt	2	teaspoons)
Cooking oil, polyunsaturated	4	tablespoons

1. Weigh out the flour and the wheat bran, and mix them together in a large bowl.
2. Place the crumbled fresh yeast* in a small bowl with the brown sugar. Add some of the warm water so that you make a creamy solution.
3. Then pour the rest of the warm water into the large bowl containing the flour. Add the yeast solution. Cover this bowl and wait about 10 or 15 minutes for the yeast to begin to work.
4. At this stage, add the salt and oil.
5. Mix the water and flour into a dough, and remove the dough from the bowl onto a smooth surface. After oiling your hands a little, knead the dough until it becomes smooth and elastic. This usually takes about 10 minutes, but it will take much less time if

---

* Yeast can be purchased in three forms: cubes of compressed yeast, premeasured packets of dried yeast, and jars of dried yeast. Where a recipe calls for compressed yeast, you may substitute one ¼-ounce packet or 7 grams (about 1½ rounded teaspoons) of dried yeast for each cube specified.

you have a food processor. If the dough is too sticky, add a little more unbleached flour until it feels right.

6. Brush the inside of two bread-baking pans with a thin coating of oil. Each pan should be about 9 inches long, 3 inches wide, and 3.5 inches high.

7. After dividing the dough into two equal parts, place the dough in each pan, press down, cover each pan with a cloth, and then leave the pans in a warm place to allow the bread to rise until about double in bulk. (This can take 1–2 hours.)

8. When the bread has risen, place it in a preheated oven set at 350°F for about 40 minutes.

9. When the bread is baked, remove the loaves from each pan and allow them to cool.

Makes 2 loaves

NUTRITIONAL ANALYSIS (per slice)			Calories 120
Nutrient	**Amount**		**% Calories**
Fat	2	g	18%
Protein	3	g	11%
Carbohydrate	17	g	68%
Fiber	2.5	g	
Cholesterol	0		
Sodium	183	mg	
Vitamin A	0		
Vitamin B_1	0.22	mg	
Vitamin B_2	0.07	mg	
Niacin	1.2	mg	
Vitamin C	0		

Approximate Food Group Equivalent

2 slices = 1 serving of Group 2 (bread)

2. *SOY PANCAKES*

The thought of using soy flour in your diet is probably new to you. But soy flour is an excellent source of protease inhibitors, which are potentially valuable anticancer agents. Whenever you make dishes with flour, always consider substituting soy flour for part of the un-bleached flour, or even part of the whole wheat flour. Although soy flour provides you with the best vegetable protein, it lacks gluten, a protein present in wheat flour that gives baked pastry its structure. So it is a good idea to combine soy flour with wheat flour in the ratio of 1:3 or 1:4 for practical reasons.

What you need:

Flour, all-purpose	¾	cup (85 grams)
Soy flour, low-fat	½	cup (45 grams)
Baking powder	3	teaspoons
Egg	1	whole
Egg white	1	
Milk, 1% fat	1½	cups
Salt	½	tablespoon

1. Mix the soy flour, all-purpose flour, baking powder, and salt together, and sift into a mixing bowl.
2. Beat the egg and the egg white together, and mix with the milk.
3. Add the egg and milk mixture to the flour and stir until all the flour is moistened, but not smooth.
4. Using a nonstick pan over low heat, add the lumpy batter so that your pancakes are about 4 or 5 inches in diameter.
5. Cook until bubbles form on the surface, then turn over and cook until underside is golden brown.

Makes 8 pancakes

NUTRITIONAL ANALYSIS (1 soy pancake)			Calories 90
Nutrient	Amount		% Calories
Fat	2	g	18%
Protein	6	g	27%
Carbohydrate	13	g	55%
Fiber	0.5	g	
Cholesterol	36	mg	
Sodium	130	mg	
Vitamin A	127	IU	
Vitamin B_1	0.14	mg	
Vitamin B_2	0.17	mg	
Niacin	0.75	mg	
Vitamin C	0.37	mg	

Approximate Food Group Equivalent

1 pancake = 1 serving of group 2 (bread)

Please note that although a soy pancake has the same protein and fat content as a Group 2 serving, it has half the calories and half the amount of carbohydrate. The fiber content is also much less than the average for Group 2 servings.

3.   *WHOLE WHEAT PANCAKES*

These pancakes can be topped with blueberry sauce or maple syrup. They are a tasty source of whole wheat flour rich in the B vitamins. Remember, you can substitute a third of the whole wheat flour with soy flour as a variation if you like. This will not change the Food Group Equivalent value.

What you need:

Whole wheat flour	1.5	cups (180 grams)
Baking powder	2	teaspoons
Egg, beaten	1	
Milk, skim	1.5	cups
Salt	¼	teaspoon
Sugar	1	tablespoon
Corn oil	3	teaspoons

1. Heat nonstick griddle.
2. While the griddle is warming, mix flour, baking powder and salt.
3. Beat egg, milk, oil, and sugar together. Then add to the flour.
4. After mixing, pour about a ¼ cup of batter onto the hot griddle. Cook on both sides until the edges are slightly dry.

Makes 8 pancakes

NUTRITIONAL ANALYSIS (1 whole wheat pancake) Calories 125		
Nutrient	**Amount**	**% Calories**
Fat	2.9 g	20%
Protein	5.2 g	16%
Carbohydrate	19.9 g	64%
Fiber	1.7 g	
Cholesterol	35 mg	
Sodium	30 mg	
Vitamin A	126 IU	
Vitamin B_1	0.15 mg	
Vitamin B_2	0.11 mg	
Niacin	1 mg	
Vitamin C	0.37 mg	

Approximate Food Group Equivalents

2 pancakes = 1 serving of Group 2 (bread)
plus 1 serving of Group 9 (fat)

Please note that 2 whole wheat pancakes will give you more calories, protein, and fat than the average amount present in a Group 2 serving.

4. *WHOLE WHEAT PITA BREAD*

This bread is ideal for filling with all sorts of vegetables, possibly mixed with a little chicken. It is also another good way to put some soy flour into your diet.

What you need:

Whole wheat pastry flour	3	cups (360 grams)
Soy flour	1	cup (90 grams)
Wheat bran	¼	cup (30 grams)
Unbleached flour, all-purpose	2	cups (230 grams)
Corn oil	1	tablespoon
Sugar	2	tablespoons
Salt	1	tablespoon
Yeast	1	cube*
Warm water	3	cups

* See footnote in Recipe 1.

1. Mix the flours together, and add the salt.
2. Prepare the yeast mixture by adding some warm water to the sugar and yeast in a small bowl. Let it stand for 10 minutes to become active.
3. Add the yeast mixture and some water to the flour to make the dough. Knead the dough for at least 10 minutes until it is smooth and elastic.
4. Leave the dough to rise for about an hour or so, and then divide it into 12 portions. Each portion should then be made into a smooth ball, and left to stand for about 10 minutes.
5. Roll out each ball into a flat round that is about 5 or 6 inches in diameter.
6. Place the rounds on a cookie sheet and bake for 10 minutes in an oven that has been preheated to 450°F.
7. When the rounds are removed from the oven they are inflated. As they cool they collapse, creating a potential space that acts like a pocket.

Makes 12 rounds

NUTRITIONAL ANALYSIS (per round)		Calories 225
Nutrient	**Amount**	**% Calories**
Fat	2.5 g	9.5%
Protein	9.5 g	17 %
Carbohydrate	41 g	73.5%
Fiber	4 g	
Cholesterol	0	
Sodium	1 mg	
Vitamin A	0	
Vitamin B_1	0.35 mg	
Vitamin B_2	0.14 mg	
Niacin	2.5 mg	
Vitamin C	0	

Approximate Food Group Equivalent

1 round of pita bread = 1 serving from group 2 (bread)

CEREALS

5.   MACARONI WITH EGGPLANT

Pasta provides you with good quality protein and safe carbohydrate. It is an excellent staple food. Whenever possible, use pasta that has not been made with whole eggs so that you avoid unnecessary cholesterol. Eggplant is a tasty source of natural fiber but only a modest source of vitamins. This is because eggplant is over 90 percent water!

What you need:

Macaroni	3½ cups (450 grams)
Tomatoes, canned	2 cups (480 grams)
Eggplant, diced	2 cups (400 grams)
Olive oil	2 tablespoons (28 grams)
Garlic, chopped	2 cloves
Green pepper, diced	½ cup
Salt and pepper to taste	

1. Salt the eggplant and leave standing in a collander for 1 hour. (This will remove the bitterness.)
2. Put the diced eggplant in a frying pan with 1 tablespoon of olive oil and fry gently over low heat (about 200°F). When cooked (approximately 10 minutes) remove the eggplant, which is now soft, from the pan and drain on a paper towel.
3. Then gently cook the tomatoes, garlic, and finely chopped green pepper with another tablespoon of olive oil and a little salt for about 25 minutes.
4. Boil the macaroni in salted water until tender (about 10 minutes). After draining, place the macaroni in a heated serving dish.
5. Then add the eggplant to the cooked tomatoes, peppers, and garlic mixture, and continue to cook for 3 minutes.
6. Finally, add the vegetables to the macaroni and serve immediately.

Serves 4

NUTRITIONAL ANALYSIS (per portion)		Calories 450
Nutrient	**Amount**	**% Calories**
Fat	8.0 g	16%
Protein	13 g	11%
Carbohydrate	82 g	73%
Fiber	7.5 g	
Cholesterol	0	
Sodium	160 mg	
Vitamin A	1,147 IU	
Vitamin B_1	0.6 mg	
Vitamin B_2	0.3 mg	
Niacin	4.7 mg	
Vitamin C	40 mg	

Approximate Food Group Equivalents

1 portion = 1 serving from Group 1 (cereals)
plus 1 serving from Group 3 (vegetables)
plus 2 servings from Group 9 (fat)

6.   *SPAGHETTI WITH TOMATOES AND BASIL SAUCE*

This dish has always been a favorite with pasta lovers. It is easy to prepare and provides a good balance of nutrients, including vitamin A.

What you need:

Spaghetti	1 pound (450 grams)
Tomatoes, canned	2 cups (480 grams)
Fresh basil leaves, chopped	2 cups
Garlic, chopped	3 cloves
Olive oil	2 tablespoons (28 grams)

1. Cook tomatoes, fresh basil, garlic, olive oil with a little salt over medium heat for 15 minutes.
2. Boil spaghetti in 5 quarts of salted water until tender but firm (*al dente*).
3. Drain spaghetti, and mix with sauce. Serve immediately.

   Serves 4

NUTRITIONAL ANALYSIS (per portion)		**Calories 500**
Nutrient	**Amount**	**% Calories**
Fat	9 g	16%
Protein	17 g	13%
Carbohydrate	93 g	71%
Fiber	4 g	
Cholesterol	0	
Sodium	160 mg	
Vitamin A	1,085 IU	
Vitamin B_1	0.58 mg	
Vitamin B_2	0.33 mg	
Niacin	4.9 mg	
Vitamin C	20.5 mg	

Approximate Food Equivalents

1 portion = 1 serving from Group 1 (cereals)
plus ½ serving from Group 3 (vegetables)
plus 2 servings from Group 9 (fat)

7. PASTA SHELLS AND BROCCOLI

The attraction of this dish is that it combines pasta with an excellent vegetable—broccoli.

What you need:

Pasta shells, dry	3½	cups (450 grams)
Fresh broccoli	1	pound (450 grams)
Onion, chopped	¼	cup (50 grams)
Garlic, chopped	2	cloves
Olive oil	1	tablespoon
Soft margarine	1	tablespoon
Swiss cheese, grated	2	tablespoons (56 grams)

1. Cook the chopped broccoli in boiling salted water until barely tender. Drain.
2. Cook the pasta shells in 5 quarts of salted boiling water until tender, but firm. Drain.
3. Gently sauté the onion and some garlic in the olive oil. Add the cooked broccoli and season with a little salt and pepper.
4. Add the broccoli to the hot pasta shells that are waiting in a heated serving dish, and then add the margarine and grated cheese. Serve immediately.

Serves 4

NUTRITIONAL ANALYSIS (per portion)			Calories 500
Nutrient	Amount	% Calories	
Fat	12 g	21%	
Protein	21 g	17%	
Carbohydrate	80 g	62%	
Fiber	9.5 g		
Cholesterol	13 mg		
Sodium	95 mg		
Vitamin A	4,037 IU		
Vitamin B_1	0.53 mg		
Vitamin B_2	0.59 mg		
Niacin	4.55 mg		
Vitamin C	140 mg		

Approximate Food Group Equivalents

1 portion = 2 servings from Group 1 (cereals)
plus ½ serving from Group 4 (vegetables)
plus 2½ servings from Group 9 (fat)

---

8.   CARROT RICE

This is an excellent dish that you can use regularly. It provides the best source of vitamin A in the form of beta-carotene, the anticancer antioxidant. It is also an excellent source of fiber.

What you need:

Rice, brown (or long grain)	3 cups (530 grams)
Carrots, grated	3 cups (450 grams)
Green pepper	½ cup (50 grams)
Salt	½ teaspoon
Lemon juice	½ cup
Olive oil	2 tablespoons
Margarine, soft	1 tablespoon

1. Boil the rice in salted water containing the lemon juice. Simmer gently for 15–20 minutes (45 minutes with brown rice).
2. Add the grated carrots to the rice and garnish with finely chopped green peppers.

Serves 6

NUTRITIONAL ANALYSIS (per portion)   **Calories 430**

Nutrient	Amount		% Calories
Fat	6.5	g	14%
Protein	7	g	7%
Carbohydrate	84	g	79%
Fiber	5	g	
Cholesterol	0		
Sodium	1,161	mg	
Vitamin A	8,184	IU	
Vitamin B$_1$	0.4	mg	
Vitamin B$_2$	0.08	mg	
Niacin	3.7	mg	
Vitamin C	26	mg	

Approximate Food Group Equivalents

1 portion = 1 serving from Group 1 (cereals)
plus ½ serving from Group 4 (vegetables)
plus 1 serving from Group 9 (fat)

9.   RICE AND ZUCCHINI

This is a very pleasant way to combine a cereal with vegetables to produce a dish that is rich in vitamin A, vitamin C, and fiber. It is also good to know that there is no cholesterol and little sodium (salt) in this recipe. Brown rice should be substituted for long grain rice if cooking time permits.

What you need:

Zucchini, diced	2 cups (420 grams)
Spanish onion, finely chopped	¼ cup (42 grams)
Garlic, finely chopped	1 clove
Tomatoes, peeled and chopped	4 small (540 grams)
Tomato paste	1 tablespoon
Rice, long grain or brown	1½ cups (280 grams)
Salt	½ teaspoon

1. Wash the zucchini and cut off the ends. Then cut the zucchini into small ¼ inch cubes. Sprinkle some salt over the cubes of zucchini and leave them to drain in a colander for 1 hour to remove the bitterness.
2. While the zucchini is draining, melt the margarine in a heavy saucepan and add the tomatoes, garlic, and chopped onion. Simmer gently for about 5 minutes, stirring frequently.
3. Instead of simmering the rice very slowly as you normally would, cook it in boiling water for a shorter period of time so that it will be slightly undercooked.
4. Rinse the zucchini cubes, and add them to the tomatoes and onions in the saucepan. Then add the tomato paste and salt. Cover the pan tightly and simmer for about 45 minutes.
5. During the last 10 minutes, add the undercooked rice to the mixture, and let simmer until all the liquid is absorbed. Serve immediately.

Serves 4

NUTRITIONAL ANALYSIS (per portion)			Calories 330
Nutrient	**Amount**	**% Calories**	
Fat	3.5 g	10%	
Protein	7 g	8%	
Carbohydrate	67 g	82%	
Fiber	6.5 g		
Cholesterol	0		
Sodium	835 mg		
Vitamin A	1,684 IU		
Vitamin B_1	0.4 mg		
Vitamin B_2	0.17 mg		
Niacin	4.37 mg		
Vitamin C	42 mg		

Approximate Food Group Equivalents

1 portion = 1 serving from Group 4 (vegetables)
plus ½ serving from Group 1 (cereals)
plus ½ serving from group 9 (fat)

VEGETABLES

10.   RATATOUILLE

This favorite dish from the south of France is an excellent way to put a variety of vegetables into your diet. When divided among four people, it becomes a main dish which is both light and satisfying. As a side dish, this recipe can serve six.

What you need:

Green peppers, diced	2	cups (200 grams)
Eggplant, diced	2	cups (400 grams)
Zucchini, sliced	4	cups (520 grams)
Tomatoes, peeled and sliced	6	small (800 grams)
Spanish onions	½	cup (55 grams)
Thyme	a	pinch
Bay leaves	2	
Garlic	2	cloves
Olive oil	2	tablespoons
Salt and pepper	to	taste

1. Fry the onions in some olive oil until they are transparent, then add eggplant, zucchini, tomatoes, green peppers, garlic, salt, bay leaves, and thyme.
2. Stir well and then cover the pan and leave the vegetables to simmer gently for about an hour and a half.
3. If the ratatouille has too much liquid, remove the lid of the pan after about 45 minutes to allow some evaporation.
4. Remove the garlic cloves and bay leaves before serving.
5. Ratatouille can be served hot with meat, or cold with a salad.

Serves 4 or 6

NUTRITIONAL ANALYSIS (per portion)
Calories 150 (4) or 100 (6)

Nutrient	Amount		% Calories
	(serving 4)	(serving 6)	
Fat	7.5 g	5 g	41%*
Protein	5 g	3.5 g	12%
Carbohydrate	19 g	13 g	47%
Fiber	10 g	7 g	
Cholesterol	0	0	
Sodium	15 mg	10 mg	
Vitamin A	1,885 IU	1,256 IU	
Vitamin B$_1$	0.20 mg	0.13 mg	
Vitamin B$_2$	0.16 mg	0.11 mg	
Niacin	1.42 mg	2.13 mg	
Vitamin C	74 mg	110 mg	

Approximate Food Group Equivalents

1 portion (serving 4) = 1½ servings from Group 4 (vegetables)
plus 2 servings from Group 9 (fat)

1 portion (serving 6) = 1 serving from Group 4 (vegetables)
plus 1 serving from Group 9 (fat)

* Although this recipe has a high percentage of "fat" calories, the total amount of fat consumed is actually quite low.

11.   LENTILS WITH CARROTS

Lentils are a concentrated source of nutrients and fiber, and this side dish is a simple and delicious way to introduce them into your diet. By combining them with carrots, you increase the amount of the potential cancer-inhibiting vitamin, beta-carotene, which is present in low amounts in lentils. However, since this combination lacks vitamin C, it would be a good idea to include a good source of vitamin C (such as an orange or broccoli) in a meal that includes lentils.

This example illustrates how you can gradually develop an awareness of the nutrient content of what you eat, and use this knowledge to plan better nutrition.

What you need:

Lentils	2	cups (400 grams)
Onion, chopped	¼	cup (40 grams)
Carrots, sliced	1½	cups (230 grams)
Clove	1	
Thyme, dried	a	pinch
Bay leaves	2	
Salt to taste		

1. Place the lentils in a large saucepan containing plenty of cold water, an onion pierced by a clove, and the carrots cut into longitudinal slices. Add the thyme and bay leaves.
2. Boil gently, adding a little salt after 30 minutes. Drain when they are soft, but still firm (about one hour). Serve immediately.

   Serves 4

NUTRITIONAL ANALYSIS (per portion)		Calories 150
Nutrient	**Amount**	**% Calories**
Fat	3 g	17%
Protein	8.5 g	21%
Carbohydrate	24.5 g	62%
Fiber	6 g	
Cholesterol	0	
Sodium	55 mg	
Vitamin A	6,242 IU	
Vitamin B_1	0.1 mg	
Vitamin B_2	0.1 mg	
Niacin	0.9 mg	
Vitamin C	4 mg	

Approximate Food Group Equivalents

1 portion = 2 servings from Group 4 (vegetables)
plus ½ serving from group 9 (fat)

12.   *VEGETARIAN DELIGHT*

This is a mixed vegetable dish that has something for everyone. However, if it doesn't contain your favorite vegetable, just add or substitute it. Then calculate the impact that this will have on the nutritional balance, and make a note of it.

What you need:

Peas	3	cups (500 grams)
Carrots	1½	cups (230 grams)
Green snap beans	1	cup (125 grams)
New potatoes, cut up	3	(400 grams)
Soft margarine	2	tablespoons
Salt and pepper	to	taste

1. Melt some of the margarine in a large saucepan at low heat, and add 2 tablespoons of water and a little salt.
2. Mix in the carrots, peas, and beans, and cover the saucepan with a large soup plate filled with cold water. Replace the water in the saucepan periodically as it evaporates.
3. After about 20 minutes, add the potatoes, which have been cut into slices or segments.
4. Maintain at low heat (about 200°F) for about another 30 minutes.
5. Add the rest of the margarine and serve.

Serves 4

NUTRITIONAL ANALYSIS (per portion)		Calories 270
Nutrient	**Amount**	**% Calories**
Fat	6.5 g	22%
Protein	9 g	13%
Carbohydrate	45 g	65%
Fiber	8 g	
Cholesterol	0	
Sodium	394 mg	
Vitamin A	7,387 IU	
Vitamin B_1	0.25 mg	
Vitamin B_2	0.17 mg	
Niacin	3 mg	
Vitamin C	34 mg	

Approximate Food Group Equivalents

1 portion = 2 servings from Group 4 (vegetables)
plus 1½ servings from Group 9 (fat)

13.   GRATED RAW CARROTS WITH VINAIGRETTE

This is a wonderful way to eat carrots, even if it does mean using up some of your scarce dietary fat in the process.

What you need:

Finely grated carrots	6	cups (675 grams)
Vinaigrette	4	tablespoons

1. Grate the carrots into fine shreds.
2. Prepare the vinaigrette (recipe 14).
3. Mix well, then serve.

Serves 4

NUTRITIONAL ANALYSIS (per portion)		Calories 166
Nutrient	**Amount**	**% Calories**
Fat	10.5 g	57 %*
Protein	1.5 g	3.0%
Carbohydrate	16.5 g	40 %
Fiber	5.5 g	
Cholesterol	5.0 mg	
Sodium	80 mg	
Vitamin A	18,150 IU	
Vitamin B$_1$	0.10 mg	
Vitamin B$_2$	0.09 mg	
Niacin	1.05 mg	
Vitamin C	13.5 mg	

Approximate Food Group Equivalents

1 portion = 1 serving from Group 4 (vegetables)
plus 2½ servings from Group 9 (fat)

* This is an example of a low-fat vegetable being converted into a high-fat food by the addition of a rich dressing. If such a dish is combined with other low-fat foods, the impact of this added fat is minimized.

14. VINAIGRETTE

This is a superb dressing for use with shredded carrots or salads. It only takes a minute, but it makes an enormous difference. This recipe is considered enough for 4 modest servings.

What you need:

Vinegar	1	tablespoon
Corn oil	3	tablespoons
Dijon mustard (prepared)	1	teaspoon
Salt and pepper	to	taste

1. Mix the mustard with the vinegar in a small dish.
2. Then add the oil slowly, beating briskly.
3. Add the vinaigrette to the salad and mix thoroughly.

Serves 4

NUTRITIONAL ANALYSIS (per portion)		Calories 95
Nutrient	**Amount**	**% Calories**
Fat	10.5 g	100%
Cholesterol	5 mg	
Approximate Food Group Equivalent		
1 portion (1 tablespoon) = 2½ servings from Group 9 (fat)		

Vinaigrette can be used to dress any salad or vegetable that is eaten raw. The use of fat to enhance the taste of important vegetables is the most valuable role fat can play in your diet.

---

15.   BRUSSELS SPROUTS WITH ALMONDS

The brussels sprout is a member of the Brassicaceae family of vegetables which includes broccoli, cauliflower, and cabbage. These are the cruciferous vegetables, which induce certain enzymes in the body to destroy some types of carcinogens, and which have been associated in epidemiological studies with the diets of populations having a lower risk of cancer, particularly cancer of the colon, lung, and esophagus.

What you need:

Brussels sprouts	4	cups (600 grams)
Almonds, flaked	7	
Soft margarine	3	teaspoons
Salt and pepper	to	taste

1. After preparing the brussels sprouts, soak them in slightly salted water for 10 minutes.
2. Add sprouts to a large saucepan containing boiling water. Simmer gently, uncovered, for 5 minutes, then cover the pan and continue to cook for about 10 minutes until they are just tender.
3. Heat the margarine in a small pan. Add the flaked almonds and saute them gently at low heat for a few minutes.
4. Drain the sprouts and add the almond sauce to them in a preheated serving dish.

   Serves 4

NUTRITIONAL ANALYSIS (per portion)			Calories 90
Nutrient	**Amount**	**% Calories**	
Fat	5 g	38%	
Protein	7.5 g	25%	
Carbohydrate	10 g	36%	
Fiber	5 g		
Cholesterol	0		
Sodium	50 mg		
Vitamin A	927 IU		
Vitamin B_1	0.12 mg		
Vitamin B_2	0.24 mg		
Niacin	1.26 mg		
Vitamin C	135 mg		

Approximate Food Group Equivalents

1 portion = 1 serving from Group 4 (vegetables)
plus 1 serving from Group 9 (fat)

16.   BAKED STUFFED TOMATOES ON BROWN RICE

Tomatoes provide a tasty and attractive way of presenting other foods. The stuffing can contain vegetables or meat, or both. Tomatoes in themselves are a good source of vitamins A and C; egg white and chicken contribute protein and a little fat; the rice provides the carbohydrate and B vitamins. The nutritional analysis for this recipe is based upon brown rice. Brown rice is preferable, not only for its nutty flavor, but also because it is higher in fiber content than enriched long-grain rice.

What you need:

Fresh tomatoes	4 large or 8 average (1,000 grams)
Onion, chopped	¼ cup (40 grams)
Garlic, chopped	1 clove
Parsley, chopped	1 tablespoon
Egg whites	2
Chicken, cooked and minced, no skin	10 ounces (280 grams)
Brown rice, cooked	4 cups (800 grams)
Wheat bran	½ cup (20 g)
Soft margarine	1 tablespoon
Salt and pepper to taste	

1. Cook the brown rice in just under twice its volume of water for about 45 minutes. Then mix in one tablespoon of soft margarine.
2. While rice is cooking, wash the tomatoes and slice off one end to make a lid. Empty the tomatoes with a spoon, taking care not to pierce the skin. Keep the pulp and discard the seeds.
3. Salt the inside of each tomato, and then turn upside down on a dish to drain away excess water.
4. Mince the chicken meat, parsley, onion, garlic, and tomato pulp.
5. Place the minced mixture in a bowl. Add two beaten egg whites and the bran. Salt and pepper to taste.
6. Then stuff each tomato case with the chicken mixture.
7. Bake in a preheated over at 400°F for 30 minutes.
8. Serve on a bed of brown rice.

   Serves 4

NUTRITIONAL ANALYSIS (per portion)		Calories 420
Nutrient	**Amount**	**% Calories**
Fat	7.5 g	17%
Protein	24 g	26%
Carbohydrate	56 g	57%
Fiber	10 g	
Cholesterol	62 mg	
Sodium	121 mg	
Vitamin A	1,821 IU	
Vitamin B_1	0.15 mg	
Vitamin B_2	0.26 mg	
Niacin	7.5 mg	
Vitamin C	43 mg	

Approximate Food Group Equivalents

1 Portion = 1 serving from Group 1 (cereal)
plus 1 serving from Group 4 (vegetables)
plus 1 serving from Group 6 (low-fat meat)
plus 1 serving from Group 9 (fat)

17. MIXED VEGETABLES

Frozen mixed vegetables are available in every supermarket and make an excellent accompaniment to any meal. Although they are unexciting when just boiled, they can be made very tasty with a little touch of ingenuity.

What you need:

Frozen mixed vegetables	20	ounces (2 boxes)
Corn oil	2	tablespoons
Turmeric	a	generous pinch
Cayenne (red pepper)	a	generous pinch
Cumin seeds about	20	

1. Pour the corn oil into a nonstick frying pan.
2. Add the turmeric, red pepper, and cumin seeds to the oil and mix while heating at about 200°F.
3. After a few minutes, place the frozen vegetables in the frying pan, and gently stir for about 5 minutes at 250°F. Then serve immediately.

Serves 4

NUTRITIONAL ANALYSIS (per portion)		**Calories 155**
Nutrient	**Amount**	**% Calories**
Fat	4 g	26%
Protein	5 g	14%
Carbohydrate	20 g	60%
Fiber	3 g	
Cholesterol	0	
Sodium	80 mg	
Vitamin A	7,388 IU	
Vitamin B_1	0.18 mg	
Vitamin B_2	0.11 mg	
Niacin	1.64 mg	
Vitamin C	12 mg	

Approximate Food Group Equivalents

1 Portion = 1 serving from Group 4 (vegetables)
plus 1 serving from Group 9 (fat)

SOUPS

18.   VEGETABLE CHOWDER

A soup that is rich in vegetables can be a gourmet's delight! Try this recipe as part of a light lunch, or to warm yourself one winter's evening. This chowder is rich in vitamin A, high in fiber, and low in fat: a great combination!

What you need:

Onion, chopped	¼ cup (40 grams)
Green pepper, chopped	¼ cup (25 grams)
Carrots, sliced	1½ cups (230 grams)
Potatoes, peeled and diced	2 (275 grams)
Margarine, soft	1 tablespoon
Water	2 cups
Marjoram, dried	⅛ teaspoon
Salt	⅛ teaspoon
Corn, whole kernel	1 cup (165 grams)
Green beans	½ cup (60 grams)
Whole wheat flour	⅓ cup (30 grams)
Milk, 2% fat	1½ cups
Garlic and pepper	as desired

1. Gently cook onion and green pepper in margarine at low heat until just tender.
2. Add potatoes, water, and seasoning to taste. Cover and simmer until the potatoes are tender—about 20 minutes.
3. Add the corn and beans.
4. Cover and simmer for another 10 minutes until the beans are tender.
5. Mix the flour with a small amount of milk and then add this to the remaining milk.
6. Stir the milk mixture into the cooked vegetable mixture.
7. Cook while stirring until the soup is slightly thickened.

Serves 4

NUTRITIONAL ANALYSIS (per portion)   Calories 140

Nutrient	Amount		% Calories
Fat	3.5	g	21%
Protein	5	g	14%
Carbohydrate	24	g	65%
Fiber	4.5	g	
Cholesterol	5	mg	
Sodium	70	mg	
Vitamin A	4,444	IU	
Vitamin B$_1$	0.15	mg	
Vitamin B$_2$	0.17	mg	
Niacin	1.6	mg	
Vitamin C	19	mg	

Approximate Food Group Equivalents

1 portion = 1 serving from Group 4 (vegetables)
plus 1 serving from Group 9 (fat)

18.   MINESTRONE

The natural creativity of the Italians is expressed in this delicious soup that is a meal in itself! Another vegetable soup that is rich in vitamin A and fiber, this too makes an excellent light lunch or first course.

What you need:

Onion, diced	¼ cup (40 grams)
Potato, peeled and diced	1 (140 grams)
Carrot, sliced	1 large (150 grams)
Corn oil	1 teaspoon
Olive oil	1 tablespoon
Water	2 cups
Zucchini, sliced	1 cup (210 grams)
Kidney beans, cooked	½ cup (80 grams)
Tomatoes, canned	1 cup (240 grams)
Macaroni, uncooked	1 cup (140 grams)
Oregano, dried	½ teaspoon
Garlic, crushed	1 clove
Basil, dried*	½ teaspoon
Salt	½ teaspoon

* Of course, if fresh basil is available, by all means substitute it for the dried herb.

1. Saute the onion, potato, and carrot in the combined corn and olive oil at low heat.
2. Add water, oregano, garlic, basil, and salt. Boil gently for 15 minutes.
3. Add the zucchini and boil gently for another 15 minutes.
4. Finally, add the beans, tomatoes, and macaroni. Boil for 12–15 minutes more until the macaroni is cooked.

   Serves 4

NUTRITIONAL ANALYSIS (per portion)		Calories 170
Nutrient	**Amount**	**% Calories**
Fat	5 g	26%
Protein	5 g	12%
Carbohydrate	25 g	62%
Fiber	7 g	
Cholesterol	130 mg	
Sodium	94 mg	
Vitamin A	4,770 IU	
Vitamin B_1	0.16 mg	
Vitamin B_2	0.12 mg	
Niacin	1.94 mg	
Vitamin C	24 mg	

Approximate Food Group Equivalents

1 portion = 1 serving from Group 4 (vegetables)
plus 1 serving from Group 9 (fat)
plus ⅙ serving from Group 1 (cereals)

With this recipe, as with others, you can choose to reduce the fat content by adjusting the recipe appropriately. For example, if you left out the olive oil, you would reduce the fat content of each serving by 3 grams and save 27 calories.

FRUIT

19.   FRUIT SALAD

This is a superb summer recipe that everyone will enjoy. Its taste is greatly enhanced by the discreet use of a teaspoon or two of Cointreau or Grand Marnier!

What you need:

Apples	2 sliced (425 grams)
Bananas	2 sliced (240 grams)
Oranges, slices	3 (400 grams)
Strawberries	1 cup (150 grams)
Sugar	4 tablespoons
Vanilla sugar*	to taste
Lemon juice	¼ cup
Grated rind from one orange	

* If you cannot find vanilla sugar in your local supermarket, it is easy to make yourself. Simply place three or four vanilla pods in a tightly closed jar of white sugar and leave for a week or more. This gives the sugar a delightful vanilla flavor.

1. Peel and cut the bananas into thin slices, and cover with lemon juice to prevent discoloration.
2. Wash apples and cut them into slices.
3. Peel the oranges and cut them into thin wheel slices.
4. Prepare and wash the strawberries. If they are large, halve them.
5. Mix the fruit together in a large bowl. Sprinkle with sugar and mix again.
6. Refrigerate.

Serves 4

NUTRITIONAL ANALYSIS (per portion)		Calories 150
Nutrient	**Amount**	**% Calories**
Fat	0.5 g	2.5%
Protein	1 g	2.5%
Carbohydrate	38 g	95 %
Fiber	4.5 g	
Cholesterol	0	
Sodium	4 mg	
Vitamin A	287 IU	
Vitamin B_1	0.11 mg	
Vitamin B_2	0.08 mg	
Niacin	0.74 mg	
Vitamin C	59 mg	

Approximate Food Group Equivalents

1 portion = 1 serving from Group 3 (fruit)
plus ½ serving from Group 10 (sugar)

Fruit varies with the seasons. Whenever possible, try to include citrus fruits. If fresh fruit is unavailable, frozen fruit such as raspberries is a good choice, providing an excellent source of nutrients and fiber.

---

20.   ORANGE AND GRAPEFRUIT IN LEMON JUICE

This is an attractive way to serve citrus fruit to your family or guests.

What you need:

Oranges	4	large (520 grams)
Grapefruit	2	large (950 grams)
Lemon juice	¼	cup
Sugar	3	tablespoons

1. With a sharp knife, slice off the top and bottom of each orange and each grapefruit. Then peel.
2. Slip your knife under the membrane of each segment and dissect it out. Be careful not to lose the juice while you do this. When you have finished, you should be able to discard the membrane skeleton of each fruit.
3. Mix the lemon juice and sugar with the orange and grapefruit segments.
4. Chill before serving.

Serves 4

NUTRITIONAL ANALYSIS (per portion)			Calories 150
Nutrient	**Amount**	**% Calories**	
Fat	0		0%
Protein	2 g		5%
Carbohydrate	38 g		95%
Fiber	3.2 g		
Cholesterol	0		
Sodium	4 mg		
Vitamin A	275 IU		
Vitamin B$_1$	0.18 mg		
Vitamin B$_2$	0.07 mg		
Niacin	0.71 mg		
Vitamin C	117 mg		

Approximate Food Group Equivalents

1 portion = 1 serving from Group 3 (fruit)
plus ½ serving from Group 10 (sugar)

21.   STRAWBERRIES WITH RASPBERRY PUREE

Some fruits are truly irresistible because they not only taste superb, but because they are also nutritious. Try strawberries combined with raspberries—they will provide you with cancer-resisting vitamins A and C as well as a lot of fiber.

What you need:

Strawberries	6	cups (900 grams)
Raspberries	6	cups (750 grams)
Lemon juice	¼	cup
Sugar	3	tablespoons

1. Wash and trim the strawberries. Drain and refrigerate.
2. Wash the raspberries, and then put them in an electric blender with lemon juice and sugar. Puree. Place the puree into a bowl and chill in the refrigerator.
3. Serve strawberries with a covering of raspberry puree.

Serves 6

NUTRITIONAL ANALYSIS (per portion)			Calories 150
Nutrient	**Amount**		**% Calories**
Fat	2	g	10%
Protein	2	g	5%
Carbohydrate	37	g	85%
Fiber	13	g	
Cholesterol	0		
Sodium	3	mg	
Vitamin A	252	IU	
Vitamin B_1	0.08	mg	
Vitamin B_2	0.21	mg	
Niacin	2	mg	
Vitamin C	123	mg	

Approximate Food Group Equivalents

1 portion = 1 serving from Group 3 (fruit)
plus ½ serving from Group 10 (sugar)

22.   *APPLE CRUMBLE*

If you are looking for a good way to combine apples with whole grain cereals, this is it.

What you need:

Tart apples, peeled and sliced	6	(1,200 grams)
Lemon juice	¼	cup
Sugar	2	tablespoons
Whole wheat flour	¼	cup (30 grams)
Rolled oats	¼	cup (60 grams)
Ground cinnamon	½	teaspoon
Ground nutmeg	¼	teaspoon
Soft margarine	2	tablespoons
Water	¼	cup

1. Place apple slices in an 8″ × 8″ × 2″ baking pan.
2. Mix the water and the apple juice and pour over the apples.
3. Mix the sugar, oats, flour, and spices.
4. Mix the margarine into the dry mixture of oats and flour until crumbly.
5. Sprinkle this dry crumble over the apples before baking them for about 45 minutes at 300°F.

Serves 4

NUTRITIONAL ANALYSIS (per portion)		Calories 300
Nutrient	**Amount**	**% Calories**
Fat	7.5 g	21%
Protein	1.4 g	2%
Carbohydrate	61 g	77%
Fiber	10 g	
Cholesterol	0	
Sodium	75 mg	
Vitamin A	520 IU	
Vitamin B_1	0.15 mg	
Vitamin B_2	0.08 mg	
Niacin	0.66 mg	
Vitamin C	19 mg	

Approximate Food Group Equivalents

1 portion = ½ serving from Group 1 (cereals)
plus 1½ servings from Group 3 (fruit)
plus 2 servings from Group 9 (fat)

---

21.   BAKED APPLES

This is an old-time family favorite that should be rediscovered.

What you need:

Cooking apples	4	large
Raisins, dried	1	cup
Sugar	2	tablespoons

1. Wash the apples and remove the core with a core parer.
2. Fill the whole you have just created with dried raisins.
3. Add half a glass of water to an oven dish and place the apples in the dish.
4. Sprinkle a little sugar over the apples.
5. Bake the apples in a preheated oven for 30 minutes at 350°F.

Serves 4

NUTRITIONAL ANALYSIS (per portion)			Calories 250
Nutrient	Amount	% Calories	
Fat	1 g	3.5%	
Protein	1 g	1.5%	
Carbohydrate	65 g	95 %	
Fiber	7.5 g		
Cholesterol	0		
Sodium	15 mg		
Vitamin A	197 IU		
Vitamin B$_1$	0.10 mg		
Vitamin B$_2$	0.07 mg		
Niacin	0.39 mg		
Vitamin C	8 mg		

Approximate Food Group Equivalents

1 portion = 1½ servings from Group 3 (fruit)
plus 1 serving from Group 10 (sugar)

POULTRY

23. SALAD OF TURKEY WITH ORANGES AND GRAPES

The light meat from a turkey is relatively low in fat and should not be used only for Thanksgiving. In this recipe, it is tastefully combined with oranges and grapes as a reminder of the importance of citrus fruit and low-fat meat in your new diet.

What you need:

Turkey breast, baked	¾	lb. (340 grams)
Onion, finely chopped	¼	cup (40 grams)
Oranges, peeled, in sections	4	cups (720 grams)
Lettuce leaves	2	cups (110 grams)
Grapes	40	(200 grams)

Dressing

Olive oil	2	tablespoons
Wine vinegar	2	teaspoons
Rosemary	a	pinch
Salt and pepper to taste		

1. Cut the baked turkey breast into bite-size pieces.
2. Marinate the turkey with the chopped onion by leaving it in the oil and vinegar dressing for about an hour and a half.
3. Add the orange segments: Toss. Serve on a bed of lettuce.
4. Garnish with grapes.

   Serves 4

NUTRITIONAL ANALYSIS (per portion)   **Calories 345**

Nutrient	Amount		% Calories
Fat	10	g	26%
Protein	30	g	36%
Carbohydrate	33	g	38%
Fiber	4	g	
Cholesterol	73	mg	
Sodium	52	mg	
Vitamin A	410	IU	
Vitamin B_1	0.27	mg	
Vitamin B_2	0.23	mg	
Niacin	10	mg	
Vitamin C	98	mg	

Approximate Food Group Equivalents

1 portion = 1½ servings from Group 6 (low-fat meat)
plus 1½ servings from Group 9 (fat)
plus 1 serving from Group 3 (fruit)

24.   MARINATED CHICKEN

This simple method of preparing poultry produces a very tasty dish, and cold leftovers make an excellent sandwich fill.

What you need:

Chicken, whole	2	lbs. (550 grams flesh)
Garlic	2	cloves
Rosemary, ground	¼	teaspoon
Oregano, dried	½	teaspoon
Paprika	½	teaspoon
Salt	½	teaspoon
Corn oil	2	tablespoons

1. Crush the garlic into a paste and mix with the ground rosemary, oregano, paprika and salt.
2. Add the corn oil to the garlic and herb mixture, mix, and insert the paste under the skin of the chicken, attempting to spread it over as much of the surface as possible. Let marinate at room temperature for at least 1 hour.
3. Place chicken in baking pan and cover completely with aluminum foil. Bake the chicken in a preheated oven at 300°F for about 45 minutes to 1 hour.
4. Remove the skin before serving.

Serves 4

NUTRITIONAL ANALYSIS (per portion)			**Calories 210**
Nutrient	**Amount**	**% Calories**	
Fat	9 g	40%*	
Protein	30 g	60%	
Carbohydrate	0		
Fiber	2 g		
Cholesterol	140 mg		
Sodium	262 mg		
Vitamin A	100 IU		
Vitamin B_1	0.07 mg		
Vitamin B_2	0.09 mg		
Niacin	11 mg		
Vitamin C	0 mg		

Approximate Food Group Equivalents

1 portion = 1½ servings from Group 6 (low-fat meat)
1½ servings from Group 9 (fat)

* Although the percent of "fat" calories appears high, it is likely that the true percentage is much lower because most fat will drain from the chicken during cooking. Be sure to bake chicken in a way that allows adequate fat drainage—and don't forget to remove the skin before serving. As with all meats, the impact of their fat content is diminished when they are combined with low-fat vegetables, fruit, or bread, as part of a complete menu.

24.   *CHICKEN CACCIATORE*

Not only is this way of preparing chicken delicious, but also each portion contributes only 10 grams of fat to your daily intake. In this recipe the chicken is boneless, but you can include bones. However, this makes it harder to estimate the amount of chicken meat per serving.

What you need:

Chicken, light meat, no skin	1¼	pounds (560 grams)
Soft margarine	1	tablespoon
Olive oil	1	tablespoon
Corn oil	1	tablespoon
Onion, chopped	2	tablespoons
Garlic, crushed	1	clove
White wine	7	ounces
Tomato paste	2	tablespoons
Chicken stock	1	cup
Bay leaf	1	
Tomatoes, peeled, seeded, and diced	4	
Thyme, dried	a	generous pinch
Tarragon, dried	a	generous pinch
Salt and pepper to taste		

1. Wrap the chicken in aluminum foil and partially cook in a pre-heated over (300 °F) for 20 minutes.
2. While the chicken is baking, heat the margarine, olive oil, and corn oil in a casserole over moderate heat.
3. Saute the chopped onions and crushed garlic in the casserole for 5 minutes.
4. Add the wine and bring it to the boil. Then stir in the tomato paste, the chicken stock, the herbs, and the seasoning.
5. When ready, take the chicken from the oven, remove the foil, and place in the casserole. Cover, and gently simmer for 1 hour.
6. Add chopped tomatoes to the casserole a few minutes before serving.

Serves 6

NUTRITIONAL ANALYSIS (per portion)			Calories 260
Nutrient	**Amount**		**% Calories**
Fat	10	g	38%
Protein	30	g	52%
Carbohydrate	6	g	10%
Fiber	1	g	
Cholesterol	140	mg	
Sodium	90	mg	
Vitamin A	950	IU	
Vitamin B₁	0.09	mg	
Vitamin B₂	0.13	mg	
Niacin	11.5	mg	
Vitamin C	20	mg	

Approximate Food Group Equivalents

1 portion = 1½ servings from Group 6 (low-fat meat)
plus 1½ servings from Group 9 (fats)

Although this recipe is reasonably low in fat for a meat dish, it is worth remembering that poultry still is an important source of cholesterol and animal fat—and should therefore be eaten in moderation. Remember, the percent of "fat" calories will decline if you serve meat dishes with generous quantities of vegetables or brown rice.

FISH DISHES

25.   FLOUNDER FLORENTINE

In this variation of flounder Florentine, broccoli is substituted for spinach.

What you need:

Flounder fillets	1	pound (450 grams)
Boiling water	1½	cups
Broccoli heads	6	cups (900 grams)
Onion, finely chopped	¼	cup (42 grams)
Flour	¼	cup (30 grams)
Milk, 1% fat	1	cup
Salt	½	teaspoon
Grated swiss cheese	2	ounces (56 grams)
Pepper to taste		

1. Lay fish fillets flat in a large frying pan. Add about 1 cup of boiling water and cook for 2 minutes. Drain.
2. Cut the heads from the broccoli. (Save the stems to add to soup, or to eat raw as a snack.) Boil the broccoli for about 2 minutes.
3. Place the broccoli in an 8″ × 8″ × 2″ baking dish with the fish layered on top.
4. Mix flour thoroughly with ¼ cup of milk.
5. Pour remaining milk into a saucepan and heat gently.
6. Add flour mixture slowly to the hot milk, stirring constantly until thickened. Stir in salt and pepper if desired.
7. Pour sauce over the fish. Sprinkle the grated cheese over the top.
8. Bake the fish and broccoli in a preheated oven at 400°F until the top is slightly browned—about 25 minutes.

Serves 4

NUTRITIONAL ANALYSIS (per portion)			**Calories 250**
Nutrient	**Amount**		**% Calories**
Fat	6	g	21%
Protein	31	g	47%
Carbohydrate	20	g	32%
Fiber	10	g	
Cholesterol	82	mg	
Sodium	97	mg	
Vitamin A	5,945	IU	
Vitamin B_1	0.29	mg	
Vitamin B_2	0.65	mg	
Niacin	2.25	mg	
Vitamin C	211	mg	

Approximate Food Group Equivalents

1 portion = 1 serving from Group 6 (low-fat fish)
plus 1 serving from Group 4 (vegetables)
plus ½ serving from Group 7 (cheese)
plus ¼ serving from group 8 (milk)

26.   FISH BAKED IN FOIL

This is an excellent way to prepare fish dishes—and it avoids the "sin" of frying!

What you need:

Fish fillets	1	pound (450 grams)
Corn oil	1	tablespoon
Onion, finely chopped	¼	cup
Garlic, crushed	1	clove
Tarragon, dried	½	teaspoon
Lemon juice	¼	cup
Almonds, chopped	1	tablespoon
Salt and pepper to taste		

1. Preheat the oven to 450 °F.
2. Mix the corn oil with the garlic, tarragon, chopped almonds, and lemon juice in a small bowl.
3. Spread the chopped onion on a piece of foil that has been brushed with a little oil. The foil must be large enough to cover the fish completely.
4. Place the fish fillets on the bed of chopped onion.
5. Sprinkle a little salt on the fish fillets.
6. Then cover the fish with the mixture of corn oil, garlic, tarragon, almonds, and lemon juice.
7. Fold the foil over the fish so that it is completely sealed in.
8. Bake the fish for about 30 minutes.

Serves 4

NUTRITIONAL ANALYSIS (per portion)*		Calories 150
Nutrient	**Amount**	**% Calories**
Fat	6.5 g	39%
Protein	20 g	52%
Carbohydrate	3 g	8%
Fiber	1 g	
Cholesterol	67 mg	
Vitamin A	3 IU	
Vitamin B_1	0.02 mg	
Vitamin B_2	0.04 mg	
Niacin	0.16 mg	
Vitamin C	8 mg	

Approximate Food Group Equivalents

1 portion = 1 serving from Group 6 (low-fat fish)
plus 1 serving from Group 9 (fats)

* In this example, the fish is sole.

Afterword

The two most important decisions you can make to prevent cancer are to stop smoking and to adopt a cancer prevention diet. If you are a smoker, these decisions will reduce your risk by up to 80%. If you are a nonsmoker, changing your diet could lower your risk by as much as 70%.

You now have the information and the means to reform your diet. Through increased understanding and this fairly simple, straightforward way of diet planning, you should be able to reduce your risk of developing many forms of cancer as well as heart disease. If this approach to nutrition were to be followed on a national scale, the reduction in premature disease and suffering among Americans could be considerable. So don't delay! Take the lead and bring immediate benefits to yourself and your family.

Remember, as much as 60 percent of cancer in women and 40 percent of cancer in men are related to a bad diet. Fortunately, simple changes in your diet can reduce not only your risk of cancer, but also your risk of heart disease. This is the encouraging news we've all been waiting for! Now you have the knowledge that could save your life.

APPENDIX

Food Tables for Diet Analysis

Although the food groups described in Chapter 15 provide a good basis for diet planning, there will be occasions when you need to know the nutrient content of a food item that is not listed in any of the groups. There may also be occasions when you would like to know the individual nutrient values for items already listed in a food group, rather than relying only upon the average nutrient value of the foods in that group.

The following food tables will help you to do this. Of course, there are so many foods in common use that it is impossible to list them all, and you may be disappointed if you can't find an old favorite. Consequently, one blank table has been added at the end so that you can record the nutrient values of commonly used recipes, menus, or new food items (using nutrient values derived from other sources).

In the real world, it is impossible to monitor your total food intake with real precision because the amount that you eat and its nutrient value can only be approximated. After all, you will not be weighing everything you eat for the rest of your life on a scientific scale! Therefore, you should not be too concerned if you cannot calculate the nutrient values of every meal precisely. The purpose of this book is to make you aware of the *balance* of your diet over a long period of time, and to encourage you to develop new habits which will shift that balance in the right direction.

Although the food tables appear to give exact amounts, remember that these values were obtained from selected foods analyzed under laboratory conditions. Many other factors can influence nutrient content, so that what you eat may not yield the values in the analysis presented here. For example, fruits and vegetables will vary depending on their ripeness or maturity, on how long they have been in storage, on the climate, and on regional variation in soil composition. This nutrient variation will not reduce the effectiveness of the Cancer Prevention Diet, nor will it reduce the benefits that your new dietary habits will bring you.

You should use these tables to calculate the approximate nutrient value of recipes and menus that you often use, or to calculate the portions of new foods that you assign to appropriate food groups. You can also use these food tables to assess your calorie intake, your fat intake, your intake of vitamins, or your intake of essential fatty acids such as oleic or linoleic acid. Although it would be much easier to use these tables with a personal computer, you should find them very useful in assessing your average nutrient intake over a period of time. If you browse through these food tables you will gradually learn to recognize foods which are high in important components such as fat, fiber, vitamin A, or cholesterol.

The foods are listed in alphabetical order. This makes it much easier to find specific foods, or to check whether a food is listed at all. If the portion size listed in the tables is not the same portion you are using, you can convert the nutrient values proportionately, using the difference in weight for the conversion. For example, if the portion size listed is 100 grams, and you wish to use 120—or 80—then multiplying all the values for that food by, respectively, 1.2 or .8 will yield the nutrient values for your portion.

My food tables are based upon "The Nutritive Value of Foods" and the "Agricultural Handbook No. 456," both published by the Department of Agriculture, and on "The Composition of Foods," revised by A. A. Paul and D. A. T. Southgate and published in London by Her Majesty's Stationary Office. Some of the fiber data were also obtained from Professor James W. Anderson, of the University of Kentucky, and from new fiber tables prepared by the National Cancer Institute. Fiber analysis is a subject of considerable interest at the present time. Old fiber data were obtained using techniques that are now thought inadequate, and the Department of Agriculture is now collecting new data on a wide range of common foods, using the most accurate and modern laboratory methods. The fiber data listed here are the most accurate currently available.

The cholesterol data were derived from "The Composition of

Foods"; from "The Cholesterol Content of Foods," by R. M. Feeley, P. E. Criner, and B. K. Watt, published in the *Journal of the American Dietetic Association,* 61: 134–139, 1972; and from the "Provisional Table on the Fatty Acid and Cholesterol Content of Selected Foods," published by the Human Nutrition Information Service of the United States Department of Agriculture, 1984.

A dash in a column for nutrients indicates a lack of reliable data for a constituent believed to be present in measurable amounts.
Notes (¹) are presented numerically at the end of the appendix.

Foods, approximate portions, nutrients, weights (28 grams = 1 ounce)	Portion size	Weight	Food Energy	Fiber	Fat	Saturated (total)	Oleic	Linoleic
							MACRO-	
						Fatty Acids		
							Unsaturated	
BEVERAGES		Grams	Calories	Grams	Grams	Grams	Grams	Grams
Beer	12 fl.oz.	375	150	0	0	0	0	0
Cocktails								
Manhattan	3.5 fl. oz.	100	164	0	0	0	0	0
Martini	3.5 fl. oz.	100	140	0	0	0	0	0
Whiskey Sour	1 drink	75	138	0	0	0	0	0
Colas								
Coke	12 fl. oz.	360	144	0	0	0	0	0
Pepsi	12 fl. oz.	360	156	0	0	0	0	0
Tonic Water	12 fl. oz.	360	132	0	0	0	0	0
Wines								
Champagne	4 fl. oz.	120	84	0	0	0	0	0
Table Wines	3.5 fl. oz.	105	85	0	0	0	0	0
DAIRY PRODUCTS (BUTTER, CHEESE, CREAM, IMITATION CREAM, MILK; RELATED PRODUCTS)								
Butter								
Regular (1 brick or 4 sticks per lb)								
Stick (½ cup)	1 stick	113	815	0	92	57.3	23.1	2.¹
Tablespoon (about ⅛ stick)	1 tbsp	14	100	0	12	7.2	2.9	.¹
Pat (1 in square, ⅓ in high; 90 per lb)	1 pat	5	35	0	4	2.5	1.0	.¹
Whipped (6 sticks or two 8-oz containers per lb)								
Stick (½ cup)	1 stick	76	540	0	61	38.2	15.4	1.¹
Tablespoon (about ⅛ stick)	1 tbsp	9	65	0	8	4.7	1.9	.¹
Pat (1¼ in square, ⅓ in high; 120 per lb)	1 pat	4	25	0	3	1.9	.8	
Cheese, natural								
Blue	1 oz	28	100	0	8	5.3	1.9	0.¹
Camembert, wedge (1.3 oz)	1 wedge	38	115	0	9	5.8	2.2	
Cheddar								
Cut pieces	1 oz	28	115	0	9	6.1	2.1	
Shredded	1 cup	113	455	0	37	24.2	8.5	
Cottage								
Creamed (4% fat)								
Large curd	1 cup	225	235	0	10	6.4	2.4	
Small curd	1 cup	210	220	0	9	6.0	2.2	
Low fat (2%)	1 cup	226	205	0	4	2.8	1.0	
Low fat (1%)	1 cup	226	165	0	2	1.5	.5	
Uncreamed (dry curd, less than 0.5% fat)	1 cup	145	125	0	1	.4	.1	Tra
Cream	1 oz	28	100	0	10	6.2	2.4	
Mozzarella								
Whole milk	1 oz	28	90	0	7	4.4	1.7	
Part skim milk	1 oz	28	80	0	5	3.1	1.2	

NUTRIENTS			VITAMINS					MINERALS				
Protein	Carbohydrate	Cholesterol	Vitamin A	Thiamin	Riboflavin	Niacin	Ascorbic Acid	Sodium	Calcium	Phosphorous	Iron	Potassium
Grams	Grams	Milli-grams	Inter-national units	Milli-grams	Milli-grams	Milli-grams	Milli-grams	Milli-grams	Milli-grams	Milli-grams	Milli-grams	Milli-grams
1	14	0	0	.01	.11	2.2	0	25	18	108	0	25
0	7.9	0	35	0	0	0	0	0	1	1	0	0
.1	.3	0	4	0	0	0	0	0	5	1	.1	0
.2	7.7	0	4	.02	0	0	8	1	2	3	0	94
0	36	0	0	0	0	0	0	1	11	61	0	4
0	39.4	0	0	0	0	0	0	1	0	52	.1	10
0	33	0	0	0	0	0	0	0	0	0	0	0
.2	3	0	0	0	0	0	0	0	0	0	0	0
0	4	0	0	0	.01	.1	0	5	9	10	.4	77
1	Trace	260	3,470	.01	.04	Trace	0	1,119	27	26	.2	29
Trace	Trace	32	430	Trace	Trace	Trace	0	46	3	3	Trace	4
Trace	Trace	11	150	Trace	Trace	Trace	0	49	1	1	Trace	1
1	Trace	175	2,310	Trace	.03	Trace	0	746	18	17	.1	20
Trace	Trace	21	290	Trace	Trace	Trace	0	93	2	2	Trace	2
Trace	Trace	9	120	0	Trace	Trace	0	38	1	1	Trace	1
6	1	24	200	0.01	0.11	0.3	0	396	150	110	0.1	73
8	Trace	25	350	.01	.19	.2	0	310	147	132	.1	71
7	Trace	30	300	.01	.11	Trace	0	176	204	145	.2	28
28	1	118	1,200	.03	.42	.1	0	700	815	579	.8	111
28	6	29	370	.05	.37	.3	Trace	910	135	297	.3	190
26	6	27	340	.04	.34	.3	Trace	850	126	277	.3	177
31	8	9	160	.05	.42	.3	Trace	918	155	340	.4	217
28	6	5	80	.05	.37	.3	Trace	913	138	302	.3	193
25	3	10	40	.04	.21	.2	0	19	46	151	.3	47
2	1	31	400	Trace	.06	Trace	0	70	23	30	.3	34
6	1	16	260	Trace	.08	Trace	0	106	163	117	.1	21
8	1	12	180	.01	.10	Trace	0	150	207	149	.1	27

A dash in a column for nutrients indicates a lack of reliable data for a constituent believed to be present in measurable amounts.
Notes (^{1}) are presented numerically at the end of the appendix.

Foods, approximate portions, nutrients, weights (28 grams = 1 ounce)	Portion size	Weight	Food Energy	Fiber	Fat	Saturated (total)	Oleic	Linoleic
		Grams	Calories	Grams	Grams	Grams	Grams	Gram
Parmesan, grated								
Cup	1 cup	100	455	0	30	19.1	7.7	
Tablespoon	1 tbsp	5	25	0	2	1.0	.4	Tra
Ounce	1 oz	28	130	0	9	5.4	2.2	
Provolone	1 oz	28	100	0	8	4.8	1.7	
Ricotta								
Whole milk	1 cup	246	430	0	32	20.4	7.1	
Part skim milk	1 cup	246	340	0	19	12.1	4.7	
Swiss	1 oz	28	105	0	8	5.0	1.7	
Cheese, pasteurized process								
American	1 oz	28	105	0	9	5.6	2.1	
Swiss	1 oz	28	95	0	7	4.5	1.7	
Cream, sweet								
Half-and-half (cream and milk)	1 cup	242	315	0	28	17.3	7.0	
	1 tbsp	15	20	0	2	1.1	.4	T
Light, coffee, or table	1 cup	240	470	0	46	28.8	11.7	
	1 tbsp	15	30	0	3	1.8	.7	
Whipping, unwhipped (volume about double when whipped)								
Light	1 cup	239	700	0	74	46.2	18.3	
	1 tbsp	15	45	0	5	2.9	1.1	
Heavy	1 cup	238	820	0	88	54.8	22.2	
	1 tbsp	15	80	0	6	3.5	1.4	
Whipped topping (pressurized)	1 cup	60	155	0	13	8.3	3.4	
	1 tbsp	3	10	0	1	.4	.2	T
Cream, sour	1 tbsp	12	25	0	3	1.6	.6	
Cream products, imitation								
Creamers, sweet								
Liquid (frozen)	1 tbsp	15	20	0	1	1.4	Trace	
Powdered	1 tsp	2	10	0	1	.7	Trace	
Whipped topping, sweet								
Frozen	1 cup	75	240	0	19	16.3	1.0	
	1 tbsp	4	15	0	1	.9	.1	
Pressurized	1 cup	70	185	0	16	13.2	1.4	
	1 tbsp	4	10	0	1	.8	.1	
Sour dressing (imitation sour cream)	1 tbsp	12	20	0	2	1.6	.2	
Ice cream and ice milk. See **Milk desserts, frozen.**								
Milk, fluid								
Whole (3.3% fat)	1 cup	244	150	0	8	5.1	2.1	
Low fat (2%)								
No milk solids added	1 cup	244	120	0	5	2.9	1.2	

MACRO

Fatty Acids

Unsaturated

NUTRIENTS			VITAMINS					MINERALS				
Protein	Carbohydrate	Cholesterol	Vitamin A	Thiamin	Riboflavin	Niacin	Ascorbic Acid	Sodium	Calcium	Phosphorous	Iron	Potassium
Grams	Grams	Milligrams	International units	Milligrams	Milligrams	Milligrams	Milligrams	Milligrams	Milligrams	Milligrams	Milligrams	Milligrams
42	4	79	700	.05	.39	.3	0	1,886	1,376	807	1.0	107
2	Trace	4	40	Trace	.02	Trace	0	93	69	40	Trace	5
12	1	22	200	.01	.11	.1	0	528	390	229	.3	30
7	1	20	230	.01	.09	Trace	0	248	214	141	.1	39
28	7	76	1,210	.03	.48	.3	0	207	509	389	.9	257
28	13	9	1,060	.05	.46	.2	0	307	669	449	1.1	308
8	1	26	240	.01	.10	Trace	0	74	272	171	Trace	31
6	Trace	27	340	.01	.10	Trace	0	406	174	211	.1	46
7	1	24	230	Trace	.08	Trace	0	388	219	216	.2	61
7	10	89	260	.08	.36	.2	2	98	254	230	.2	314
Trace	1	6	20	.01	.02	Trace	Trace	6	16	14	Trace	19
6	9	160	1,730	.08	.36	.1	2	96	231	192	.1	292
Trace	1	10	110	Trace	.02	Trace	Trace	6	14	12	Trace	18
5	7	265	2,690	0.06	0.30	0.1	1	82	166	146	0.1	231
Trace	Trace	17	170	Trace	.02	Trace	Trace	5	10	9	Trace	15
5	7	326	3,500	.05	.26	.1	1	89	154	149	.1	179
Trace	Trace	20	220	Trace	.02	Trace	Trace	6	10	9	Trace	11
2	7	420	550	.02	.04	Trace	0	30	61	54	Trace	88
Trace	Trace	21	30	Trace	Trace	Trace	0	20	3	3	Trace	4
Trace	1	5	90	Trace	.02	Trace	Trace	6	14	10	Trace	17
Trace	2	0	10	0	0	0	0	196	1	10	Trace	29
Trace	1	0	Trace	0	Trace	0	0	12	Trace	8	Trace	16
1	17	0	650	0	0	0	0	38	5	6	.1	14
Trace	1	0	30	0	0	0	0	2	Trace	Trace	Trace	1
1	11	0	330	0	0	0	0	35	4	13	Trace	13
Trace	1	0	20	0	0	0	0	2	Trace	1	Trace	1
Trace	1	0	Trace	.01	.02	Trace	Trace	12	14	10	Trace	19
8	11	33	¹310	.09	.40	.2	2	120	291	228	.1	370
8	12	18	500	.10	.40	.2	2	122	297	232	.1	377

A dash in a column for nutrients indicates a lack of reliable data for a constituent believed to be present in measurable amounts.
Notes (¹) are presented numerically at the end of the appendix.

Foods, approximate portions, nutrients, weights (28 grams = 1 ounce)	Portion size	Weight	Food Energy	Fiber	Fat	MACRO- Fatty Acids Saturated (total)	Unsaturated Oleic	Linoleic
		Grams	Calories	Grams	Grams	Grams	Grams	Grams
Milk solids added								
Less than 10 grams of protein per cup	1 cup	245	125	0	5	2.9	1.2	
10 or more grams of protein per cup	1 cup	246	135	0	5	3.0	1.2	
Low fat (1%)								
No milk solids added	1 cup	244	100	0	3	1.6	.7	
Milk solids added								
Less than 10 grams of protein per cup	1 cup	245	105	0	2	1.5	.6	
10 or more grams of protein per cup	1 cup	246	120	0	3	1.8	.7	
Nonfat (skim)								
No milk solids added	1 cup	245	85	0	Trace	.3	.1	Tra
Milk solids added								
Less than 10 grams of protein per cup	1 cup	245	90	0	1	0.4	0.1	Tra
10 or more grams of protein per cup	1 cup	246	100	0	1	.4	.1	Tra
Buttermilk	1 cup	245	100	0	2	1.3	.5	Tra
Milk, canned								
Evaporated, unsweetened								
Whole milk	1 cup	252	340	0	19	11.6	5.3	
Skim milk	1 cup	255	200	0	1	.3	.1	Tra
Sweetened, condensed	1 cup	306	980	0	27	16.8	6.7	
Milk, dried, nonfat instant								
Cup	1 cup	68	245	0	Trace	.3	.1	Tr
Milk beverages								
Chocolate milk (commercial)								
Regular	1 cup	250	210	0	8	5.3	2.2	
Low fat (2%)	1 cup	250	180	0	5	3.1	1.3	
Low fat (1%)	1 cup	250	160	0	3	1.5	.7	
Eggnog (commercial)	1 cup	254	340	0	19	11.3	5.0	
Milk desserts, frozen								
Ice cream								
Regular (about 11% fat)								
Hardened	1 cup	133	270	0	14	8.9	3.6	
Soft serve (frozen custard)	1 cup	173	375	0	23	13.5	5.9	
Rich (about 16% fat), hardened	1 cup	148	350	0	24	14.7	6.0	
Ice milk								
Hardened (about 4.3% fat)	1 cup	131	185	0	6	3.5	1.4	
Soft serve (about 2.6% fat)	1 cup	175	225	0	5	2.9	1.2	
Sherbet (about 2% fat)	1 cup	193	270	0	4	2.4	1.0	
Milk desserts, other								
Custard, baked	1 cup	265	305	0	15	6.8	5.4	
Puddings								
From home recipe								
Starch base								
Chocolate	1 cup	260	385	0	12	7.6	3.3	
Vanilla (blancmange)	1 cup	255	285	0	10	6.2	2.5	

NUTRIENTS			VITAMINS					MINERALS				
Protein	Carbohydrate	Cholesterol	Vitamin A	Thiamin	Riboflavin	Niacin	Ascorbic Acid	Sodium	Calcium	Phosphorous	Iron	Potassium
Grams	Grams	Milli-grams	Inter-national units	Milli-grams	Milli-grams	Milli-grams	Milli-grams	Milli-grams	Milli-grams	Milli-grams	Milli-grams	Milli-grams
9	12	18	500	.10	.42	.2	2	122	313	245	.1	397
10	14	18	500	.11	.48	.2	3	122	352	276	.1	447
8	12	10	500	.10	.41	2	2	122	300	235	.1	381
9	12	10	500	10	.42	2	2	122	313	245	.1	397
10	14	10	500	.11	.47	.2	3	122	349	273	.1	444
8	12	5	500	.09	.34	.2	2	126	302	247	.1	406
9	12	5	500	0.10	0.43	0.2	2	126	316	255	0.1	418
10	14	5	500	.11	.48	.2	3	126	352	275	.1	446
8	12	9	[1]80	.08	.38	1	2	257	285	219	.1	371
17	25	74	[1]610	.12	.80	.5	5	266	657	510	.5	764
19	29	10	[2]1,000	.11	.79	.4	3	294	738	497	.7	845
24	166	104	[1]1,000	.28	1.27	.6	8	389	868	775	.6	1,136
24	35	24	[2]1,610	.28	1.19	.6	4	398	837	670	.2	1,160
8	26	30	300	.09	.41	.3	2	149	280	251	.6	417
8	26	20	500	.10	.42	.3	2	147	284	254	.6	422
8	26	——	500	.10	.40	.2	2	149	287	257	.6	426
10	34	149	890	.09	.48	.4	4	138	330	278	.5	420
5	32	60	540	.05	.33	.1	1	84	176	134	.1	257
7	38	——	790	.08	.45	.2	1	109	236	199	.4	338
4	32	88	900	.04	.28	.1	1	49	151	115	.1	221
5	29	18	210	.08	.35	.1	1	105	176	129	.1	265
8	38	13	180	0.12	0.54	0.2	1	119	274	202	0.3	412
2	59	14	190	.03	.09	.1	4	19	103	74	.3	198
14	29	278	930	.11	.50	.3	1	209	297	1.1	310	387
8	67	——	390	.05	.36	.3	1	146	250	1.3	255	445
9	41	——	410	.08	.41	.3	2	166	298	Trace	232	352

A dash in a column for nutrients indicates a lack of reliable data for a constituent believed to be present in measurable amounts.
Notes ([1]) are presented numerically at the end of the appendix.

Foods, approximate portions, nutrients, weights (28 grams = 1 ounce)	Portion size	Weight	Food Energy	Fiber	Fat	Saturated (total)	Unsaturated Oleic	Unsaturated Linoleic
		Grams	Calories	Grams	Grams	Grams	Grams	Grams
Tapioca cream	1 cup	165	220	0	8	4.1	2.5	.5
From mix (chocolate) and milk								
Regular (cooked)	1 cup	260	320	0	8	4.3	2.6	.2
Instant	1 cup	260	325	0	7	3.6	2.2	.3
Yogurt								
With added milk solids								
Made with low-fat milk								
Fruit flavored[3]	8-oz container	227	230	0	3	1.8	.6	.1
Plain	8-oz container	227	145	0	4	2.3	.8	.1
Made with nonfat milk	8-oz container	227	125	0	Trace	.3	.1	Trace
Without added milk solids								
Made with whole milk	8-oz container	227	140	0	7	4.8	1.7	
EGGS								
Eggs, large (24 oz per dozen)								
Raw								
Whole, without shell (medium)	1 egg	50	80	0	6	1.7	2.0	
White	1 white	33	15	0	Trace	0	0	
Yolk	1 yolk	17	65	0	6	1.7	2.1	
Cooked								
Fried in butter	1 egg	46	85	0	6	2.4	2.2	
Hard-cooked, shell removed	1 egg	50	80	0	6	1.7	2.0	
Poached	1 egg	50	80	0	6	1.7	2.0	
Scrambled (milk added) in butter	1 egg	64	95	0	7	2.8	2.3	
FATS, OILS; RELATED PRODUCTS								
Fats, cooking (vegetable shortenings)	1 tbsp	13	110	0	13	3.2	5.7	3
Lard	1 tbsp	13	115	0	13	5.1	5.3	1
Margarine								
Regular (4 sticks per lb)								
Stick (½ cup)	1 stick	113	815	0	92	16.7	42.9	24
Tablespoon (about ⅛ stick)	1 tbsp	14	100	0	12	2.1	5.3	3
Pat (1 in square, ⅓ in high)	1 pat	5	35	0	4	.7	1.9	1
Soft	1 tbsp	14	100	0	12	2.0	4.5	4
Whipped (6 sticks per lb)								
Stick (½ cup)	1 stick	76	545	0	61	11.2	28.7	1
Tablespoon (about ⅛ stick)	1 tbsp	9	70	0	8	1.4	3.6	
Pat (1 in square, ⅓ in thick)	1 pat	4	25	0	.3	1.9	.8	
Oils, salad or cooking								
Corn	1 tbsp	14	120	0	14	1.7	3.3	
Olive	1 tbsp	14	120	0	14	1.9	9.7	
Peanut	1 tbsp	14	120	0	14	2.3	6.2	
Safflower	1 tbsp	14	120	0	14	1.3	1.6	1
Soybean, hydrogenated (partially hardened)	1 tbsp	14	120	0	14	2.0	5.8	
Soybean-cottonseed blend, hydrogenated	1 tbsp	14	120	0	14	2.4	3.9	

NUTRIENTS			VITAMINS					MINERALS				
Protein	Carbohydrate	Cholesterol	Vitamin A	Thiamin	Riboflavin	Niacin	Ascorbic Acid	Sodium	Calcium	Phosphorous	Iron	Potassium
Grams	Grams	Milli-grams	Inter-national units	Milli-grams	Milli-grams	Milli-grams	Milli-grams	Milli-grams	Milli-grams	Milli-grams	Milli-grams	Milli-grams
8	28	—	480	.07	.30	.2	2	257	173	.7	180	223
9	59	—	340	.05	.39	.3	2	335	265	.8	247	354
8	63	—	340	.08	.39	.3	2	322	374	1.3	237	335
10	42	10	[1]120	.08	.40	.2	1	121	343	.2	269	439
12	16	14	[1]150	.10	.49	.3	2	159	415	.2	326	531
13	17	4	[1]20	.11	.53	.3	2	174	452	.2	355	579
8	11	29	280	.07	.32	.2	1	105	274	.1	215	351
6	1	274	260	.04	.15	Trace	0	63	28	90	1.0	65
3	Trace	0	0	Trace	.14	.03	0	54	2	11	.03	45
3	Trace	274	310	.04	.07	Trace	0	9	26	86	.9	15
5	1	312	290	.03	.13	Trace	0	144	26	80	.9	58
6	1	274	260	.04	.14	Trace	0	54	28	90	1.0	65
6	1	274	260	.04	.13	Trace	0	61	28	90	1.0	65
6	1	314	310	.04	.16	Trace	0	164	47	97	9	85
0	0	0	—	0	0	0	0	Trace	0	0	0	0
0	0	12	0	0	0	0	0	Trace	0	0	0	0
1	Trace	0	[4]3,750	.01	.04	Trace	0	1,119	27	26	.2	29
Trace	Trace	0	[4]470	Trace	Trace	Trace	0	140	3	3	Trace	4
Trace	Trace	0	[4]170	Trace	Trace	Trace	0	45	1	1	Trace	1
Trace	Trace	0	[4]470	Trace	Trace	Trace	0	140	3	3	Trace	4
Trace	Trace	0	[4]2,500	Trace	.03	Trace	0	746	18	17	.1	20
Trace	Trace	0	[4]310	Trace	Trace	Trace	0	93	2	2	Trace	2
Trace	Trace	0	[4]120	Trace	Trace	Trace	0	38	1	1	Trace	1
0	0	0	—	0	0	0	0	0	0	0	0	0
0	0	0	—	0	0	0	0	0	0	0	0	0
0	0	0	—	0	0	0	0	0	0	0	0	0
0	0	0	—	0	0	0	0	0	0	0	0	0
0	0	0	—	0	0	0	0	0	0	0	0	0
0	0	0	—	0	0	0	0	0	0	0	0	0

A dash in a column for nutrients indicates a lack of reliable data for a constituent believed to be present in measurable amounts.
Notes (^{1}) are presented numerically at the end of the appendix.

Foods, approximate portions, nutrients, weights (28 grams = 1 ounce)	Portion size	Weight	Food Energy	Fiber	Fat	Saturated (total)	Oleic	Linoleic
		Grams	Calories	Grams	Grams	Grams	Grams	Grar
Salad dressings, commercial								
Blue cheese								
Regular	1 tbsp	15	75	0	8	1.6	1.7	
Low calorie (5 cal per tsp)	1 tbsp	16	10	0	1	.5	.3	Tr
French								
Regular	1 tbsp	16	65	0	6	1.1	1.3	
Low calorie (5 cal per tsp)	1 tbsp	16	15	0	1	.1	.1	
Italian								
Regular	1 tbsp	15	85	0	9	1.6	1.9	
Low calorie (2 cal per tsp)	1 tbsp	15	10	0	1	.1	.1	
Mayonnaise	1 tbsp	14	100	0	11	2.0	2.4	
Mayonnaise type								
Regular	1 tbsp	15	65	0	6	1.1	1.4	
Low calorie (8 cal per tsp)	1 tbsp	16	20	0	2	.4	.4	
Tartar sauce, regular	1 tbsp	14	75	0	8	1.5	1.8	
Thousand Island								
Regular	1 tbsp	16	80	0	8	1.4	1.7	
Low calorie (10 cal per tsp)	1 tbsp	15	25	0	2	.4	.4	
FISH, SHELLFISH, MEAT, POULTRY; RELATED PRODUCTS								
Fish and Shellfish								
Bluefish, baked with butter or margarine	3 oz	85	135	0	4	—	—	
Clams								
Raw, meat only	3 oz	85	65	0	1	—	—	
Canned, meat and liquid	3 oz	85	45	0	1	0.2	Trace	
Crabmeat (white or king, canned)	1 cup	135	135	0	3	.6	0.4	
Fish sticks, frozen, breaded, cooked, reheated (stick, 4 by 1 by ½ in)	1 stick	28	50	0	3	—	—	
Haddock, breaded, fried	3 oz	85	140	0	5	1.4	2.2	
Ocean perch, breaded, fried	1 fillet	85	195	0	11	2.7	4.4	
Oysters, raw (13–19 medium)	1 cup	240	160	0	4	1.3	.2	
Salmon, pink, canned, meat, bones, and liquid	3 oz	85	120	0	5	.9	.8	
Sardines, Atlantic, canned in oil, drained	3 oz	85	175	0	9	3.0	2.5	
Scallops, frozen, breaded, fried, reheated	6 scallops	90	175	0	8	—	—	
Shad, baked with butter or margarine, bacon	3 oz	85	170	0	10	—	—	
Shrimp								
Breaded, French fried	3 oz	85	190	0	9	2.3	3.7	
Canned	3 oz	85	100	0	1	.1	.1	
Tuna, canned in oil, drained	3 oz	85	170	0	7	1.7	1.7	

NUTRIENTS			VITAMINS					MINERALS				
Protein	Carbohydrate	Cholesterol	Vitamin A	Thiamin	Riboflavin	Niacin	Ascorbic Acid	Sodium	Calcium	Phosphorous	Iron	Potassium
Grams	Grams	Milli-grams	Inter-national units	Milli-grams	Milli-grams	Milli-grams	Milli-grams	Milli-grams	Milli-grams	Milli-grams	Milli-grams	Milli-grams
1	1	——	30	Trace	.02	Trace	Trace	164	12	11	Trace	6
Trace	1	——	30	Trace	.01	Trace	Trace	177	10	8	Trace	5
Trace	3	——	——	——	——	——	——	126	2	2	.1	13
Trace	2	——	——	——	——	——	——	140	2	2	.1	13
Trace	1	——	Trace	Trace	Trace	Trace	——	314	2	1	Trace	2
Trace	Trace	——	Trace	Trace	Trace	Trace	——	118	Trace	1	Trace	2
Trace	Trace	10	40	Trace	.01	Trace	——	84	3	4	.1	5
Trace	2	8	30	Trace	Trace	Trace	——	88	2	4	Trace	1
Trace	2	——	40	Trace	Trace	Trace	——	19	3	4	Trace	1
Trace	1	——	30	Trace	Trace	Trace	Trace	99	3	4	.1	11
Trace	2	——	50	Trace	Trace	Trace	Trace	112	2	3	.1	18
Trace	2	——	50	Trace	Trace	Trace	Trace	105	2	3	.1	17
22	0	——	40	0.09	0.08	1.6	——	87	25	244	0.6	——
11	2	42	90	.08	.15	1.1	8	174	59	138	5.2	154
7	2	42	——	.01	.09	.9	——	174	47	116	3.5	119
24	1	85	——	.11	.11	2.6	——	675	61	246	1.1	149
5	2	——	0	.01	.02	.5	——	50	3	47	.1	——
17	5	51	——	.03	.06	2.7	2	150	34	210	1.0	296
16	6	——	——	.10	.10	1.6	——	129	28	192	1.1	242
20	8	120	740	.34	.43	6.0	——	175	226	343	13.2	290
17	0	30	60	.03	.16	6.8	——	329	167	243	.7	307
20	0	60	190	.02	.17	4.6	——	699	372	424	2.5	502
16	9	32	——				——	229	——	——		——
20	0	——	30	.11	.22	7.3	——	46	20	266	.5	320
17	9	128	——	.03	.07	2.3	——	119	61	162	1.7	195
21	1	127	50	.01	.03	1.5	——	53	98	224	2.6	104
24	0	55	70	.04	.10	10.1	——	680	7	199	1.6	——

A dash in a column for nutrients indicates a lack of reliable data for a constituent believed to be present in measurable amounts.
Notes (^{1}) are presented numerically at the end of the appendix.

Foods, approximate portions, nutrients, weights (28 grams = 1 ounce)	Portion size	Weight	Food Energy	Fiber	Fat	Saturated (total)	Oleic	Linoleic
		Grams	Calories	Grams	Grams	Grams	Grams	Gram
Meat and Meat Products								
Bacon (20 slices per lb) broiled or fried, crisp ...	2 slices	15	85	0	8	2.5	3.7	
Beef, trimmed, cooked								
Cuts, braised, simmered, or pot roasted								
Lean and fat (piece, 2½ by 2½ by ¾ in)	3 oz	85	245	0	16	6.8	6.5	
Lean only	2.5 oz	72	140	0	5	2.1	1.8	
Ground beef, broiled								
Lean with 10% fat (patty, 3 by ⅝ in)	1 patty	85	185	0	10	4.0	3.9	
Lean with 21% fat (patty, 3 by ⅝ in)	1 patty	82	235	0	17	7.0	6.7	
Roast, oven cooked								
Relatively fat, such as rib								
Lean and fat (2 pieces, 4 by 2¼ by ¼ in) ...	3 oz	85	375	0	33	14.0	13.6	
Lean only	1.8 oz	51	125	0	7	3.0	2.5	
Relatively lean, such as heel of round								
Lean and fat (2 pieces, 4 by 2¼ by ¼ in) ...	3 oz	85	165	0	7	2.8	2.7	
Lean only	2.8 oz	78	125	0	3	1.2	1.0	
Steak								
Relatively fat, sirloin, broiled								
Lean and fat (piece, 2½ by 2½ by ¾ in)	3 oz	85	330	0	27	11.3	11.1	
Lean only	2 oz	56	115	0	4	1.8	1.6	
Relatively lean, round, braised								
Lean and fat (piece, 4 by 2¼ by ½ in)	3 oz	85	220	0	13	5.5	5.2	
Lean only	2.4 oz	68	130	0	4	1.7	1.5	
Beef, corned, canned								
Hash	1 cup	220	400	0	25	11.9	10.9	
Meat	3 oz	85	185	0	10	4.9	4.5	
Beef, dried, chipped (2½-oz jar)	1 jar	71	145	0	4	2.1	2.0	
Lamb, cooked								
Chop, rib (cut 3 per lb with bone), broiled								
Lean and fat	3.1 oz	89	360	0	32	14.8	12.1	
Lean only	2 oz	57	120	0	6	2.5	2.1	
Leg, roasted								
Lean and fat (2 pieces, 4 by 2½ by ¼ in)	3 oz	85	235	0	16	7.3	6.0	
Lean only	2.5 oz	71	130	0	5	2.1	1.8	
Shoulder, roasted								
Lean and fat (3 pieces, 2½ by 2½ by ¼ in) ...	3 oz	85	285	0	23	10.8	8.8	
Lean only	2.3 oz	64	130	0	6	3.6	2.3	
Liver, beef, fried in margarine (slice, 6½ by 2½ by ½ in)	3 oz	85	195	0	9	2.5	3.5	
Pork, cured, cooked								
Ham, light cure, trimmed, lean and fat, roasted (2 pieces, 4 by 2¼ by ¼ in)	3 oz	85	245	0	19	6.8	7.9	
Luncheon meat. See also **Sausage.**								
Boiled ham, slice (8 per 8-oz pkg)	1 oz	28	65	0	5	1.7	2.0	

370

NUTRIENTS			VITAMINS					MINERALS				
Protein	Carbohydrate	Cholesterol	Vitamin A	Thiamin	Riboflavin	Niacin	Ascorbic Acid	Sodium	Calcium	Phosphorous	Iron	Potassium
Grams	Grams	Milli-grams	Inter-national units	Milli-grams	Milli-grams	Milli-grams	Milli-grams	Milli-grams	Milli-grams	Milli-grams	Milli-grams	Milli-grams
4	Trace	33	0	.08	.05	.8	——	102	2	34	.5	35
23	0	70	30	.04	.18	3.6	——	24	10	114	2.9	184
22	0	59	10	.04	.17	3.3	——	38	10	108	2.7	176
23	0	70	20	.08	.20	5.1	——	57	10	196	3.0	261
20	0	67	30	.07	.17	4.4	——	49	9	159	2.6	221
17	0	70	70	.05	.13	3.1	——	45	8	158	2.2	189
14	0	42	10	.04	.11	2.6	——	36	6	131	1.8	161
25	0	70	10	.06	.19	4.5	——	59	11	208	3.2	279
24	0	64	Trace	0.06	0.18	4.3	——	60	10	199	3.0	268
20	0	70	50	.05	.15	4.0	——	49	9	162	2.5	220
18	0	46	10	.05	.14	3.6	——	40	7	146	2.2	202
24	0	70	20	.07	.19	4.8	— —	52	10	213	3.0	272
21	0	56	10	.05	.16	4.1	——	62	9	182	2.5	238
19	24	——	——	.02	.20	4.6	——	1,188	29	147	4.4	440
22	0	——	——	.01	.20	2.9	——	800	17	90	3.7	——
24	0	58	——	.05	.23	2.7	0	3,047	14	287	3.6	142
18	0	98	——	.11	.19	4.1	——	49	8	139	1.0	200
16	0	63	——	.09	.15	3.4	——	39	6	121	1.1	174
22	0	93	——	.13	.23	4.7	——	53	9	177	1.4	241
20	0	78	——	.12	.21	4.4	——	50	9	169	1.4	227
18	0	93	——	.11	.20	4.0	——	45	9	146	1.0	206
17	0	70	——	.10	.18	3.7	——	42	8	140	1.0	193
22	5	280	[5]45,390	.22	3.56	14.0	23	156	9	405	7.5	323
18	0	28	0	.40	.15	3.1	——	637	8	146	2.2	199
5	0	15	0	.12	.04	.7	——	367	3	47	.8	——

A dash in a column for nutrients indicates a lack of reliable data for a constituent believed to be present in measurable amounts.
Notes (^{1}) are presented numerically at the end of the appendix.

Foods, approximate portions, nutrients, weights (28 grams = 1 ounce)	Portion size	Weight	Food Energy	Fiber	Fat	Saturated (total)	Oleic	Linoleic
		Grams	Calories	Grams	Grams	Grams	Grams	Gram
Canned, spiced or unspiced, slice (approx 3 by 2 by ½ in)	1 slice	60	175	0	15	5.4	6.7	1
Pork, fresh, trimmed, cooked								
Chop, loin (cut 3 per lb with bone), broiled								
Lean and fat	2.7 oz	78	305	0	25	8.9	10.4	2
Lean only	2 oz	56	150	0	9	3.1	3.6	
Roast, oven cooked								
Lean and fat (piece, 2½ by 2½ by ¾ in)	3 oz	85	310	0	24	8.7	10.2	
Lean only	2.4 oz	68	175	0	10	3.5	4.1	
Shoulder cut, simmered								
Lean and fat (3 pieces, 2½ by 2½ by ¼ in)	3 oz	85	320	0	26	9.3	10.9	
Lean only	2.2 oz	63	135	0	6	2.2	2.6	
Sausage. See also **Pork, cured** Luncheon meat.								
Bologna, slice (8 per 8-oz pkg)	1 slice	28	85	0	8	3.0	3.4	
Braunschweiger, slice (6 per 6-oz pkg)	1 slice	28	90	0	8	2.6	3.4	
Brown and serve (10-11 per 8-oz pkg), cooked	1 link	17	70	0	6	2.3	2.8	
Deviled ham, canned	1 tbsp	13	45	0	4	1.5	1.8	
Frankfurter (8 per 1-lb pkg), heated	1 frankfurter	56	170	0	15	5.6	6.5	
Pork link (16 per 1-lb pkg), cooked	1 link	13	60	0	6	2.1	2.4	
Salami								
Dry, slice (12 per 4-oz pkg)	1 slice	10	45	0	4	1.6	1.6	
Cooked, slice (8 per 8-oz pkg)	1 slice	28	90	0	7	3:1	3.0	
Vienna sausage (7 per 4-oz can)	1 sausage	16	40	0	3	1.2	1.4	
Veal, medium fat, cooked, bone removed								
Cutlet (4 by 2¼ by ½ in), braised or broiled	3 oz	85	185	0	9	4.0	3.4	
Rib (2 pieces, 4 by 2¼ by ¼ in), roasted	3 oz	85	230	0	14	6.1	5.1	
Poultry and Poultry Products								
Chicken, cooked								
Breast, fried in vegetable shortening								
½ breast (3.3 oz with bones)	2.8 oz	79	160	0	5	1.4	1.8	
Drumstick, fried in vegetable shortening (2 oz with bones)	1.3 oz	38	90	0	4	1.1	1.3	
Half broiler, broiled (10.4 oz with bones)	6.2 oz	176	240	0	7	2.2	2.5	
Roast, light meat, skinless	5 oz	140	255	0	6.9	2.2	2.6	
Turkey, roasted								
Dark meat (4 pieces, 2½ by 1⅝ by ¼ in)	3 oz	85	175	0	7	2.1	1.5	
Light meat (2 pieces, 4 by 2 by ¼ in)	3 oz	85	150	0	3	.9	.6	
Light and dark meat, chopped or diced	1 cup	140	265	0	9	2.5	1.7	
FRUITS AND FRUIT PRODUCTS								
Apples, fresh, unpeeled, cored								
2¾-in diam (about 3 per lb with cores)	1 apple	138	80	3.3	1	—	—	
3¼-in diam (about 2 per lb with cores)	1 apple	212	125	5	1	—	—	

Protein	Carbohydrate	Cholesterol	Vitamin A	Thiamin	Riboflavin	Niacin	Ascorbic Acid	Sodium	Calcium	Phosphorous	Iron	Potassium
Grams	Grams	Milligrams	International units	Milligrams	Milligrams	Milligrams	Milligrams	Milligrams	Milligrams	Milligrams	Milligrams	Milligrams
9	1	32	0	.19	.13	1.8	—	740	5	65	1.3	133
19	0	86	0	0.75	0.22	4.5	—	47	9	209	2.7	216
17	0	62	0	.63	.18	3.8	—	42	7	181	2.2	192
21	0	93	0	.78	.22	4.8	—	51	9	218	2.7	233
20	0	75	0	.73	.21	4.4	—	49	9	211	2.6	224
20	0	93	0	.46	.21	4.1	—	47	9	118	2.6	158
18	0	69	0	.42	.19	3.7	—	41	8	111	2.3	146
3	Trace	—	—	.05	.06	.7	—	369	2	36	.5	65
4	1	—	1.850	.05	.41	2.3	—	324	3	69	1.7	—
3	Trace	—	—	—	—	—	—	219	—	—	—	—
2	0	—	0	.02	.01	.2	—	117	1	12	.3	—
7	1	—	—	.08	.11	1.4	—	627	3	57	.8	—
2	Trace	—	0	.10	.04	.5	—	125	1	21	.3	35
2	Trace	—	—	.04	.03	.5	—	226	1	28	.4	—
5	Trace	—	—	.07	.07	1.2	—	298	3	57	.7	—
2	Trace	—	—	.01	.02	.4	—	152	1	24	.3	—
23	0	47	—	.06	.21	4.6	—	55	9	196	2.7	258
23	0	47	—	.11	.26	6.6	—	57	10	211	2.9	259
26	1	58	70	.04	.17	11.6	—	53	9	218	1.3	—
12	Trace	46	50	.03	.15	2.7	—	31	6	89	.9	—
42	0	134	160	.09	.34	15.5	—	116	16	355	3.0	483
5.2	0	119	150	.11	.14	16.5	0	92	15	381	1.8	575
26	0	86	—	.03	.20	3.6	—	84	—	—	2.0	338
28	0	65	—	.04	.12	9.4	—	70	—	—	1.0	349
44	0	124	—	.07	.25	10.8	—	126	11	351	2.5	514
ce	20	0	120	.04	.03	.1	6	1	10	14	.4	152
ice	31	0	190	.06	.04	.2	8	1	15	21	.6	233

A dash in a column for nutrients indicates a lack of reliable data for a constituent believed to be present in measurable amounts.
Notes (¹) are presented numerically at the end of the appendix.

Foods, approximate portions, nutrients, weights (28 grams = 1 ounce)	Portion size	Weight	Food Energy	Fiber	Fat	MACRO Fatty Acids Saturated (total)	Unsaturated Oleic	Linoleic
		Grams	Calories	Grams	Grams	Grams	Grams	Gram
Apple juice, bottled or canned	1 cup	248	120	0	Trace	——	——	—
Applesauce, canned								
Sweetened	1 cup	255	230	5	Trace	——	——	—
Unsweetened.................................	1 cup	244	100	5	Trace	——	——	—
Apricots								
Fresh, without pits (about 12 per lb with pits) ..	3 apricots	107	55	2.1	Trace	——	——	—
Canned in heavy syrup (halves and syrup)	1 cup	258	220	4.4	Trace	——	——	—
Dried (28 large or 37 medium halves per cup)								
Uncooked	1 cup	130	340	10	1	——	——	—
Cooked, unsweetened (fruit and liquid)	1 cup	250	215	10	1	——	——	—
Apricot nectar, canned	1 cup	251	145	0	Trace	——	——	—
Avocados, fresh, whole, without skins and pits								
California, mid and late winter (3-in diam)	1 avocado	216	370	4.3	37	5.5	22.0	
Florida, late summer and fall (4-in diam)	1 avocado	304	390	6.1	33	6.7	15.7	
Bananas (about 2-6 per lb)	1 banana	119	100	4	Trace	——	——	
Blackberries, fresh	1 cup	144	85	10.5	1	——	——	
Blueberries, fresh	1 cup	145	90	3.8	1	——	——	
Cantaloupe. See **Muskmelons.**								
Cherries								
Sour, canned, red, pitted, water pack	1 cup	244	105	3.9	Trace	——	——	
Sweet, fresh, without pits or stems	10 cherries	68	45	1.1	Trace	——	——	
Cranberry juice cocktail, bottled, sweetened ...	1 cup	253	165	0	Trace	——	——	
Cranberry sauce, canned, sweetened	1 cup	277	405	.5	1	——	——	
Dates								
Whole, without pits	10 dates	80	220	7	Trace	——	——	
Chopped.....................................	1 cup	178	490	15.5	1	——	——	
Fruit cocktail, canned in heavy syrup	1 cup	255	195	2.8	Trace	——	——	
Grapefruit								
Fresh, medium, 3¾-in diam, with peel								
Pink or red..................................	½ grapefruit	241	50	1.5	Trace	——	——	
White.......................................	½ grapefruit	241	45	1.5	Trace	——	——	
Canned, sections with syrup	1 cup	254	180	1.0	Trace	——	——	
Grapefruit juice								
Fresh, pink or red	1 cup	246	95	0	Trace	——	——	
White..	1 cup	246	95	0	Trace	——	——	
Canned, white								
Unsweetened	1 cup	247	100	0	Trace	——	——	
Sweetened.................................	1 cup	250	135	0	Trace	——	——	
Frozen concentrate, unsweetened, diluted with								
3 parts water by volume.....................	1 cup	247	100	0	Trace	——	——	

NUTRIENTS			VITAMINS					MINERALS				
Protein	Carbohydrate	Cholesterol	Vitamin A	Thiamin	Riboflavin	Niacin	Ascorbic Acid	Sodium	Calcium	Phosphorous	Iron	Potassium
Grams	Grams	Milligrams	International units	Milligrams	Milligrams	Milligrams	Milligrams	Milligrams	Milligrams	Milligrams	Milligrams	Milligrams
Trace	30	0	—	.02	.05	.2	[6]2	3	15	22	1.5	250
1	61	0	100	.05	.03	.1	[6]3	5	10	13	1.3	166
Trace	26	0	100	.05	.02	.1	[6]2	5	10	12	1.2	190
1	14	0	2,890	.03	.04	.6	11	1	18	25	.5	301
2	57	0	4,490	.05	.05	1.0	10	2	28	39	.8	604
7	86	0	14,170	.01	.21	4.3	16	34	87	140	7.2	1,273
4	54	0	7,500	.01	.13	2.5	8	20	55	88	4.5	795
1	37	0	2,380	.03	.03	.5	36	0	23	30	.5	379
5	13	0	630	.24	.43	3.5	30	5	22	91	1.3	1,303
4	27	0	880	.33	.61	4.9	43	5	30	128	1.8	1,836
1	26	0	230	.06	.07	.8	12	1	10	31	.8	440
2	19	0	290	0.04	0.06	0.6	30	1	46	.09	.71.3	245
1	22	0	150	.04	.09	.7	20	1	22	19	1.5	117
2	26	0	1,660	.07	.05	.5	12	5	37	32	.7	317
1	12	0	70	.03	.04	.3	7	1	15	13	.3	129
Trace	42	0	Trace	.03	.03	.1	81	1	13	8	.8	25
Trace	104	0	60	.03	.03	.1	6	1	17	11	.6	83
2	58	0	40	.07	.08	1.8	0	1	47	50	2.4	518
4	130	0	90	.16	.18	3.9	0	2	105	112	5.3	1,153
1	50	0	360	.05	.03	1.0	5	5	23	31	1.0	411
1	13	0	540	.05	.02	.2	44	1	20	20	.5	166
1	12	0	10	.05	.02	.2	44	1	19	19	.5	159
2	45	0	30	.08	.05	.5	76	4	33	36	.8	343
1	23	0	1,080	10	.05	.5	93	1	22	37	.5	399
1	23	0	20	10	.05	.5	93	1	22	37	.5	399
1	24	0	20	.07	.05	.5	84	2	20	35	1.0	400
1	32	0	30	.08	.05	.5	78	2	20	35	1.0	405
1	24	0	20	.10	.04	.5	96	2	25	42	.2	420

A dash in a column for nutrients indicates a lack of reliable data for a constituent believed to be present in measurable amounts.
Notes (^{1}) are presented numerically at the end of the appendix.

Foods, approximate portions, nutrients, weights (28 grams = 1 ounce)	Portion size	Weight	Food Energy	Fiber	Fat	Saturated (total)	Oleic	Linoleic
		Grams	Calories	Grams	Grams	Grams	Grams	Gram
Grapes, fresh								
Thompson Seedless (green)	10 grapes	50	35	0.5	Trace	——	——	—
Tokay and Emperor (red), seeded	10 grapes	60	40	0.5	Trace	——	——	—
Grape juice								
Bottled or canned	1 cup	253	165	0	Trace	——	——	—
Frozen concentrate, sweetened, diluted with 3 parts water by volume	1 cup	250	135	0	Trace	——	——	—
Grape drink, canned	1 cup	250	135	0	Trace	——	——	—
Lemon, fresh, without peel and seeds	1 lemon	74	20	5.2	Trace	——	——	—
Lemon juice	1 tbsp	15	4	0	Trace	——	——	—
Fresh	1 cup	244	60	0	Trace	——	——	—
Bottled or canned, unsweetened	1 cup	244	55	0	Trace	——	——	—
Lemonade, frozen concentrate, diluted with 4⅓ parts water by volume	1 cup	248	105	0	Trace	——	——	—
Limeade, frozen concentrate, diluted with 4⅓ parts water by volume	1 cup	247	100	0	Trace	——	——	—
Lime juice								
Fresh	1 cup	246	65	0	Trace	——	——	—
Canned, unsweetened	1 cup	246	65	0	Trace	——	——	—
Muskmelons, fresh, with rind, without seed cavity								
Cantaloupe, orange-fleshed (5-in diam)	½ melon	477	80	7.6	Trace	——	——	
Honeydew (6½-in diam)	1/10 melon	226	50	2	Trace	——	——	
Oranges, all varieties, fresh								
Whole, 3-in diam, without peel and seeds	1 orange	131	65	2.7	Trace	——	——	
Sections, without membranes	1 cup	180	90	3.7	Trace	——	——	
Orange juice								
Fresh, all varieties	1 cup	248	110	0	Trace	——	——	
Canned, unsweetened	1 cup	249	120	0	Trace	——	——	
Frozen concentrate, unsweetened, diluted with 3 parts water by volume	1 cup	249	120	0	Trace	——	——	
Papayas, fresh, ½-in cubes	1 cup	140	55	——	Trace	——	——	
Peaches								
Fresh, yellow-fleshed								
Whole, 2½-in diam, peeled, pitted (about 4 per lb with peels and pits)	1 peach	100	40	1.4	Trace	——	——	
Sliced	1 cup	170	65	2.4	Trace	——	——	
Canned, fruit and liquid (halves or slices)								
Syrup pack	1 cup	256	200	2.5	Trace	——	——	
Water packed	1 cup	244	75	2.4	Trace	——	——	

NUTRIENTS			VITAMINS					MINERALS				
Protein	Carbohydrate	Cholesterol	Vitamin A	Thiamin	Riboflavin	Niacin	Ascorbic Acid	Sodium	Calcium	Phosphorous	Iron	Potassium
Grams	Grams	Milli-grams	Inter-national units	Milli-grams	Milli-grams	Milli-grams	Milli-grams	Milli-grams	Milli-grams	Milli-grams	Milli-grams	Milli-grams
Trace	9	0	50	.03	.02	.2	2	1	6	10	.2	87
Trace	10	0	60	.03	.02	.2	2	1	7	11	.2	99
1	42	0	—	.10	.05	.5	[6]Trace	5	28	30	.8	293
1	33	0	10	.05	.08	.5	[6]10	7	8	10	.3	85
Trace	35	0	—	(⁷)	(⁷)	.3	11	2	8	10	.3	88
1	6	0	10	.03	.01	.1	39	2	19	12	.4	102
.1	1.2	0	Trace	Trace	Trace	Trace	7	Trace	1	2	Trace	21
1	20	0	50	.07	.02	.2	112	1	17	24	.5	344
1	19	0	50	.07	.02	.2	102	1	17	24	.5	344
Trace	28	0	10	.01	.02	.2	17	Trace	2	3	.1	40
Trace	27	0	Trace	Trace	Trace	Trace	6	Trace	3	3	Trace	32
1	22	0	20	.05	.02	.2	79	1	22	27	.5	256
1	22	0	20	.05	.02	.2	52	1	22	27	.5	256
2	20	0	9,240	.11	.08	1.6	90	57	38	44	1.1	682
1	11	0	60	.06	.04	.9	34	27	21	24	.6	374
1	16	0	260	.13	.05	.5	66	1	54	26	.5	263
2	22	0	360	.18	.07	.7	90	1	74	36	.7	360
2	26	0	500	.22	.07	1.0	124	1	27	42	.5	496
2	28	0	500	.17	.05	.7	100	1	25	45	1.0	496
2	29	0	540	.23	.03	.9	120	1	25	42	.2	503
1	14	0	2,450	.06	.06	.4	78	3	28	22	.4	328
1	10	0	1,330	.02	.05	1.0	7	1	9	19	.5	202
1	16	0	2,260	.03	.09	1.7	12	1	15	32	.9	343
1	51	0	1,100	.03	.05	1.5	8	5	10	31	.8	333
1	20	0	1,100	.02	.07	1.5	7	5	10	32	.7	334

A dash in a column for nutrients indicates a lack of reliable data for a constituent believed to be present in measurable amounts.
Notes (¹) are presented numerically at the end of the appendix.

Foods, approximate portions, nutrients, weights (28 grams = 1 ounce)	Portion size	Weight	Food Energy	Fiber	Fat	Saturated (total)	Unsaturated Oleic	Unsaturated Linoleic
		Grams	Calories	Grams	Grams	Grams	Grams	Grams
Dried								
Uncooked	1 cup	160	420	23.4	1	—	—	—
Frozen, sliced, sweetened, ascorbic acid added								
10-oz container	1 container	284	250	—	Trace	—	—	—
Cup	1 cup	250	220	—	Trace	—	—	—
Pears								
Fresh, with skin, cored								
Bartlett, 2½-in diam (about 2½ per lb with cores and stems)	1 pear	164	100	2.8	1	—	—	—
Bosc, 2½-in diam (about 3 per lb with cores and stems)	1 pear	141	85	3.4	1	—	—	—
D'Anjou, 3-in diam (about 2 per lb with cores and stems)	1 pear	200	120	4.9	1	—	—	—
Canned in heavy syrup (fruit and liquid)	1 cup	255	195	4.2	1	—	—	—
Pineapple								
Fresh, diced	1 cup	155	80	1.6	Trace	—	—	—
Canned in heavy syrup (fruit and liquid)								
Crushed, chunks, tidbits	1 cup	255	190	2.6	Trace	—	—	—
Slices and liquid, medium	1 slice	58	45	.6	Trace	—	—	—
Pineapple juice, unsweetened, canned	1 cup	250	140	0	Trace	—	—	—
Plums								
Fresh, without pits								
Japanese and hybrid (2-in diam, about 6½ per lb with pits)	1 plum	66	30	1.4	Trace	—	—	—
Prune-type (1½-in diam, about 15 per lb with pits)	1 plum	28	20	.6	Trace	—	—	—
Canned in heavy syrup								
Cup	1 cup	272	215	5.9	Trace	—	—	—
Portion	3 plums	140	110	3.1	Trace	—	—	—
Prunes, dried, "softenized," with pits								
Uncooked, large	5 prunes	49	110	7.8	Trace	—	—	—
Cooked, unsweetened, all sizes, fruit and liquid	1 cup	250	255	20	1	—	—	—
Prune juice, bottled or canned	1 cup	256	195	0	Trace	—	—	—
Raisins, seedless								
Cup	1 cup	145	420	10.4	Trace	—	—	—
Packet, ½ oz (1½ tbsp)	1 packet	14	40	1	Trace	—	—	—
Raspberries, red								
Fresh, hulled, whole	1 cup	123	70	9.1	1	—	—	—
Frozen, sweetened, 10-oz container	1 container	284	280	21	1	—	—	—
Rhubarb, cooked, added sugar								
Fresh	1 cup	270	380	7	Trace	—	—	—
Frozen, sweetened	1 cup	270	385	7	1	—	—	—

378

NUTRIENTS			VITAMINS					MINERALS				
Protein	Carbohydrate	Cholesterol	Vitamin A	Thiamin	Riboflavin	Niacin	Ascorbic Acid	Sodium	Calcium	Phosphorous	Iron	Potassium
Grams	Grams	Milli-grams	Inter-national units	Milli-grams	Milli-grams	Milli-grams	Milli-grams	Milli-grams	Milli-grams	Milli-grams	Milli-grams	Milli-grams
5	109	0	6,240	.02	.30	8.5	29	24	77	187	9.6	1,520
1	64	0	1,850	0.03	0.11	2.0	116	5	11	37	1.4	352
1	57	0	1,630	.03	.10	1.8	103	5	10	33	1.3	310
1	25	0	30	.03	.07	.2	7	3	13	18	.5	213
1	22	0	30	.03	.06	.1	6	1	11	16	.4	83
1	31	0	40	.04	.08	.2	8	1	16	22	.6	260
1	50	0	10	.03	.05	.3	3	1	13	18	.5	214
1	21	0	110	.14	.05	.3	26	1	26	12	.8	226
1	49	0	130	.20	.05	.5	18	2	28	13	.8	245
Trace	11	0	30	.05	.01	.1	4	Trace	6	3	.2	56
1	34	0	130	.13	.05	.5	80	3	38	23	.8	373
Trace	8	0	160	.02	.02	.3	4	2	8	12	.3	112
Trace	6	0	80	.01	.01	.1	1	1	3	5	.1	48
1	56	0	3,130	.05	.05	1.0	5	3	23	26	2.3	367
1	29	0	1,610	.03	.03	.5	3	1	12	13	1.2	189
1	29	0	690	.04	.07	.7	1	5	22	34	1.7	298
2	67	0	1,590	.07	.15	1.5	2	10	51	79	3.8	695
1	49	0	——	.03	.03	1.0	5	6	36	51	1.8	602
4	112	0	30	.16	.12	.7	1	50	90	146	5.1	1,106
Trace	11	0	Trace	.02	.01	1	Trace	5	9	14	.5	107
1	17	0	160	.04	.11	1.1	31	1	27	27	1.1	207
2	70	0	200	.06	.17	1.7	60	1	37	48	1.7	284
1	97	0	220	.05	.14	.8	16	2	211	41	1.6	548
1	98	0	190	.05	.11	.5	16	4	211	32	1.9	475

A dash in a column for nutrients indicates a lack of reliable data for a constituent believed to be present in measurable amounts.
Notes ([1]) are presented numerically at the end of the appendix.

Foods, approximate portions, nutrients, weights (28 grams = 1 ounce)	Portion size	Weight	Food Energy	Fiber	Fat	Saturated (total)	Oleic	Linoleic
MACRO- / Fatty Acids / Unsaturated								
		Grams	Calories	Grams	Grams	Grams	Grams	Grams
Strawberries								
Fresh, whole berries, hulled	1 cup	149	55	3.2	1	—	—	—
Frozen, sweetened								
Sliced, 10-oz container	1 container	284	310	6.1	1	—	—	—
Whole, 1 lb-container	1 container	454	415	9.8	1	—	—	—
Tangerine, fresh, 2½-in diam	1 tangerine	86	40	1.7	Trace	—	—	—
Tangerine juice, canned, sweetened	1 cup	249	125	0	Trace	—	—	—
Watermelon, fresh, with rind and seeds, 4 by 8 in wedge	1 wedge	926	110	8.1	1	—	—	—
GRAIN PRODUCTS; RELATED PRODUCTS								
Bagel, 3-in diam								
Egg	1 bagel	55	165	1.1	2	0.5	0.9	0
Water	1 bagel	55	165	1.1	1	.2	.4	
Biscuits, baking powder, 2-in diam (enriched flour, vegetable shortening)								
From home recipe	1 biscuit	28	105	.6	5	1.2	2.0	1
From mix	1 biscuit	28	90	.6	3	.6	1.1	
Breadcrumbs (enriched)								
Dry, grated	1 cup	100	390	3.4	5	1.0	1.6	1
Soft	1 cup	45	120	1.5	1	.3	.5	
Breads								
Boston brown bread (white cornmeal), canned, slice (½-in)	1 slice	45	95	1.6	1	.1	.2	
Cracked-wheat bread (¾ enriched wheat flour, ¼ cracked wheat), slice (18 per 1-lb loaf) ...	1 slice	25	65	1.3	1	.1	.2	
French bread (enriched), slice (5 by 2½ in)	1 slice	35	100	1	1	.2	.4	
Raisin bread (enriched), slice (18 per 1-lb loaf)	1 slice	25	65	.5	1	.2	.3	
Rye bread								
American, light (⅔ enriched wheat flour, ⅓ rye flour), slice (4¾ by 3¾ in)	1 slice	25	60	.8	Trace	Trace	Trace	
Pumpernickel (⅔ rye flour, ⅓ enriched wheat flour), slice (5 by 4 in).....................	1 slice	32	80	1.5	Trace	.1	Trace	
White bread (enriched)								
Soft-crumb type								
Slice (18 per 1-lb loaf)	1 slice	25	70	.7	1	.2	.3	
Slice (22 per 1-lb loaf)	1 slice	20	55	.5	1	.2	.2	
Cubes	1 cup	30	80	.8	1	.2	.3	
Firm-crumb type								
Slice (20 per 1-lb loaf)	1 slice	23	65	.6	1	.2	.3	
Slice (34 per 2-lb loaf)	1 slice	27	75	.7	1	.2	.3	
Whole-wheat bread								
Soft-crumb type								
Slice (16 per 1-lb loaf).....................	1 slice	28	65	1.4	1	.1	.2	

NUTRIENTS			VITAMINS					MINERALS				
Protein	Carbohydrate	Cholesterol	Vitamin A	Thiamin	Riboflavin	Niacin	Ascorbic Acid	Sodium	Calcium	Phosphorous	Iron	Potassium
Grams	Grams	Milligrams	International units	Milligrams	Milligrams	Milligrams	Milligrams	Milligrams	Milligrams	Milligrams	Milligrams	Milligrams
1	13	0	90	0.04	0.10	0.9	88	1	31	31	1.5	244
1	79	0	90	.06	.17	1.4	151	2	40	48	2.0	318
2	107	0	140	.09	.27	2.3	249	4	59	73	2.7	472
1	10	0	360	.05	.02	.1	27	2	34	15	.3	108
1	30	0	1,040	.15	.05	.2	54	2	44	35	.5	440
2	27	0	2,510	.13	.13	.9	30	9	30	43	2.1	426
6	28	—	30	.14	.10	1.2	0	205	9	43	1.2	41
6	30	0	0	.15	.11	1.4	0	205	8	41	1.2	42
2	13	0	Trace	.08	.08	.7	Trace	175	34	49	.4	33
2	15	0	Trace	.09	.08	.8	Trace	272	19	65	.6	32
13	73	0	Trace	.35	.35	4.8	Trace	736	122	141	3.6	152
4	23	0	Trace	.18	.11	1.5	Trace	331	38	44	1.1	47
2	21	0	0	.06	.04	.7	0	120	41	72	.9	131
2	13	0	Trace	.08	.06	.8	Trace	125	22	32	.5	34
3	19	0	Trace	.14	.08	1.2	Trace	203	15	30	.8	32
2	13	0	Trace	.09	.06	.6	Trace	85	18	22	.6	58
2	13	0	0	.07	.05	.7	0	128	19	37	.5	36
3	17	0	0	.09	.07	.6	0	182	27	73	.8	145
2	13	0	Trace	.10	.06	.8	Trace	127	21	24	.6	26
2	10	0	Trace	.08	.05	.7	Trace	102	17	19	.5	21
3	15	0	Trace	.12	.07	1.0	Trace	153	25	29	.8	32
2	12	0	Trace	.09	.06	.8	Trace	117	22	23	.6	28
2	14	0	Trace	.11	.06	.9	Trace	120	26	28	.7	33
3	14	0	Trace	.09	.03	.8	Trace	121	24	71	.8	72

A dash in a column for nutrients indicates a lack of reliable data for a constituent believed to be present in measurable amounts.
Notes (¹) are presented numerically at the end of the appendix.

Foods, approximate portions, nutrients, weights (28 grams = 1 ounce)	Portion size	Weight	Food Energy	Fiber	Fat	MACRO- Fatty Acids Saturated (total)	Unsaturated Oleic	Linoleic
		Grams	Calories	Grams	Grams	Grams	Grams	Grams
Firm-crumb type								
Slice (18 per 1-lb loaf)	1 slice	25	60	1.3	1	.1	.2	.3
Breakfast cereals								
Hot, cooked								
Corn (hominy) grits, white variety, degermed								
Enriched	1 cup	245	125	4	Trace	Trace	Trace	
Farina, quick cooking, enriched, without								
disodium phosphate	1 cup	245	105	.9	Trace	Trace	Trace	
Oatmeal or rolled oats	1 cup	240	130	5.4	2	.4	.8	
Wheat, rolled	1 cup	240	180	6	1	—	—	—
Wheat, whole meal	1 cup	245	110	5.2	1	—	—	—
Ready to eat								
Bran flakes (40% bran), added sugar, salt,								
iron, vitamins	1 cup	35	105	6	1	—	—	—
Bran flakes with raisins, added sugar, salt,								
iron, vitamins, added nutrients	1 cup	50	145	10.2	1	—	—	—
Corn flakes								
Plain, added sugar, salt, iron, vitamins	1 cup	25	95	3.1	Trace	—	—	—
Sugar coated, added salt, iron, vitamins	1 cup	40	155	3.1	Trace	—	—	—
Corn, puffed, plain, added sugar, salt, iron,								
vitamins	1 cup	20	80	4.5	1	—	—	—
Corn, shredded, added sugar, salt, iron,								
thiamin, niacin	1 cup	25	95	3.1	Trace	—	—	—
Oats, puffed, added sugar, salt, minerals,								
vitamins	1 cup	25	100	3	1	—	—	—
Rice, puffed								
Plain, added iron, thiamin, niacin	1 cup	15	60	.7	Trace	—	—	—
Presweetened, added salt, iron, vitamins	1 cup	28	115	.7	0	—	—	—
Wheat flakes, added sugar, salt, iron, vitamins	1 cup	30	105	1.5	Trace	—	—	—
Wheat, puffed								
Plain, added iron, thiamin, niacin	1 cup	15	55	2.5	Trace	—	—	—
Presweetened, added salt, iron, vitamins	1 cup	38	140	2.5	Trace	—	—	—
Wheat, shredded, plain	1 biscuit	25	90	3.3	1	—	—	—
Wheat germ, without salt and sugar, toasted ..	1 tbsp	6	25	.6	1	—	—	—
Buckwheat flour, light, sifted	1 cup	98	340	1.6	1	0.2	0.4	
Bulgur (parboiled wheat), canned, seasoned	1 cup	135	245	1.2	4	—	—	—
Cake icings. See **Sugars and Sweets.**								
Cakes, made from cake mixes (enriched flour)								
Angel food (9¾-in diam tube cake), piece (1/12								
of cake)	1 piece	53	135	0	Trace	—	—	—
Coffee cake (7¾ by 6 in), piece (1/6 of cake)	1 piece	72	230	.1	7	2.0	2.7	
Cupcakes, made with egg, milk (2½-in diam)								
Without icing	1 cupcake	25	90	<1	3	.8	1.2	
With chocolate icing	1 cupcake	36	130	<1	5	2.0	1.6	

382

NUTRIENTS			VITAMINS					MINERALS				
Protein	Carbohydrate	Cholesterol	Vitamin A	Thiamin	Riboflavin	Niacin	Ascorbic Acid	Sodium	Calcium	Phosphorous	Iron	Potassium
Grams	Grams	Milli-grams	Inter-national units	Milli-grams	Milli-grams	Milli-grams	Milli-grams	Milli-grams	Milli-grams	Milli-grams	Milli-grams	Milli-grams
3	12	0	Trace	.06	.03	.7	Trace	119	25	57	.8	68
3	27	0	Trace	.10	.07	1.0	0	500	2	25	.7	27
3	22	0	0	(7)	.07	1.0	0	2	147	113	12	25
5	23	0	0	.19	.05	.2	0	5	22	137	1.4	146
5	41	0	0	.17	.07	2.2	0	3	19	182	1.7	202
4	23	0	0	.15	.05	1.5	0	3	17	127	1.2	118
4	28	0	1,540	.46	.52	6.2	0	425	19	125	5.6	137
4	40	0	[8]2,200	(7)	(7)	(7)	0	667	28	146	7.9	154
2	21	0	(7)	(7)	(7)	(7)	[8]13	229	(7)	9	(7)	30
2	37	0	1,760	.53	.60	7.1	21	391	1	10	(7)	27
2	16	0	880	.26	.30	3.5	11	220	4	18	5.7	——
2	22	0	0	.33	.05	4.4	13	277	1	10	.6	——
3	19	0	1,100	.33	.38	4.4	13	271	44	102	4.0	——
1	13	0	0	.07	.01	.7	0	1	3	14	.3	15
1	26	0	1,240	(7)	(7)	(7)	[8]15	377	3	14	(7)	43
3	24	0	1,320	.40	.45	5.3	16	380	12	83	4.8	81
2	12	0	0	.08	.03	1.2	0	1	4	48	.6	51
3	33	0	1,680	.50	.57	6.7	[8]20	62	7	52	(7)	63
2	20	0	0	.06	.03	1.1	0	3	11	97	.9	87
2	3	0	10	.11	.05	.3	1	1	3	70	.5	57
6	78	0	0	.08	.04	.4	0	1	11	86	1.0	314
8	44	0	0	.08	.05	4.1	0	810	27	263	1.9	151
3	32	0	0	.03	.08	.3	0	1,792	50	63	.2	32
5	38	——	120	.14	.15	1.3	Trace	310	44	125	1.2	78
1	14	——	40	.05	.05	.4	Trace	120	40	.4	.3	21
2	21	——	60	.05	.06	.4	Trace	134	47	71	.4	42

A dash in a column for nutrients indicates a lack of reliable data for a constituent believed to be present in measurable amounts.
Notes (¹) are presented numerically at the end of the appendix.

Foods, approximate portions, nutrients, weights (28 grams = 1 ounce)	Portion size	Weight	Food Energy	Fiber	Fat	Saturated (total)	Oleic	Linoleic
		Grams	Calories	Grams	Grams	Grams	Grams	Grams
Devil's food with chocolate icing (2-layer cake, 8- or 9-in diam)								
Piece (1/16 of cake)	1 piece	69	235	<1	8	3.1	2.8	1
Cupcake (2½-in diam)	1 cupcake	35	120	<1	4	1.6	1.4	
Gingerbread (8-in square), piece (1/9 of cake)	1 piece	63	175	<1	4	1.1	1.8	1
White (2-layer with chocolate icing, 8- or 9-in diam), piece (1/16 of cake)	1 piece	71	250	<1	8	3.0	2.9	1
Yellow (2-layer with chocolate icing, 8- or 9-in diam), piece (1/16 of cake)	1 piece	69	235	<1	8	3.0	3.0	1
Boston cream pie with custard filling (8-in diam), piece (1/12 of cake)	1 piece	69	210	<1	6	1.9	2.5	1
Fruitcake, dark (loaf, 1-lb, 7½ by 2 by 1½ in), slice (1/30 of loaf)	1 slice	15	55	<1	2	.5	1.1	
Plain, sheet cake (9-in square)								
Without icing, piece (1/9 of cake)	1 piece	86	315	<1	12	3.3	4.9	2
With uncooked white icing, piece (1/9 of cake)	1 piece	121	445	<1	14	4.7	5.5	2
Pound (loaf, 8½ by 3½ by 3¼ in), slice (1/17 of loaf)	1 slice	33	160	<1	10	2.5	4.3	
Sponge cake with butter icing (9¾-in diam tube cake), piece (1/12 of cake)	1 piece	66	195	<1	4	1.1	1.3	
Cookies (enriched flour, except for macaroons)								
Brownies, with nuts (1¾ by 1¾ by 1 in)								
From home recipe	1 brownie	20	95	<1	6	1.5	3.0	
From mix	1 brownie	20	85	<1	4	.9	1.4	
Frozen, with chocolate icing made with butter (1½ by 1¾ by 1 in)	1 brownie	25	105	<1	5	2.0	2.2	
Chocolate chip								
Commercial (2½-in diam, ⅜ in thick)	4 cookies	42	200	0	9	2.8	2.9	
From home recipe (2⅓-in diam)	4 cookies	40	205	0	12	3.5	4.5	
Fig bars, square (1⅝ by 1⅝ by ⅜ in)	4 cookies	56	200	2	3	.8	1.2	
Gingersnaps (2-in diam, ¼-in thick)	4 cookies	28	90	0	2	.7	1.0	
Macaroons (2¾-in diam, ¼ in thick)	2 cookies	38	180	0	9	—	—	
Oatmeal, with raisins (3-in diam, ¼ in thick)	4 cookies	52	235	1.5	8	2.0	3.3	
Plain, from commercial chilled dough (2½-in diam, ¼ in thick)	4 cookies	48	240	0	12	3.0	5.2	
Sandwich type (chocolate or vanilla, 1¾-in diam, ⅜ in thick)	4 cookies	40	200	0	9	2.2	3.9	
Vanilla wafers (1¾-in diam, ¼ in thick)	10 cookies	40	185	0	6	—	—	
Cornmeal, yellow variety								
Whole ground, unbolted, dry form	1 cup	122	435	18.6	5	.5	1.0	
Bolted (nearly whole grain), dry form	1 cup	122	440	18.7	4	.5	.9	
Degermed, enriched								
Dry form	1 cup	138	500	13	2	.2	.4	
Cooked	1 cup	240	120	3.1	Trace	Trace	.1	

MACRO-

Fatty Acids

Unsaturated

NUTRIENTS			VITAMINS					MINERALS				
Protein	Carbohydrate	Cholesterol	Vitamin A	Thiamin	Riboflavin	Niacin	Ascorbic Acid	Sodium	Calcium	Phosphorous	Iron	Potassium
Grams	Grams	Milli-grams	International units	Milli-grams	Milli-grams	Milli-grams	Milli-grams	Milli-grams	Milli-grams	Milli-grams	Milli-grams	Milli-grams
3	40	——	100	.07	.10	.6	Trace	181	41	72	1.0	90
2	20	——	50	.03	.05	.3	Trace	92	21	37	.5	46
2	32	——	Trace	.09	.11	.8	Trace	192	57	63	.9	173
3	45	——	40	.09	.11	.8	Trace	161	70	127	.7	82
3	40	——	100	.08	.10	.7	Trace	157	63	126	.8	75
3	34	——	140	.09	.11	.8	Trace	120	46	70	.7	61
1	9	——	20	.02	.02	.2	Trace	24	11	17	.4	74
4	48	——	150	.13	.15	1.1	Trace	279	55	88	.9	68
4	77	——	240	.14	.16	1.1	Trace	340	61	91	.8	74
2	16	——	80	.05	.06	.4	0	30	6	24	.5	20
5	36	——	300	.09	.14	.6	Trace	111	20	74	1.1	57
1	10	——	40	.04	.03	.2	Trace	50	8	30	.4	38
1	13	——	20	.03	.02	.2	Trace	55	9	27	.4	34
1	15	——	50	.03	.03	.2	Trace	50	10	31	.4	44
2	29	——	50	.10	.17	.9	Trace	168	16	48	1.0	56
2	24	——	40	.06	.06	.5	Trace	168	14	40	.8	47
2	42	0	60	.04	.14	.9	Trace	0	44	34	1.0	111
2	22	0	20	.08	.06	.7	0	161	20	13	.7	129
2	25	——	0	.02	.06	.2	0	14	10	32	.3	176
3	38	0	30	.15	.10	1.0	Trace	85	11	53	1.4	192
2	31	——	30	0.10	0.08	0.9	0	264	17	35	0.6	23
2	28	——	0	.06	.10	.7	0	195	10	96	.7	15
2	30	——	50	.10	.09	.8	0	102	16	25	.6	29
11	90	——	620	.46	.13	2.4	0	1,690	24	312	2.9	346
11	91	——	590	.37	.10	2.3	0	1,690	21	272	2.2	303
11	108	——	610	.61	.36	4.8	0	1,690	8	137	4.0	166
3	26	——	140	.14	.10	1.2	0	0	2	34	1.0	38

A dash in a column for nutrients indicates a lack of reliable data for a constituent believed to be present in measurable amounts.
Notes (^{1}) are presented numerically at the end of the appendix.

Foods, approximate portions, nutrients, weights (28 grams = 1 ounce)	Portion size	Weight	Food Energy	Fiber	Fat	MACRO- Fatty Acids Saturated (total)	Unsaturated Oleic	Linoleic
		Grams	Calories	Grams	Grams	Grams	Grams	Grams
Degermed, unenriched								
Dry form	1 cup	138	500	13	2	.2	.4	.9
Cooked	1 cup	240	120	3.1	Trace	Trace	.1	.2
Crackers, made with vegetable shortening								
Graham, plain (2½-in square)	2 crackers	14	55	<1	1	.3	.5	.3
Rye wafers, whole grain (1⅞ by 3½ in)	2 wafers	13	45	<1	Trace	—	—	—
Saltines, made with enriched flour	4 crackers	11	50	0	1	.3	.5	.4
Danish pastry, plain, without fruit or nuts (enriched flour, vegetable shortening, butter), (round pieces, about 4¼-in diam by 1 in)	1 pastry	65	275	<1	15	4.7	6.1	3.2
Doughnuts, made with enriched flour and vegetable shortening								
Cake type, plain (2½-in diam, 1 in high)	1 doughnut	25	100	<1	5	1.2	2.0	1.
Yeast leavened, glazed (3¾-in diam, 1¼ in high)	1 doughnut	50	205	<1	11	3.3	5.8	3.
Flours								
All-purpose white flour	100 g.	100	365.4	3	.87	.17	.09	.4
Soy flours	100 g.	100	420.2	11.9	20.2	0	0	
Wheat flours								
All-purpose or family flour, enriched, sifted, spooned	1 cup	115	420	4	1	.2	.1	
All-purpose or family flour, enriched, unsifted, unspooned	1 cup	125	455	4	1	.2	.1	
Cake or pastry flour, enriched, sifted, spooned	1 cup	96	350	3	1	.1	.1	
Self-rising, enriched, unsifted, unspooned	1 cup	125	440	5	1	.2	.1	
Whole wheat bread flour	1 cup	120	400	9	2	.4	.2	
Macaroni, enriched, cut lengths, elbows, shells								
Cooked, firm stage, "al dente"	1 cup	130	190	2	1	—	—	—
Cooked, tender stage	1 cup	140	155	2	1	—	—	—
Muffins, made with enriched flour and vegetable shortening								
From home recipe								
Blueberry (2-in diam, 1½ in high)	1 muffin	40	110	1	4	1.1	1.4	
Bran	1 muffin	40	105	3.3	4	1.2	1.4	
Corn (enriched, degermed yellow cornmeal and flour, 3-in diam, 1½ in high)	1 muffin	40	125	1	4	1.2	1.6	
Plain (3-in diam, 1½ in high)	1 muffin	40	120	1	4	1.0	1.7	
From mix (degermed yellow cornmeal, enriched flour), egg, milk								
Corn (3-in diam, 1½ in high)	1 muffin	40	130	1	4	1.2	1.7	
Noodles (egg noodles), enriched, cooked	1 cup	160	200	2	2	—	—	—

NUTRIENTS			VITAMINS					MINERALS				
Protein	Carbohydrate	Cholesterol	Vitamin A	Thiamin	Riboflavin	Niacin	Ascorbic Acid	Sodium	Calcium	Phosphorous	Iron	Potassium
Grams	Grams	Milli-grams	Inter-national units	Milli-grams	Milli-grams	Milli-grams	Milli-grams	Milli-grams	Milli-grams	Milli-grams	Milli-grams	Milli-grams
11	108	——	610	.19	.07	1.4	0	1,690	8	137	1.5	166
3	26	——	140	.05	.02	.2	0	0	2	34	.5	38
1	10	——	0	.02	.08	.5	0	94	6	21	.5	55
2	10	——	0	.04	.03	.2	0	124	7	50	.5	78
1	8	——	0	.05	.05	.4	0	132	2	10	.5	13
5	30	——	200	.18	.19	1.7	Trace	1,243	33	71	1.2	73
1	13	10	20	.05	.05	.4	Trace	125	10	48	.4	23
3	22	13	25	.10	.10	.8	0	117	16	33	.6	34
10.4	76.6	0	0	.64	.4	5.3	0	1.7	15.7	87	2.9	87
36.6	30.3	0	110	.85	.31	2.1	0	1.1	198.7	556.8	8.4	1660
12	88	0	0	.74	.46	6.1	0	2	18	100	3.3	109
13	95	0	0	.8	.5	6.6	0	2	20	109	3.6	119
7	76	0	0	.61	.38	5.1	0	2	16	70	2.8	91
12	93	0	0	.80	.5	6.6	0	1,348	331	583	3.6	——
16	85	0	0	.66	.14	5.2	0	2	49	446	4	458.4
7	39	——	0	.23	.13	1.8	0	1	14	85	1.4	103
5	32	——	0	.20	.11	1.5	0	1	11	70	1.3	85
3	17	0	90	.09	.10	.7	Trace	253	34	53	.6	46
3	17	0	90	.07	.10	1.7	Trace	179	57	162	1.5	172
3	19	0	120	.10	.10	.7	Trace	192	42	68	.7	54
3	17	0	40	0.09	0.12	0.9	Trace	176	42	60	0.6	50
3	20	0	100	.08	.09	.7	Trace	192	96	152	.6	44
7	37	——	110	.22	.13	1.9	0	3	16	94	1.4	70

A dash in a column for nutrients indicates a lack of reliable data for a constituent believed to be present in measurable amounts.
Notes (^{1}) are presented numerically at the end of the appendix.

Foods, approximate portions, nutrients, weights (28 grams = 1 ounce)	Portion size	Weight	Food Energy	Fiber	Fat	Saturated (total)	Unsaturated Oleic	Linoleic
		Grams	Calories	Grams	Grams	Grams	Grams	Grams
Pancakes, made with vegetable shortening (4-in diam)								
Buckwheat, made from mix (buckwheat and enriched flours), egg, milk	1 cake	27	55	1	2	.8	.9	
Plain								
From mix (enriched flour), egg, milk	1 cake	27	60	1	2	.7	.7	
Pies, piecrust made with enriched flour, vegetable shortening (9-in diam)								
Apple, sector (1/7 of pie)	1 sector	135	345	2	15	3.9	6.4	3
Banana cream, sector (1/7 of pie)	1 sector	130	285	1.5	12	3.8	4.7	2
Blueberry, sector (1/7 of pie)................	1 sector	135	325	3	15	3.5	6.2	3
Cherry, sector (1/7 of pie)	1 sector	135	350	1	15	4.0	6.4	3
Custard, sector (1/7 of pie)	1 sector	130	285	<1	14	4.8	5.5	2
Lemon meringue, sector (1/7 of pie)	1 sector	120	305	<1	12	3.7	4.8	2
Mince, sector (1/7 of pie)	1 sector	135	365	2	16	4.0	6.6	3
Peach, sector (1/7 of pie)	1 sector	135	345	3	14	3.5	6.2	3
Pecan, sector (1/7 of pie)	1 sector	118	495	3	27	4.0	14.4	
Pumpkin, sector (1/7 of pie)	1 sector	130	275	3	15	5.4	5.4	
Piecrust, home recipe, made with enriched flour and vegetable shortening (9-in diam)	1 pie shell	180	900	2	60	14.8	26.1	1
Piecrust mix, with enriched flour and vegetable shortening, 10-oz pkg (9-in diam) .	Piecrust for 2-crust pie	320	1,485	2	93	22.7	39.7	2
Pizza, cheese (4¾-in sector)	1 sector	60	145	<1	4	1.7	1.5	
Popcorn, popped								
Plain, large kernel	1 cup	6	25	1	Trace	Trace	.1	
With oil (coconut) and salt added, large kernel .	1 cup	9	40	1	2	1.5	.2	
Sugar coated................................	1 cup	35	135	1	1	.5	.2	
Pretzels (enriched flour)								
Dutch, twisted (2¾ by 2⅝ in)	1 pretzel	16	60	0	1	——	——	
Thin, twisted (3¼ by 2¼ by ¼ in)	10 pretzels	60	235	1	3	——	——	
Stick (2¼ in long)	10 pretzels	3	10	0	Trace	——	——	
Rice (white, enriched)								
Instant, ready-to-serve	1 cup	165	180	1.5	Trace	Trace	Trace	
Long grain, cooked	1 cup	205	225	2	Trace	.1	.1	
Parboiled, cooked	1 cup	175	185	2	Trace	.1	.1	
Brown, cooked	1 cup	195	232	4.8	1.2	0	0	
Rolls (enriched, made with vegetable shortening) Commercial								
Brown-and-serve (12 per 12-oz pkg), browned	1 roll	26	85	<1	2	.4	.7	
Cloverleaf or pan (2½-in diam)	1 roll	28	85	<1	2	.4	.6	
Frankfurter and hamburger (8 per 11½-oz pkg)	1 roll	40	120	<1	2	.5	.8	

MACRO-

NUTRIENTS			VITAMINS					MINERALS				
Protein	Carbohydrate	Cholesterol	Vitamin A	Thiamin	Riboflavin	Niacin	Ascorbic Acid	Sodium	Calcium	Phosphorous	Iron	Potassium
Grams	Grams	Milli-grams	Inter-national units	Milli-grams	Milli-grams	Milli-grams	Milli-grams	Milli-grams	Milli-grams	Milli-grams	Milli-grams	Milli-grams
2	6	0	60	.04	.05	.2	Trace	125	59	91	.4	66
2	9	0	70	.04	.06	.2	Trace	152	58	70	.3	42
3	51	0	40	.15	.11	1.3	2	407	11	30	.9	108
6	40	0	330	.11	.22	1.0	1	195	86	107	1.0	264
3	47	0	40	.15	.11	1.4	4	361	15	31	1.4	88
4	52	0	590	.16	.12	1.4	Trace	410	19	34	.9	142
8	30	0	300	.11	.27	.8	0	373	125	147	1.2	178
4	45	0	200	.09	.12	.7	4	339	17	59	1.0	60
3	56	0	Trace	.14	.12	1.4	1	604	38	51	1.9	240
3	52	0	990	.15	.14	2.0	4	201	14	39	1.2	201
6	61	0	190	.26	.14	1.0	Trace	261	55	122	3.7	145
5	32	0	3,210	.11	.18	1.0	Trace	278	66	90	1.0	208
11	79	0	0	.47	.40	5.0	0	1,100	25	90	3.1	89
20	141	0	0	1.07	.79	9.9	0	2,602	131	272	6.1	179
6	22	25	230	0.16	0.18	1.6	4	421	86	89	1.1	67
1	5	0	—	—	.01	.1	0	0	1	17	.2	—
1	5	0	—	—	.01	.2	0	75	1	19	.2	—
2	30	0	—	—	.02	.4	0	0	2	47	.5	—
2	12	0	0	.05	.04	.7	0	268	4	21	.2	21
6	46	0	0	.20	.15	2.5	0	1,006	13	79	.9	78
Trace	2	0	0	.01	.01	.1	0	50	1	4	Trace	4
4	40	0	0	.21	(^{7})	1.7	0	450	5	31	1.3	—
4	50	0	0	.23	.02	2.1	0	735	21	57	1.8	57
4	41	0	0	.19	.02	2.1	0	628	33	100	1.4	75
4.9	49.7	0	0	.18	.04	2.7	0	550	23	142	1	137
2	14	0	Trace	.10	.06	.9	Trace	146	20	23	.5	25
2	15	0	Trace	.11	.07	.9	Trace	193	21	24	.5	27
3	21	0	Trace	.16	.10	1.3	Trace	203	30	34	.8	38

A dash in a column for nutrients indicates a lack of reliable data for a constituent believed to be present in measurable amounts.
Notes (¹) are presented numerically at the end of the appendix.

Foods, approximate portions, nutrients, weights (28 grams = 1 ounce)	Portion size	Weight	Food Energy	Fiber	Fat	Saturated (total)	Oleic	Linoleic
		Grams	Calories	Grams	Grams	Grams	Grams	Grams
Hard (3¾-in diam)	1 roll	50	155	<1	2	.4	.6	.5
Hoagie or submarine (11½ by 3 by 2½ in)	1 roll	135	390	<1	4	.9	1.4	1.4
From home recipe								
Cloverleaf (2½-in diam)	1 roll	35	120	<1	3	.8	1.1	.7
Spaghetti (enriched)								
Cooked, firm stage, "al dente"	1 cup	130	190	<1	1	—	—	—
Cooked, tender stage	1 cup	140	155	<1	1	—	—	—
Waffles (enriched, made with vegetable shortening, 7-in diam)								
From home recipe	1 waffle	75	210	1	7	2.3	2.8	1.
From mix, egg and milk added	1 waffle	75	205	1	8	2.8	2.9	1
Wheat bran	100 g.	100	206	44	5.5	1.1	.84	3
Yeast (baker's, dry, active)	1 pkg.	7	20	.2	0	0	0	
LEGUMES, NUTS, SEEDS; RELATED PRODUCTS								
Almonds, shelled								
Chopped (about 130 almonds)	1 cup	130	775	18.6	70	5.6	47.7	12
Slivered (about 115 almonds)	1 cup	115	690	16.2	62	5.0	42.2	11
Beans								
Dry, cooked, drained								
Great Northern	1 cup	180	210	16.8	1	—	—	—
Lima	1 cup	190	260	16.6	1	—	—	—
Navy (pea)	1 cup	190	225	16	1	—	—	—
Canned, beans and liquid								
White, with pork and tomato sauce	1 cup	255	310	14	7	2.4	2.8	
Red kidney	1 cup	255	230	19.5	1	—	—	
Black-eyed peas, dry, cooked	1 cup	250	190	19	1	—	—	
Brazil nuts, shelled (6–8 large kernels)	1 oz	28	185	11.5	19	4.8	6.2	
Cashew nuts, roasted in oil	1 cup	140	785	—	64	12.9	36.8	1
Coconut meat, fresh								
Piece (about 2 by 2 by ½ in)	1 piece	45	155	6.1	16	14.0	.9	
Shredded or grated	1 cup	80	276	10.9	28	24.8	1.6	
Filberts (hazelnuts), chopped (about 80 kernels)	1 cup	115	730	7	72	5.1	55.2	
Lentils, whole, cooked	1 cup	200	210	7.4	Trace	—	—	—
Peanuts, roasted in oil, salted, chopped	1 cup	144	840	13.4	72	13.7	33.0	
Peanut butter	1 tbsp	16	95	1.2	8	1.5	3.7	
Peas, split, dry, cooked	1 cup	200	230	10.2	1	—	—	—
Pecans, chopped or pieces (about 120 large halves)	1 cup	118	810	8.5	84	7.2	50.5	

NUTRIENTS			VITAMINS					MINERALS				
Protein	Carbohydrate	Cholesterol	Vitamin A	Thiamin	Riboflavin	Niacin	Ascorbic Acid	Sodium	Calcium	Phosphorous	Iron	Potassium
Grams	Grams	Milligrams	International units	Milligrams	Milligrams	Milligrams	Milligrams	Milligrams	Milligrams	Milligrams	Milligrams	Milligrams
5	30	0	Trace	.20	.12	1.7	Trace	313	24	46	1.2	49
12	75	0	Trace	.54	.32	4.5	Trace	675	58	115	3.0	122
3	20	0	30	.12	.12	1.2	Trace	240	16	36	.7	41
7	39	0	0	.23	.13	1.8	0	1	14	85	1.4	103
5	32	0	0	.20	.11	1.5	0	2	11	70	1.3	85
7	28	0	250	.17	.23	1.4	Trace	356	85	130	1.3	109
7	27	45	170	.14	.22	.9	Trace	515	179	257	1.0	146
14.1	26.8	0	4700	.89	.36	29.6	0	28	110	1200	12.9	777
3	3	0	0	1.6	.38	2.6	0	4	3	90	1.1	140
24	25	0	0	.31	1.20	4.6	Trace	4	304	655	6.1	1,005
21	22	0	0	.28	1.06	4.0	Trace	3	269	580	5.4	889
14	38	0	0	.25	.13	1.3	0	13	90	266	4.9	749
16	49	0	—	.25	.11	1.3	—	2	55	293	5.9	1,163
15	40	0	0	.27	.13	1.3	0	13	95	281	5.1	790
16	48	<10	330	.20	.08	1.5	5	1,300	138	235	4.6	536
15	42	0	10	.13	.10	1.5	—	8	74	278	4.6	673
13	35	0	30	.40	.10	1.0	—	2	43	238	3.3	573
4	3	0	Trace	.27	.03	.5	—	1	53	196	1.0	203
24	41	0	140	.60	.35	2.5	—	21	53	522	5.3	650
2	4	0	0	.02	.01	.2	1	9	6	43	.8	115
3	8	0	0	.04	.02	.4	2	13	10	76	1.4	205
14	19	0	—	.53	—	1.0	Trace	1	240	388	3.9	810
16	39	0	40	.14	.12	1.2	0	24	50	238	4.2	498
37	27	0	—	.46	.19	24.8	0	633	107	577	3.0	971
4	3	0	—	.02	.02	2.4	0	18	9	61	.3	100
16	42	0	80	.30	.18	1.8	—	2	22	178	3.4	592
11	17	0	150	1.01	.15	1.1	2	1	86	341	2.8	712

A dash in a column for nutrients indicates a lack of reliable data for a constituent believed to be present in measurable amounts.
Notes (^{1}) are presented numerically at the end of the appendix.

Foods, approximate portions, nutrients, weights (28 grams = 1 ounce)	Portion size	Weight	Food Energy	Fiber	Fat	Fatty Acids Saturated (total)	Unsaturated Oleic	Unsaturated Linoleic
		Grams	Calories	Grams	Grams	Grams	Grams	Grams
Pumpkin and squash seeds, dry, hulled	1 cup	140	775	9	65	11.8	23.5	27.?
Sunflower seeds, dry, hulled	1 cup	145	810	17	69	8.2	13.7	43.?
Walnuts								
Black								
Chopped or broken kernels	1 cup	125	785	6.5	74	6.3	13.3	45.
Ground (finely)	1 cup	80	500	4.2	47	4.0	8.5	29.
Persian or English, chopped (about 60 halves)	1 cup	120	780	6.2	77	8.4	11.8	42.
SUGARS, SWEETS, SALT								
Cake icings								
Boiled, white								
Plain	1 cup	94	295	0	0	0	0	
With coconut	1 cup	166	605	0	13	11.0	.9	Trac
Uncooked								
Chocolate, made with milk and butter	1 cup	275	1,035	0	38	23.4	11.7	1
Creamy fudge, from mix and water	1 cup	245	830	4	16	5.1	6.7	3
White	1 cup	319	1,200	0	21	12.7	5.1	
Candy								
Caramels, plain or chocolate	1 oz	28	115	0	3	1.6	1.1	
Chocolate								
Milk, plain	1 oz	28	145	0	9	5.5	3.0	
Semisweet, small pieces (60 per oz)	1 cup	170	860	0	61	36.2	19.8	
Chocolate-coated peanuts	1 oz	28	160	0	12	4.0	4.7	
Fondant, uncoated (mints, candy corn, other)	1 oz	28	105	0	1	.1	.3	
Fudge, chocolate, plain	1 oz	28	115	0	3	1.3	1.4	
Gumdrops	1 oz	28	100	0	Trace	—	—	—
Hard	1 oz	28	110	0	Trace	—	—	—
Marshmallows	1 oz	28	90	0	Trace	—	—	—
Chocolate-flavored beverage powders (about 4 heaping tsp per oz)								
With nonfat dry milk	1 oz	28	100	0	1	.5	.3	T
Without milk	1 oz	28	100	0	1	.4	.2	T
Honey, strained or extracted	1 tbsp	21	65	0	0	0	0	
Jams and preserves	1 tbsp	20	55	0	Trace	—	—	—
Jellies	1 tbsp	18	50	0	Trace	—	—	—
	1 packet	14	40	0	Trace	—	—	—
Salt	1 tbsp	17	0	0	0	0	0	
Syrups								
Chocolate-flavored syrup or topping								
Thin type	1 fl oz or 2 tbsp	38	90	0	1	.5	.3	T
Fudge type	1 fl oz or 2 tbsp	38	125	0	5	3.1	1.6	

NUTRIENTS			VITAMINS					MINERALS				
Protein	Carbohydrate	Cholesterol	Vitamin A	Thiamin	Riboflavin	Niacin	Ascorbic Acid	Sodium	Calcium	Phosphorous	Iron	Potassium
Grams	Grams	Milli-grams	Inter-national units	Milli-grams	Milli-grams	Milli-grams	Milli-grams	Milli-grams	Milli-grams	Milli-grams	Milli-grams	Milli-grams
41	21	0	100	.34	.27	3.4	—	0	71	1,602	15.7	1,386
35	29	0	70	2.84	.33	7.8	—	44	174	1,214	10.3	1,334
26	19	0	380	.28	.14	.9	—	4	Trace	713	7.5	575
16	12	0	240	.18	.09	.6	—	3	Trace	456	4.8	368
18	19	0	40	.40	.16	1.1	2	2	119	456	3.7	540
1	75	—	0	Trace	0.03	Trace	0	1,321	2	2	Trace	17
3	124	—	0	0.02	.07	0.3	0	199	10	50	0.8	277
9	185	—	580	.06	.28	.6	1	165	165	305	3.3	536
7	183	—	Trace	.05	.20	.7	Trace	564	96	218	2.7	238
2	260	—	860	Trace	.06	Trace	Trace	160	48	38	Trace	57
1	22	0	Trace	.01	.05	.1	Trace	63	42	35	.4	54
2	16	—	80	.02	.10	.1	Trace	26	65	65	.3	109
7	97	—	30	.02	.14	.9	0	6	51	255	4.4	553
5	11	0	Trace	.10	.05	2.1	Trace	17	33	84	.4	143
Trace	25	0	0	Trace	Trace	Trace	0	52	4	2	.3	1
1	21	0	Trace	.01	.03	.1	Trace	66	22	24	.3	42
Trace	25	0	0	0	Trace	Trace	0	10	2	Trace	.1	1
0	28	0	0	0	0	0	0	9	6	2	.5	1
1	23	0	0	0	0	Trace	0	14	5	2	.5	2
5	20	0	10	.04	.21	.2	1	153	167	155	5	227
1	25	0	—	.01	.03	.1	0	108	9	48	.6	142
Trace	17	0	0	Trace	.01	.1	Trace	1	1	1	.1	11
Trace	14	0	Trace	Trace	.01	Trace	Trace	1	4	2	.2	18
Trace	13	0	Trace	Trace	.01	Trace	1	3	4	1	.3	14
Trace	10	0	Trace	Trace	Trace	Trace	1	3	3	1	.2	11
0	0	0	0	0	0	0	0	6589	0	0	0	0
1	24	0	Trace	.01	.03	.2	0	20	6	35	.6	106
2	20	0	60	.02	.08	.2	Trace	34	48	60	.5	107

A dash in a column for nutrients indicates a lack of reliable data for a constituent believed to be present in measurable amounts.
Notes (^{1}) are presented numerically at the end of the appendix.

Foods, approximate portions, nutrients, weights (28 grams = 1 ounce)	Portion size	Weight	Food Energy	Fiber	Fat	Saturated (total)	Oleic	Linoleic
		Grams	Calories	Grams	Grams	Grams	Grams	Grams
Molasses, cane								
Light (first extraction)	1 tbsp	20	50	0	—	—	—	—
Blackstrap (third extraction)	1 tbsp	20	45	0	—	—	—	—
Sorghum	1 tbsp	21	55	0	—	—	—	—
Table blends, chiefly corn, light and dark	1 tbsp	21	60	0	0	0	0	0
Sugars								
Brown	1 tbsp	13.2	49.2	0	0	0	0	
White								
Granulated	1 cup	200	770	0	0	0	0	
	1 tbsp	12	45	0	0	0	0	
Powdered, sifted, spooned into cup	1 cup	100	385	0	0	0	0	
VEGETABLES AND VEGETABLE PRODUCTS								
Asparagus								
Cooked, drained								
Cuts and tips, 1½- to 2-in lengths								
Fresh	1 cup	145	30	2.5	Trace	—	—	—
Frozen	1 cup	180	40	3	Trace	—	—	—
Spears, ½-in diam at base								
Fresh	4 spears	60	10	1	Trace	—	—	—
Frozen	4 spears	60	15	1	Trace	—	—	—
Canned, spears, ½-in diam at base	4 spears	80	15	1.5	Trace	—	—	—
Beans								
Lima, frozen, cooked, drained								
Thick-seeded types (Fordhooks)	1 cup	170	170	15.8	Trace	—	—	—
Thin-seeded types (baby limas)	1 cup	180	210	16.7	Trace	—	—	—
Snap, green								
Cooked, drained								
Fresh (cuts and French style)	1 cup	125	30	4	Trace	—	—	—
Frozen (French style)	1 cup	130	35	4.1	Trace	—	—	—
Canned, drained vegetables	1 cup	135	30	4.3	Trace	—	—	—
Yellow or wax								
Cooked, drained								
Fresh (cuts and French style)	1 cup	125	30	6.4	Trace	—	—	—
Frozen (cuts)	1 cup	135	35	6.9	Trace	—	—	—
Canned, drained vegetables (cuts)	1 cup	135	30	6.9	Trace	—	—	—
Bean sprouts (mung)								
Raw	1 cup	105	35	23.1	Trace	—	—	—
Cooked, drained	1 cup	125	35	8	Trace	—	—	—
Beets								
Cooked, drained, peeled								
Whole beets, 2-in diam	2 beets	100	30	2.5	Trace	—	—	
Diced or sliced	1 cup	170	55	4.5	Trace	—	—	

NUTRIENTS			VITAMINS					MINERALS				
Protein	Carbohydrate	Cholesterol	Vitamin A	Thiamin	Riboflavin	Niacin	Ascorbic Acid	Sodium	Calcium	Phosphorous	Iron	Potassium
Grams	Grams	Milli-grams	Inter-national units	Milli-grams	Milli-grams	Milli-grams	Milli-grams	Milli-grams	Milli-grams	Milli-grams	Milli-grams	Milli-grams
—	13	0	—	.01	.01	Trace	—	16	33	9	.9	183
—	11	0	—	.02	.04	.4	—	0	137	17	3.2	585
—	14	0	—	—	.02	Trace	—	4	35	5	2.6	—
0	15	0	0	0	0	0	0	14	9	3	.8	1
0	12.7	0	0	0	0	.02	0	3.2	11.2	2.5	.45	45
0	199	0	0	0	0	0	0	0	0	0	.2	6
0	12	0	0	0	0	0	0	0	0	0	Trace	Trace
0	100	0	0	0	0	0	0	0	0	0	.1	3
3	5	0	1,310	0.23	0.26	2.0	38	1	30	73	0.9	265
6	6	0	1,530	.25	.23	1.8	41	0	40	115	2.2	396
1	2	0	540	.10	.11	.8	16	0	13	30	.4	110
2	2	0	470	.10	.08	.7	16	1	13	40	.7	143
2	3	0	640	.05	.08	.6	12	189	15	42	1.5	133
10	32	0	390	.12	.09	1.7	29	219	34	153	2.9	724
13	40	0	400	.16	.09	2.2	22	182	63	227	4.7	709
2	7	0	680	.09	.11	.6	15	5	63	46	.8	189
2	8	0	690	.08	.10	.4	9	1	49	39	1.2	177
2	7	0	630	.04	.07	.4	5	319	61	34	2.0	128
2	6	0	290	.09	.11	.6	16	9	63	46	.8	189
2	8	0	140	.09	.11	.5	8	1	47	42	.9	221
2	7	0	140	.04	.07	.4	7	379	61	34	2.0	128
4	7	0	20	.14	.14	.8	20	5	20	67	1.4	234
4	7	0	30	.11	.13	.9	8	5	21	60	1.1	195
1	7	0	20	.03	.04	.3	6	43	14	23	.5	208
2	12	0	30	.05	.07	.5	10	71	24	39	.9	354

A dash in a column for nutrients indicates a lack of reliable data for a constituent believed to be present in measurable amounts.
Notes (^{1}) are presented numerically at the end of the appendix.

Foods, approximate portions, nutrients, weights (28 grams = 1 ounce)	Portion size	Weight	Food Energy	Fiber	Fat	MACRO- Fatty Acids Saturated (total)	Unsaturated Oleic	Linoleic
		Grams	Calories	Grams	Grams	Grams	Grams	Grams
Canned, drained vegetables								
Whole beets, small	1 cup	160	60	4	Trace	—	—	—
Diced or sliced	1 cup	170	65	4.2	Trace	—	—	—
Beet greens, leaves and stems, cooked, drained	1 cup	145	25	5.2	Trace	—	—	—
Black-eyed peas, cooked and drained								
Fresh	1 cup	165	180	—	1	—	—	—
Frozen	1 cup	170	220	—	1	—	—	—
Broccoli, cooked, drained								
Fresh								
Stalk, medium size	1 stalk	180	45	7.4	1	—	—	—
Stalks cut into ½-in pieces	1 cup	155	40	6.4	Trace	—	—	—
Frozen								
Stalk, 4½ to 5 in long	1 stalk	30	10	1.2	Trace	—	—	—
Chopped	1 cup	185	50	7.6	1	—	—	—
Fresh, raw, cut into ½-in pieces	1 cup	155	36	5.6	Trace	—	—	—
Brussels sprouts, cooked, drained								
Fresh, 7–8 sprouts (1¼- to 1½-in diam)	1 cup	155	55	4.5	1	—	—	—
Frozen	1 cup	155	50	4.5	Trace	—	—	—
Cabbage								
Common varieties								
Raw, coarsely shredded or sliced	1 cup	70	15	2.5	Trace	—	—	—
Cooked, drained	1 cup	145	30	3.6	Trace	—	—	—
Red, raw, coarsely shredded or sliced	1 cup	70	20	2.4	Trace	—	—	—
Savoy, raw, coarsely shredded or sliced	1 cup	70	15	2.2	Trace	—	—	—
Cabbage, white mustard (also called bokchoy or pakchoy), cooked, drained	1 cup	170	25	5.8	Trace	—	—	—
Carrots								
Raw, trimmed, scraped								
Whole, 7½ by 1⅛ in	1 carrot	72	30	2.4	Trace	—	—	—
Grated	1 cup	110	45	3.6	Trace	—	—	—
Cooked (crosswise cuts), drained	1 cup	155	50	4.8	Trace	—	—	—
Canned, sliced, drained vegetables	1 cup	155	45	4.8	Trace	—	—	—
Cauliflower								
Raw, chopped	1 cup	115	31	2.4	Trace	—	—	—
Cooked, drained								
Fresh (flower buds)	1 cup	125	30	2.2	Trace	—	—	—
Frozen (flowerets)	1 cup	180	30	3.2	Trace	—	—	—
Celery, Pascal, raw								
Stalk, large outer, 8 in long	1 stalk	40	6	.7	Trace	—	—	—
Pieces, diced	1 cup	120	20	2.2	Trace	—	—	—

NUTRIENTS			VITAMINS					MINERALS				
Protein	Carbohydrate	Cholesterol	Vitamin A	Thiamin	Riboflavin	Niacin	Ascorbic Acid	Sodium	Calcium	Phosphorous	Iron	Potassium
Grams	Grams	Milligrams	International units	Milligrams	Milligrams	Milligrams	Milligrams	Milligrams	Milligrams	Milligrams	Milligrams	Milligrams
2	14	0	30	.02	.05	.2	5	400	30	29	1.1	267
2	15	0	30	.02	.05	.2	5	401	32	31	1.2	284
2	5	0	7,400	.10	.22	.4	22	110	144	36	2.8	481
13	30	0	580	.50	.18	2.3	28	0	40	241	3.5	625
15	40	0	290	.68	.19	2.4	15	0	43	286	4.8	573
6	8	0	4,500	.16	.36	1.4	162	18	158	112	1.4	481
5	7	0	3,880	.14	.31	1.2	140	16	136	96	1.2	414
1	1	0	570	.02	.03	.2	22	5	12	17	.2	66
5	9	0	4,810	.11	.22	.9	105	28	100	104	1.3	392
5	3.9	0	3,800	.15	.46	1.55	170	18	155	104	2.3	527
7	10	0	810	.12	.22	1.2	135	16	50	112	1.7	423
5	10	0	880	.12	.16	.9	126	22	33	95	1.2	457
1	4	0	90	0.04	0.04	0.2	33	14	34	20	0.3	163
2	6	0	190	.06	.06	.4	48	20	64	29	.4	236
1	5	0	30	.06	.04	.3	43	18	29	25	.6	188
2	3	0	140	.04	.06	.2	39	15	47	38	.6	188
2	4	0	5,270	.07	.14	1.2	26	11	252	56	1.0	364
1	7	0	7,930	.04	.04	.4	6	34	27	26	.5	246
1	11	0	12,100	.07	.06	.7	9	52	41	40	.8	375
1	11	0	16,280	.08	.08	.8	9	51	51	48	.9	344
1	10	0	23,250	.03	.05	.6	3	366	47	34	1.1	186
3	6	0	70	.13	.12	.8	90	15	29	64	1.3	339
3	5	0	80	.11	.10	.8	69	11	26	53	.9	258
3	6	0	50	.07	.09	.7	74	18	31	68	.9	373
Trace	2	0	110	.01	.01	.1	4	50	16	11	.1	136
1	5	0	320	.04	.04	.4	11	151	47	34	.4	409

A dash in a column for nutrients indicates a lack of reliable data for a constituent believed to be present in measurable amounts.
Notes (^{1}) are presented numerically at the end of the appendix.

Foods, approximate portions, nutrients, weights (28 grams = 1 ounce)	Portion size	Weight	Food Energy	Fiber	Fat	MACRO- Fatty Acids Saturated (total)	Unsaturated Oleic	Linoleic
		Grams	Calories	Grams	Grams	Grams	Grams	Grams
Collards, cooked, drained								
Fresh (leaves without stems)	1 cup	190	65	4	1	—	—	—
Frozen (chopped)	1 cup	170	50	3.6	1	—	—	—
Corn, yellow sweet								
Cooked, drained								
Fresh, ear 5 by 1³⁄₄ in	1 ear	140	70	8	1	—	—	—
Frozen								
Ear, 5 in long	1 ear	229	120	13	1	—	—	—
Kernels	1 cup	165	130	9.4	1	—	—	—
Cucumber slices, ⅛ in thick (large, 2⅛-in diam)								
With peel	8 slices	28	5	.4	Trace	—	—	—
Without peel	6½ pieces	28	5	.1	Trace	—	—	—
Dandelion greens, cooked, drained	1 cup	105	35	—	1	—	—	—
Endive, curly (including escarole), raw, small								
pieces	1 cup	50	10	1.1	Trace	—	—	—
Kale, cooked, drained								
Fresh (leaves without stems and midribs)	1 cup	110	45	2.2	1	—	—	—
Frozen (leaf style)	1 cup	130	40	2.6	1	—	—	—
Lettuce								
Butterhead, as Boston types								
Head, 5-in diam	1 head	220	25	3.3	Trace	—	—	—
Leaves, outer	1 leaf	15	Trace	.2	Trace	—	—	—
Crisphead, as Iceberg								
Head, 6-in diam	1 head	567	70	8.5	1	—	—	—
Wedge, ¼ of head	1 wedge	135	20	2	Trace	—	—	—
Pieces, chopped or shredded	1 cup	55	5	.8	Trace	—	—	—
Loose-leaf (bunching varieties including								
Romaine), chopped or shredded	1 cup	55	10	.8	Trace	—	—	—
Mushrooms, raw, sliced or chopped	1 cup	70	20	1.7	Trace	—	—	—
Mustard greens, without stems and midribs,								
cooked, drained	1 cup	140	30	5.2	1	—	—	—
Okra pods, 3 in long, cooked	10 pods	106	30	3.4	Trace	—	—	—
Onions								
Mature, white-fleshed								
Raw								
Chopped	1 cup	170	65	3.6	Trace	—	—	—
Sliced	1 cup	115	45	2.4	Trace	—	—	—
Cooked (whole or sliced), drained	1 cup	210	60	2.7	Trace	—	—	—
Young green, bulb and white portion of top	6 onions	30	15	.6	Trace	—	—	—
Parsley, fresh, chopped	1 tbsp	4	Trace	.4	Trace	—	—	—
Parsnips, cooked, diced	1 cup	155	100	6.2	1	—	—	—

Protein	Carbohydrate	Cholesterol	Vitamin A	Thiamin	Riboflavin	Niacin	Ascorbic Acid	Sodium	Calcium	Phosphorous	Iron	Potassium
			VITAMINS					MINERALS				
Grams	Grams	Milli-grams	Inter-national units	Milli-grams	Milli-grams	Milli-grams	Milli-grams	Milli-grams	Milli-grams	Milli-grams	Milli-grams	Milli-grams
7	10	0	14,820	.21	.38	2.3	144	48	357	99	1.5	498
5	10	0	11,560	.10	.24	1.0	56	27	299	87	1.7	401
2	16	0	310	.09	.08	1.1	7	0	2	69	.5	151
4	27	0	440	.18	.10	2.1	9	2	4	121	1.0	291
5	31	0	580	.15	.10	2.5	8	0	5	120	1.3	304
Trace	1	0	70	.01	.01	.1	3	2	7	8	.3	45
Trace	1	0	Trace	0.01	0.01	0.1	3	2	5	5	0.1	45
2	7	0	12,290	.14	.17	—	19	46	147	44	1.9	244
1	2	0	1,650	.04	.07	.3	5	7	41	27	.9	147
5	7	0	9,130	.11	.20	1.8	102	47	206	64	1.8	243
4	7	0	10,660	.08	.20	.9	49	27	157	62	1.3	251
2	4	0	1,580	.10	.10	.5	13	20	57	42	3.3	430
Trace	Trace	0	150	.01	.01	Trace	1	1	5	4	.3	40
5	16	0	1,780	.32	.32	1.6	32	51	108	118	2.7	943
1	4	0	450	.08	.08	.4	8	12	27	30	.7	236
Trace	2	0	180	.03	.03	.2	3	5	11	12	.3	96
1	2	0	1,050	.03	.04	.2	10	5	37	14	.8	145
2	3	0	Trace	.07	.32	2.9	2	2	4	81	.6	290
3	6	0	8,120	.11	.20	.8	67	25	193	45	2.5	308
2	6	0	520	.14	.19	1.0	21	2	98	43	.5	184
3	15	0	Trace	.05	.07	.3	17	17	46	61	.9	267
2	10	0	Trace	.03	.05	.2	12	12	31	41	.6	181
3	14	0	Trace	.06	.06	.4	15	15	50	61	.8	231
Trace	3	0	Trace	.02	.01	.1	8	2	12	12	.2	69
Trace	Trace	0	300	Trace	.01	Trace	6	2	7	2	.2	25
2	23	0	50	.11	.12	.2	16	12	70	96	.9	587

A dash in a column for nutrients indicates a lack of reliable data for a constituent believed to be present in measurable amounts.
Notes (¹) are presented numerically at the end of the appendix.

Foods, approximate portions, nutrients, weights (28 grams = 1 ounce)	Portion size	Weight	Food Energy	Fiber	Fat	Saturated (total)	Oleic	Linoleic
		Grams	Calories	Grams	Grams	Grams	Grams	Grams
Peas, green								
Canned								
Whole, drained vegetables	1 cup	170	150	8.6	1	—	—	—
Frozen, cooked, drained	1 cup	160	110	8.2	Trace	—	—	—
Peppers, sweet (about 5 per lb, whole), stem and seeds removed								
Raw	1 pod	74	15	1.4	Trace	—	—	—
Cooked, boiled, drained	1 pod	73	15	1.1	Trace	—	—	—
Potatoes, cooked								
Baked, peeled after baking (about 2 per lb)	1 potato	156	145	3.9	Trace	—	—	—
Boiled (about 3 per lb)								
Peeled after boiling	1 potato	137	105	2.7	Trace	—	—	—
Peeled before boiling	1 potato	135	90	2.7	Trace	—	—	—
French-fried, strip, 2 to 3½ in long								
Prepared from raw	10 strips	50	135	1	7	1.7	1.2	3.
Frozen, oven heated	10 strips	50	110	1	4	1.1	.8	2.
Hashed brown, prepared from frozen	1 cup	155	345	2	18	4.6	3.2	9
Mashed, prepared from raw								
Milk added.................................	1 cup	210	135	1.9	2	.7	.4	Trac
Potato chips, 1¾ by 2½ in	10 chips	20	115	0	8	2.1	1.4	4
Pumpkin, canned	1 cup	245	80	1.2	1	—	—	—
Radishes, raw (prepackaged), trimmed	4 radishes	18	5	.2	Trace	—	—	—
Sauerkraut, canned, solids and liquid	1 cup	235	40	3	Trace	—	—	—
Spinach								
Fresh, chopped.............................	1 cup	55	15	2	Trace	—	—	—
Cooked, drained								
Fresh..................................	1 cup	180	40	11.3	1	—	—	—
Frozen								
Chopped	1 cup	205	45	12.9	1	—	—	—
Leaf...................................	1 cup	190	45	14.3	1	—	—	—
Canned, drained	1 cup	205	50	12.9	1	—	—	—
Squash, cooked								
Summer (all varieties), diced, drained	1 cup	210	30	4.6	Trace	—	—	—
Winter (all varieties), baked, mashed	1 cup	205	130	5.9	1	—	—	—
Sweet potatoes								
Cooked (raw, 5 by 2 in)								
Baked in skin, peeled	1 potato	114	160	3.2	1	—	—	—
Boiled in skin, peeled	1 potato	151	170	4.2	1	—	—	—
Canned								
Solid pack (mashed)	1 cup	255	275	7	1	—	—	—
Vacuum pack, 2¾ by 1-in piece	1 piece	40	45	1.1	Trace	—	—	—

MACRO-

Fatty Acids

Unsaturated

NUTRIENTS			VITAMINS					MINERALS				
Protein	Carbohydrate	Cholesterol	Vitamin A	Thiamin	Riboflavin	Niacin	Ascorbic Acid	Sodium	Calcium	Phosphorous	Iron	Potassium
Grams	Grams	Milli-grams	Inter-national units	Milli-grams	Milli-grams	Milli-grams	Milli-grams	Milli-grams	Milli-grams	Milli-grams	Milli-grams	Milli-grams
8	29	0	1,170	.15	.10	1.4	14	401	44	129	3.2	163
8	19	0	960	.43	.14	2.7	21	184	30	138	3.0	216
1	4	0	310	.06	.06	.4	94	10	7	16	.5	157
1	3	0	310	.05	.05	.4	70	10	7	12	.4	109
4	33	0	Trace	.15	.07	2.7	31	6	14	101	1.1	782
3	23	0	Trace	.12	.05	2.0	22	4	10	72	.8	556
3	20	0	Trace	.12	.05	1.6	22	3	8	57	.7	385
2	18	0	Trace	.07	.04	1.6	11	3	8	56	.7	427
2	17	0	Trace	.07	.01	1.3	11	2	5	43	.9	326
3	45	0	Trace	.11	.03	1.6	12	446	28	78	1.9	439
4	27	Trace	40	.17	.11	2.1	21	6	50	103	.8	548
1	10	0	Trace	.04	.01	1.0	3	250	8	28	.4	226
2	19	0	15,680	.07	.12	1.5	12	4	61	64	1.0	588
Trace	1	0	Trace	.01	.01	.1	5	3	5	6	.2	58
2	9	0	120	.07	.09	.5	33	1,501	85	42	1.2	329
2	2	0	4,460	.06	.11	.3	28	39	51	28	1.7	259
5	6	0	14,580	.13	.25	.9	50	90	167	68	4.0	583
6	8	0	16,200	.14	.31	.8	39	107	232	90	4.3	683
6	7	0	15,390	.15	.27	1.0	53	93	200	84	4.8	688
6	7	0	16,400	.04	.25	.6	29	483	242	53	5.3	513
2	7	0	820	.11	.17	1.7	21	2	53	53	.8	296
4	32	0	8,610	.10	.27	1.4	27	2	57	98	1.6	945
2	37	0	9,230	.10	.08	.8	25	14	46	66	1.0	342
3	40	0	11,940	.14	.09	.9	26	13	48	71	1.1	367
5	63	0	19,890	.13	.10	1.5	36	122	64	105	2.0	510
1	10	0	3,120	.02	.02	.2	6	24	10	16	.3	80

A dash in a column for nutrients indicates a lack of reliable data for a constituent believed to be present in measurable amounts.
Notes (^{1}) are presented numerically at the end of the appendix.

Foods, approximate portions, nutrients, weights (28 grams = 1 ounce)	Portion size	Weight	Food Energy	Fiber	Fat	MACRO- Fatty Acids Saturated (total)	Unsaturated Oleic	Linoleic
		Grams	Calories	Grams	Grams	Grams	Grams	Grams
Tomatoes Fresh, including cores and stem ends, 2½-in								
diam	1 tomato	135	25	2	Trace	—	—	—
Canned, solids and liquid	1 cup	241	50	3.6	Trace	—	—	—
Tomato catsup	1 tbsp	15	15	0	Trace	—	—	—
Tomato juice, canned	1 cup	243	45	0	Trace	—	—	—
Turnips, cooked, diced	1 cup	155	35	——	Trace	—	—	—
Turnip greens, cooked, drained Fresh (leaves and stems)	1 cup	145	30	3.4	Trace	—	—	—
Frozen (chopped)	1 cup	165	40	3.6	Trace	—	—	—
Vegetables, mixed, frozen, cooked	1 cup	182	115	——	1	—	—	—

NOTES:
^{1} Applies to products without added vitamin A.
^{2} Applies to products with added vitamin A.
^{3} Fat, carbohydrate, and vitamin A content vary with product. Consult label.
^{4} Based on the average vitamin A content of fortified margarine.
^{5} Value varies widely.
^{6} Applies to products without added ascorbic acid.
^{7} Varies with brand. Consult label.
^{8} Applies to products with added nutrient. Without added nutrient, value is trace.
^{9} Without calcium salts added.

NUTRIENTS			VITAMINS					MINERALS				
Protein	Carbohydrate	Cholesterol	Vitamin A	Thiamin	Riboflavin	Niacin	Ascorbic Acid	Sodium	Calcium	Phosphorous	Iron	Potassium
Grams	Grams	Milli-grams	Inter-national units	Milli-grams	Milli-grams	Milli-grams	Milli-grams	Milli-grams	Milli-grams	Milli-grams	Milli-grams	Milli-grams
1	6	0	1,110	.07	.05	.9	28	4	16	33	.6	300
2	10	0	2,170	.12	.07	1.7	41	313	[9]14	46	1.2	523
Trace	4	0	210	.01	.01	.2	2	156	3	8	.1	54
2	10	0	1,940	.12	.07	1.9	39	486	17	44	2.2	552
1	8	0	Trace	.06	.08	.5	34	310	54	37	.6	291
3	5	0	8,270	.15	.33	.7	68	51	252	49	1.5	——
4	6	0	11,390	.08	.15	.7	31	56	195	64	2.6	246
6	24	0	9,010	.22	.13	2.0	15	96	46	115	2.4	348

Foods, approximate portions, nutrients, weights (28 grams = 1 ounce)	Portion size	Weight	Food Energy	Fiber	Fat	Saturated (total)	Oleic	Linoleic
							MACRO-	
						Fatty Acids		
							Unsaturated	
		Grams	Calories	Grams	Grams	Grams	Grams	Grams

NUTRIENTS			VITAMINS					MINERALS				
Protein	Carbohydrate	Cholesterol	Vitamin A	Thiamin	Riboflavin	Niacin	Ascorbic Acid	Sodium	Calcium	Phosphorous	Iron	Potassium
Grams	Grams	Milli-grams	Inter-national units	Milli-grams	Milli-grams	Milli-grams	Milli-grams	Milli-grams	Milli-grams	Milli-grams	Milli-grams	Milli-grams

Notes

INTRODUCTION

1. J. Higginson. 1969. In: *Proceedings of the Eighth Canadian Cancer Research Conference* (Oxford: Pergamon Press), pp. 40–75.
2. E. L. Wynder and G. B. Gori. 1977. *Journal of the National Cancer Institute,* 58:825–32.
3. Diet, Nutrition and Cancer. 1982. (Washington, D.C.: National Academy of the Sciences)
4. *Nutrition and Cancer: Cause and Prevention: An American Cancer Society Special Report.* 1984. (New York: American Cancer Society)
5. R. Doll and R. Peto. 1981. *Journal of the National Cancer Institute,* 66:1192–1308.

CHAPTER 2

1. D. G. Milller. 1980. *Cancer,* 46:1307.
2. H. A. Kahn. 1966. In: *National Cancer Institute Monograph* 19. (Washington, D.C.: U.S. Government Printing Office)
3. E. L. Wynder and G. B. Gori. 1977. *Journal of the National Cancer Institute,* 58:825–32.
4. R. Doll and R. Peto. 1981. *Journal of the National Cancer Institute,* 66:1192–1308.
5. Surgeon-General. 1982. *Health Consequences of Smoking.* (Rockville, Maryland: U.S. Dept. of Health and Human Services)
6. P. Buell. 1973. *Journal of the National Cancer Institute,* 51:1479–83.
7. W. Haenszel. 1961. *Journal of the National Cancer Institute,* 26:37–132.
8. W. Haenszel, M. Kurihara, M. Segi, and R. K. C. Lee. 1972. *Journal of the National Cancer Institute,* 49:969–88.
9. E. Silverberg. 1983 *Cancer Statistics.* (New York: American Cancer Society)
10. J. R. Daling, N. S. Weiss, L. L. Klopfenstein, L. E. Cochran, W. H. Chow, and R. Daifuku. 1982. *Journal of the American Medical Association,* 247:1988.
11. W. P. Tseng, H. M. Chu, S. W. How, J. M. Fong, C. S. Lin, and S. Yeh. 1968. *Journal of the National Cancer Institute,* 40:453–63.

CHAPTER 3

1. T. Hirayama, 1977. In: *Origins of Human Cancer, Book A,* eds. H. H. Hiatt, J. D. Watson, and J. A. Winston. (Cold Spring Harbor, New York: Cold Spring Harbor Laboratory), pp. 55–75.

CHAPTER 4

1. D. S. Siscovick, N. S. Weiss, R. H. Fletcher, and T. Lasky, 1984. *New England Journal of Medicine,* 311:874–77.
2. B. Armstrong and R. Doll. 1975. *International Journal of Cancer,* 15:617–31.
3. S. P. Gaskill, W. L. McGuire, C. K. Osborne, and M. P. Stern. 1979. *Cancer Research,* 39:3628–37.
4. G. Hems. 1978. *British Journal of Cancer,* 37:974–82.
5. R. L. Phillips. *Cancer Research,* 35:3513–22.
6. J. H. Lubin, P. E. Burns, W. J. Blot, R. G. Ziegler, A. W. Lees, and J. F. Fraumeni, Jr. 1981. *International Journal of Cancer,* 28:685–89.
7. A. Nomura, B. E. Henderson, and J. Lee. 1978. *American Journal of Clinical Nutrition,* 31:2020–25.
8. R. MacLennan, O. M. Jensen, J. Mosbech, and H. Vouri. 1978. *American Journal of Clinical Nutrition,* 31:5227–30.
9. B. S. Reddy, A. R. Hedges, K. Laakso, and E. L. Wynder. 1978. *Cancer,* 42:2832–38.
10. J. Higginson, 1966. *Journal of the National Cancer Institute,* 37:527–45.
11. A. J. Lea. 1967. *Annals of the Royal College of Surgeons of England,* 41:432–38.
12. T. Hirayama. 1977. In: *Origins of Human Cancer, Book A,* eds. H. H. Hiatt, J. D. Watson, and J. A. Winston. (Cold Spring Harbor, New York: Cold Spring Harbor Laboratory), p. 55–76.
13. M. A. Howell. 1974. *British Journal of Cancer,* 29:328–36.
14. L. N. Kolonel, J. H. Hankin, J. Lee, S. Y. Chu, A. M. Y. Nomura, and M. W. Hinds. 1981. *British Journal of Cancer,* 44:332–39.
15. A. Blair, and J. F. Fraumeni, Jr. 1978. *Journal of the National Cancer Institute,* 61:1379–84.
16. I. D. Rotkin. 1977. *Cancer Treatment Reports,* 61:173–80.
17. L. M. Schuman, J. S. Mandell, A. Radke, U. Seal, and F. Halberg. 1982. In: *Trends in Cancer Incidence: Causes and Practical Implications* (Washington, New York, and London: Hemisphere Publishing Corporation)
18. A. F. Watson and E. Mellanby. 1930. *British Journal of Experimental Pathology,* 11:311–22.
19. P. S. Lavik and C. A. Baumann. 1943. *Cancer Research,* 3:749–56.
20. A. Tannenbaum. 1942. *Cancer Research,* 2:468–75.
21. A. Tannenbaum and H. Silverstone. 1957: In: *Cancer,* Vol 1, ed. R. W. Raven. (London: Butterworth and Co., Ltd.), pp. 306–34.
22. K. K. Carroll. 1980. *Journal of Environmental Pathology and Toxicology,* 3(4):253–71.
23. K. K. Carroll and G. J. Hopkins. 1979. *Lipids* 14:155–58.
24. J. Silverman, C. J. Shellabarger, S. Holtzman, J. P. Stone, and J. H.

Weisburger. 1980. *Journal of the National Cancer Institute,* 64:631–34.

25. P. B. McCay, M. King, L. E. Rikans, and J. V. Pitha. 1980. *Journal of Environmental Pathology and Toxicology,* 3(4):451–65.

26. N. D. Nigro, D. V. Singh, R. L. Campbell, and M. S. Pak. 1975. *Journal of the National Cancer Institute,* 54:439–42.

27. B. S. Reddy, J. H. Weisburger, and E. L. Wynder. 1974. *Journal of the National Cancer Institute,* 52:507–11.

28. B. R. Bansal, J. E. Rhoads, Jr., and S. C. Bansal. 1978. *Cancer Research,* 3 832 93 –3 03.

29. P. M. Newberne and E. Ziegler. 1978. In: *Advances in Modern Toxicology,* Vol. 5, eds. Wh. Flamm & M. A. Mehlman. *Mutagenesis.* (New York, London, Sidney and Toronto: John Wiley and Sons), pp. 52–84.

30. P. M. Newberne, J. Weigert, and N. Kula. 1979. *Cancer Research,* 39:3986–91.

31. B. D. Roebuck, J. D. Yager, Jr., and D. S. Longnecker, 1981. *Cancer Research,* 41:888–93.

32. K. Liu, J. Stamler, D. Moss, D. Garside, V. Persky, and I. Soltero. 1979. *Lancet,* 2:782–85.

33. G. Rose, H. Blackburn, A. Keys, H. L. Taylor, W. B. Kannel, O. Paul, D. D. Reid, and J. Stamler. 1974. *Lancet,* 1:181–83.

34. A. Kagan, D. L. McGee, K. Yano, G. G. Rhoads, and A. Nomura. 1981. *American Journal of Epidemiology,* 114:11–20.

35. L. A. Cohen. 1981. *Cancer Research,* 41:3808–10.

36. W. J. Cave and M. J. Erickson-Lucas. 1982. *Journal of the National Cancer Institute,* 68:219–24.

37. A. E. Rogers. 1983. *Cancer Research Supplement,* 43:2477–84.

CHAPTER 5

1. B. Armstrong and R. Doll. 1975. *International Journal of Cancer,* 15:617–31.

2. E. G. Knox. 1977. *British Journal of Preventive Society of Medicine,* 31:71–80.

3. G. Hems. 1978. *British Journal of Cancer,* 37:974–82.

4. G. Gray, M. C. Pike, and B. E. Henderson. 1979. *British Journal of Cancer,* 39:1–7.

5. L. N. Kolonel, J. H. Hankins, J. Lee, S. Y. Chu, A. M. Y. Nomura, and M. W. Hinds. 1981. *British Journal of Cancer,* 44:332–39.

6. A. B. Miller, A. Kelly, N. W. Choi, V. Matthews, R. W. Morgan, L. Munan, J. D. Burch, J. Feather, G. R. Howe, and M. Jain. 1978. *American Journal of Epidemiology,* 107:499–509.

7. R. L. Phillips. 1975. *Cancer Research,* 35:3513–22.

8. J. H. Lubin, J. Blot, and P. E. Burns. 1981. *American Journal of Epidemiology,* 114:422.

9. O. Gregor, R. Toman, and F. Prusova. 1969. *Gut,* 10:1031–34.
10. M. Jain, G. M. Cook, F. G. Davis, M. G. Grace, G. R. Howe, and A. B. Miller. 1980. *International Journal of Cancer* 26:757–68.
11. J. W. Berg and M. A. Howell. 1974. *Cancer,* 34:805–14.
12. M. A. Howell. 1975. *Journal of Chronic Disease,* 28:67–80.
13. E. G. Knox. 1977. *British Journal of Preventive Society of Medicine,* 31:71–80.
14. J. E. Enstrom. 1975. *British Journal of Cancer,* 32:432–39.
15. A. J. Lea. 1967. *Annals of the Royal College of Surgeons of England,* 41:432–38.
16. K. Ishii, K. Nakamura, H. Ozaki, N. Yamada, and T. Takeuchi. 1968. *Japanese Journal of Clinical Medicine,* 26:1839–42.
17. T. Hirayama. 1977. In: *Origins of Human Cancer, Book A,* eds. H. H. Hiatt, J. D. Watson, and J. A. Winsten. (Cold Spring Harbor, New York: Cold Spring Harbor Laboratory), pp. 55–76.
18. B. Armstrong, A. Garrod, and R. Doll. 1976. *British Journal of Cancer,* 33:127–36.
19. L. N. Kolonel, J. H. Hankin, J. Lee, S. Y. Chu, A. M. Y. Nomura, and M. W. Hinds. 1981. *British Journal of Cancer,* 44:332–39.
20. M. H. Ross, G. Bras, and M. S. Ragbeer. 1970. *Journal of Nutrition,* 100:177–89.
21. A. Tannenbaum. 1945 a, b,. *Cancer Research,* 5:609–25.
22. M. H. Ross and G. Bras. 1973. *Journal of Nutrition,* 103:944–63.
23. H. Silverstone and A. Tannenbaum. 1951. *Cancer Research,* 11:442–46.
24. K. K. Carrol. 1975. *Cancer Research,* 35:3374–83.
25. C. D. Larsen and W. E. Heston. 1945. *Journal of the National Cancer Institute,* 6(1):31–40.
26. J. White and H. B. Andervont. 1943. *Journal of the National Cancer Institute,* 3:449–51.
27. F. R. White and J. White. 1944. *Journal of the National Cancer Institute,* 5:41–42.
28. J. White, F. R. White, and G. B. Mider. 1947. *Journal of the National Cancer Institute,* 7:199–202.
29. R. W. Engel and D. H. Copeland. 1952. *Cancer Research,* 12:211–15.

CHAPTER 6

1. D. H. Calloway. 1971. *Environmental Biological Medicine,* 1:175–86.
2. B. Armstrong and R. Doll. 1975. *International Journal of Cancer,* 15:617–31.
3. G. Hems. 1978. *British Journal of Cancer,* 37:974–82.
4. G. Hems and A. Stuart. 1975. *British Journal of Cancer,* 3:118–23.
5. B. Draser and D. Irving. 1973. *British Journal of Cancer,* 27:167–72.
6. M. Hakama and E. A. Saxen. 1967. *International Journal of Cancer,* 2:265–68.

7. B. Modan, F. Lubin, V. Barrell, R. A. Greenberg, M. Modan and S. Graham. 1974. *Cancer,* 34:2087–92.
8. U. W. de Jong, N. Breslow, J. G. E. Hong, M. Sridharan, and K. Shanmugaratnam. 1974. *International Journal of Cancer,* 13:291–303.
9. S. K. Hoehn and K. K. Carroll. 1979. *Nutrition and Cancer,* 1(3):27–30.
10. G. Kolata. 1983. "Dietary Dogma Disproved." *Science.* 220:487–88.
11. D. J. A. Jenkins, R. H. Taylor, and T. M. S. Wolever. 1982. *Diabetologica,* 23:477.
12. Dietary Goals for the United States (2nd ed.). 1977. (Washington, D.C.: U.S. Government Printing Office)

CHAPTER 7

1. D. P. Burkitt. 1971. *Cancer,* 28:3
2. J. Perisse, F. Sigaret, and P. Francois. 1969. *Nutrition Newsletter,* (FAO) 7:1–9.
3. S. Bingham, D. R. R. Williams, T. J. Cole, and W. P. T. James. 1979. *British Journal of Cancer,* 40:456–63.
4. A. M. Stephen and J. H. Cummings. 1980. *Nature,* 284:283–84.
5. R. MacLennan, O. M. Jensen, J. Mosbech, and H. Vuori. 1978. *American Journal of Clinical Nutrition,* 31:S239–42.
6. S. L. Malhotra. 1977. *Medical Hypotheses,* 3:122–26.
7. B. S. Reddy, H. Morig, and M. Nicolais. 1981. *Journal of the National Cancer Institute,* 66:553–57.

CHAPTER 8

1. R. MacLennan, J. Da Costa, N. E. Day, C. H. Law, Y. K. Ng, and K. Shannugaratnam. 1977. *International Journal of Cancer,* 20:854–60.
2. A. Gregor, P. N. Lee, F. J. C. Roe, M. J. Wilson, and A. Melton. 1980. *Nutrition and Cancer,* 2:93–97.
3. P. G. Smith and H. Jick. 1978. *Cancer,* 42:808–11.
4. R. B. Shekelle, S. Liu, W. J. Raynor, M. Lepper, C. Maliza, and A. H. Rossof. 1981. *Lancet,* 2:1185–89.
5. S. Graham, J. Marshall, C. Mettlin, T. Rzepka, T. Nemoto, and T. Byers. 1982. *American Journal of Epidemiology,* 116:68–75.
6. I. D. Capel and D. C. Williams. 1979. *ICRS Medical Sciences,* 7:361.
7. S. Graham, C. Mettlin, J. Marshall, R. Priore, T. Rzepka, and D. Shedd. 1981. *American Journal of Epidemiology,* 113:675–80.
8. C. Mettlin, S. Graham, and M. Swanson. 1979. *Journal of the National Cancer Institute,* 62:1435–1438.
9. E. L. Wynder and I. J. Bross. 1961. *Cancer,* 14:389–413.
10. C. Mettlin, S. Graham, R. Priore, J. Marshall, and M. Swanson. 1981. *Nutrition and Cancer,* 2:143–47.
11. T. Hirayama. 1977. In: *Origins of Human Cancer,* eds. H. H. Hiatt,

J. D. Watson, and J. A. Winston. (Cold Spring Harbor, New York: Cold Spring Harbor Laboratory)

12. E. Bjelke. 1978. *Aktuel. Ernaehrungsmed. Klin. Prax. Suppl.,* 2:10–17.
13. L. M. Schumann, J. S. Mandell, A. Radke, U. Seal, and F. Halburg. 1982. In: *Trends in Cancer Incidence: Causes and Practical Implications,* ed. K. Magnus. (New York: Hemisphere Publishing Corp.), pp. 345–54.
14. P. Nettesheim and M. L. Williams. 1976. *International Journal of Cancer,* 17:351–57.
15. U. Saffiotti, R. Montesano, A. R. Sellakumar, and S. A. Borg. 1967. *Cancer,* 20:857–864.
16. M. B. Sporn, N. M. Dunlop, D. L. Newton, J. M. Smith. 1976. *Federation Proceedings,* 35:1332–38.
17. D. L. McCormick, F. J. Burns, and R. E. Albert. 1981. *Journal of the National Cancer Institute,* 66:559–64.
18. M. M. Mathews-Roth, 1982. *Oncology,* 39:33–37.
19. E. Siefter, F. Wong, F. Stratford, S. M. Levenson, G. Rettura. 1982. National Meeting of American Chemical Society, Las Vegas.
20. H. Rosenberg and A. N. Felzman. 1974. In: *The Book of Vitamin Therapy.* (New York: Berkley Publishing Corporation).
21. K. Guggenheim and E. Beuchler. 1946. *Proceedings of the Society of Experimental and Biological Medicine,* 61:413.
22. H. Schaumberg, J. Kaplan, A. Windebank, N. Vick, S. Rasmus, D. Pleasure, and M. J. Brown. 1983. *New England Journal of Medicine,* No. 8, 309:445–48.
23. V. Herbert and E. Jacob. 1974. *Journal of the American Medical Association,* 230:241–42.
24. J. D. Hines. 1975. *Journal of the American Medical Association,* 234:24.
25. J. J. Kunis and A. L. Sereng. 1984. *Science,* 226:1199–2103.
26. P. J. Cook-Mozaffari, F. Azordegan, N. E. Day, A. Ressicand, C. Sabai, and B. Aramesh. 1979. *British Journal of Cancer,* 39:293–309.
27. L. Meinsma. 1964. *Nutrition and Cancer,* 25:357–65.
28. E. Bjelke. 1974. *Scandinavian Journal of Gastroenterology* [suppl.], 31:1–235.
29. S. Wasserthiel-Smoller, S. L. Romney, J. Wylie-Rosset, S. Slagle, G. Miller, D. Lucido, C. Duttagupta, and P. R. Palan. 1981. *American Journal of Epidemiology,* 114:714–24.
30. S. S. Mirvish, L. Wallcave, M. Eagan, and P. Shubick. 1972. *Science,* 177:65–68.
31. E. Cameron and L. Pauling. 1979. In: *Cancer and Vitamin C,* p. 116.
32. J. J. DeCosse, M. B. Adams, J. F. Kuzma, P. Logerfo, and R. E. London. 1975. *Surgery,* 78:608–12.

33. H. P. Leis and C. S. Kwon. 1979. *Journal of Reproductive Medicine,* 22:291.
34. R. R. Monson, S. Yen, and B. MacMahon. 1976. *Lancet,* 2:224.
35. W. C. Willett, B. F. Polk, B. A. Underwood et al. 1984. *New England Journal of Medicine,* 310:430–34.
36. M. C. Cook and P. McNamara. 1980. *Cancer Research,* 40:1329–31.
37. M. C. Weinstein. 1983. "Cost-Effective Priorities for Cancer Prevention." *Science,* 221:17–23.

CHAPTER 9

1. R. J. Shamberger and C. E. Willis. 1971. *Critical Revue of Clinical Laboratory Science,* 2:211–21.
2. R. J. Shamberger, S. A. Tytko and C. E. Willis. 1976. *Archives of Environmental Health,* 31:231–35.
3. G. N. Schrauzer. 1976. *Bioinorganic Chemistry,* 5:275–281.
4. G. N. Schrauzer, D. A. White, and C. J. Schneider. 1977. *Bioinorganic Chemistry,* 7:23–34.
5. G. N. Schrauzer, D. A. White, and C. J. Schneider. 1977. *Bioinorganic Chemistry,* 7:35–56.
6. W. Willet, B. F. Polk, et al. 1983. *Lancet,* 2:130–34.
7. G. N. Schrauzer and D. A. White. 1978. *Bioinorganic Chemistry,* 8:303.
8. C. Ip and D. K. Sinha. 1981. *Cancer Research,* 41:31–34.
9. H. B. Demopolous, D. D. Pietronigro, E. S. Flamm, M. L. Seligman. 1980. *Journal of Environmental Pathology and Toxicology,* 3, 273.
10. M. V. Marshall, M. A. Arnott, M. M. Jacobs, A. C. Griffin, 1979. *Cancer Letters,* 7:331–38.
11. J. E. Spallholz. 1981. In: *Selenium in Biology and Medicine,* ed. J. E. Spallholz, J. L. Martin, H. E. Gauther. Westport, Conn: AVI Publishing: 103–17.
12. P. Kurkela. 1977. 22nd General Conference, International Federation of Agricultural Producers. Helsinki, Finland.
13. Chinese Academy of Medical Sciences. 1977. Keshan Disease Group. Beijing. *Chinese Medical Journal,* 92:477.
14. G. Yang, S. Wang, R. Zhou, and S. Sun. 1983. *The American Journal of Nutrition,* 37:872–81.
15. H. Sakurai and K. Tsuchiya. 1975. *Environmental Physiology and Biochemistry,* 5:107.
16. V. R. Young and D. Richardson. 1979. *Cancer,* 43:2125.
17. P. Frost, J. C. Chen, I. Rabbini, et al. 1977. *Proceedings of Clinical Biological Research,* 14:143.
18. P. Stocks and R. I. Davies. 1964. *British Journal of Cancer,* 18:14–24.
19. S. J. van Rensburg. 1981. *Journal of the National Cancer Institute,* 67:243–51.

20. L. G. Larsson, A. Sandstrom, and P. Wrestling. 1975. *Cancer Research,* 35:3308–16.

21. S. A. Broitman, H. Velez, and J. J. Vitale. 1981. *Advances in Experimental Medical Biology,* 91:155–81.

22. E. D. Williams, I. Doniach, O. Bjarnason, and W. Michie. 1977. *Cancer,* 39:215–22.

23. Coordinating Group for Research on Etiology of Esophageal Cancer in North China. 1975. *Chinese Medical Journal* (Peking, English edition), 1:167–83.

24. R. J. W. Burrell, W. A. Roach, and A. Shadwell. 1966. *Journal of the National Cancer Institute,* 36:201–14.

25. J. W. Berg, W. Haenszel, and S. S. Devesa. 1973. *Seventh National Cancer Conference Proceedings,* J. B. Lippincott, Philadelphia.

26. X. M. Luo, H. J. Wei, G. G. Hu, A. L. Shang, Y. Y. Liu, S. M. Lu, and S. P. Yang. 1981. *Federation Proceedings, Federation of American Society of Experimental Biology,* 40:928.

27. V. V. Koval'skiy and G. A. Yarovaya. 1966. *Agrokhimiya,* 8:68–91.

28. J. W. Berg and F. Burbank. 1972. *Annals of the New York Academy of Sciences,* 199:249–64.

29. L. N. Kolonel. 1976. *Cancer,* 37:1782–87.

30. P. Galy, R. Touraine, J. Brune, P. Gallois, P. Roudier, R. Loire, P. Leheureux, and T. Weisendanger. 1963. *Lyon Médecine* 210:735–44.

31. W. P. Tseng, H. M. Chu, S. W. How, J. M. Fong, C. S. Lin, and S. Yeh. 1968. *Journal of the National Cancer Institute,* 40:453–63.

CHAPTER 10

1. B. N. Ames. 1983. "Dietary Carcinogens and Anticarcinogens." *Science,* 221:1256–64.

2. U.S. Food and Drug Administration. 1981. *FDA Consumer Update* 18:1–3.

3. *Diet, Nutrition and Cancer.* 1982. (Washington, D.C.: National Academy of the Sciences).

4. H. Bulow. H. K. Wullstein, G. Bottger, and F. H. Schroeder. 1973. *Urologe A,* 12:249–53.

5. W. Lijinsky and A. E. Ross. 1967. *Food Cosmetic Toxicology,* 5:343–47.

6. C. Lintas, M. C. de Matthaeis, and F. Merli. 1979. *Food Cosmetic Toxicology,* 17:325–28.

7. J. W. Howard and T. Fazio. 1980. *Journal of the Association of Analytical Chemistry,* 63:1077–1104.

8. P. Dolara, B. Commoner, A. Vithayathil, G. Cuca, E. Tuley, P. Madyastha, S. Nair, and D. Kriebel. 1979. *Mutation Research,* 60:231–37.

9. N. E. Spingarn, H. Kasai, L. L. Vuolo, S. Nishimura, Z. Yamaizumi, T. Sugimura, T. Matsushima, and J. H. Weisburger. *Cancer Letters,* 9:177–83.

10. M. Nagao, Y. Takahashi, K. Wakabayashi, and T. Sugimura. 1981. *Mutation Research,* 88:147–54.

11. K. Morita, M. Hara, and T. Kada. 1978. *Agricultural Biological Chemistry* 42:1235–38.

12. C. N. Lai. 1979. *Nutrition and Cancer,* 1(3):19–21.

13. R. H. McKee and A. M. Tometsko. 1979. *Journal of the National Cancer Institute,* 63:473–77.

14. R. J. Shamberger, C. L. Corlett, K. D. Beaman, and B. L. Kasten. 1979. *Mutation Research,* 66:349–55.

15. S. J. Van Rensburg, J. J. van der Watt, I. F. H. Purchase, L. P. Coutinho, and R. Markham. 1974. *South African Medical Journal* 48:2508a–2508d.

16. B. Armstrong. 1980. *International Journal of Epidemiology,* 9:305–15.

17. C. S. Yang. 1980. *Cancer Research,* 40:2633–44.

18. B. MacMahon, S. Yen, D. Trichopoulos, K. Warren, and G. Nardi. 1981. *New England Journal of Medicine,* 304:630–33.

19. S. Graham, W. Schotz, and P. Martino. 1972. *Cancer,* 30:927–38.

20. W. Haenszel, M. Kurihara, F. B. Locke, and M. Segi. 1976. *Journal of the National Cancer Institute,* 56:265–74.

21. T. Hirayama. 1977. In: *Origins of Human Cancer, Book A,* eds. H. H. Hiatt, J. D. Watson, and J. A. Winston. (Cold Spring Harbor, New York: Cold Spring Harbor Laboratory), pp. 55–75.

22. S. Graham, H. Dayal, M. Swanson, A. Mittelman, and G. Wilkinson. 1978. *Journal of the National Cancer Institute,* 51:709–14.

23. W. Troll. 1981. In: *Cancer: Achievements, Challenges, and Prospects for the 1980's,* eds. J. H. Burchenal and H. F. Oettgen. Vol. 1. (New York: Grune and Stratton), pp. 549–55.

24. A. M. Novi. 1981. *Science,* 212:541.

25. E. J. Pantuck, C. B. Pantuck, W. A. Garland, B. H. Min, L. W. Wattenberg, K. E. Anderson, A. Kappas, and A. H. Conney. 1979. *Clinical Pharmacology Therapeutics,* 25:88–95.

CHAPTER 11

1. S. Kono and M. Ikeda. 1979. *British Journal of Breast Cancer,* 40:449–55.

2. P. Cook. 1971. *British Journal of Cancer,* 25:853–80.

3. A. J. Tuyns, G. Pequignot, and J. S. Abbatucci. 1979. *Bulletin of Cancer,* 64:45–60.

4. A. J. Tuyns and L. M. F. Masse. 1973. *International Journal of Epidemiology,* 2:241–45.

5. L. Lamy. 1910. *Arch. Mal. Appar. Dig. Mal. Nutr.* 4:451–75.

6. J. Hoey, C. Montvernay, and R. Lambert. 1981. *American Journal of Epidemiology,* 113:668–74.

7. O. M. Jensen. 1979. *International Journal of Cancer,* 23:454–63.

8. J. E. Enstrom. 1975. *Cancer,* 36:825–41.

9. E. L. Wynder, F. R. Lemon, and I. J. Bross. 1959. *Cancer,* 12:1016–28.

10. P. Stocks. 1957. *British Empire Cancer Research Campaign 35th Annual Report.* Supplement to Part II.

11. G. Dean, R. MacLennan, H. McLoughlin, and E. Shelley. 1979. *British Journal of Cancer,* 40:581–89.

12. E. Bjelke. 1973. (Ph.D. diss., University of Minnesota).

13. K. W. Kwan. 1937. *Chinese Medical Journal* (Beijing), 52:237–54.

14. J. J. Vitale, S. A. Broitman, and L. S. Gottlieb. 1981. In: *Nutrition and Cancer,* eds. G. R. Newell and N. M. Ellison. (New York: Raven Press), pp. 291–301.

15. R. Doll and R. Peto. 1981. *The Causes of Cancer.* (Oxford: Oxford University Press).

CHAPTER 12

1. J. W. Berg. 1975. *Cancer Research,* 35:3345–50.

2. M. Hill, R. MacLennan, and K. Newcombe. 1979. *Lancet,* 1:436.

3. B. Armstrong and R. Doll. 1975. *International Journal of Cancer,* 15:617–31.

4. F. de Waard, J. P. Cornelis, K. Aoki, and M. Yoshida. 1977. *Cancer,* 40:1269–75.

5. E. A. Lew and L. Garfinkel. 1979. *Journal of Chronic Disease,* 32:749–56.

6. A. Tannenbaum. 1945. *Cancer Research,* 5:609–15.

CHAPTER 13

1. E. L. Wynder and G. B. Gori. 1977. *Journal of the National Cancer Institute,* 58:825–32.

2. R. Doll and R. Peto. 1981. *Journal of the National Cancer Institute,* 66:1192–1308.

3. Senate Committee on Nutrition and Human Needs. 1977. *Dietary Goals for the United States.* (Washington, D.C.: U.S. Gov't. Printing Office)

4. A. C. Upton. 1979. "Statement on Diet, Nutrition and Cancer before the U.S. Committee on Agriculture, Nutrition and Forestry." (Washington, D.C.: U.S. Gov't. Printing Office)

5. Diet, Nutrition and Cancer. 1982. (Washington, D.C.: National Academy of the Sciences)

Glossary

Age-adjusted cancer incidence (or mortality): The incidence of (or mortality rate for) cancer after adjusting for differences in the age distribution of the populations being compared.

Anticarcinogen: A substance that inhibits or prevents the activity of a carcinogen. Many exist in fruits and vegetables.

Antimutagen: A substance that inhibits or prevents the action of a mutagen. Many exist in fruits and vegetables.

Antioxidant: A substance that retards oxidation and can inhibit carcinogenesis. Examples of antioxidants include beta-carotene, vitamin C, and vitamin E. Selenium can function as an antioxidant indirectly by stimulating the activity of the enzyme glutathione peroxidase. Antioxidants can inhibit the action of free radicals that may cause cancer, blood vessel disease, and aging. They are also used to prevent food spoilage.

Benign tumor: An abnormal growth of cells that are not cancerous, and which do not spread beyond their natural boundaries.

Cancer: An abnormal, uncontrolled growth of cells that can spread beyond their natural boundaries to other parts of the body. Cancers can develop in many different parts of the body. Sometimes a cancer is called a malignant tumor or neoplasm.

Carcinogen: A chemical, physical, or biological agent that can increase the risk of developing cancer. For example, carcinogenic chemicals are found in some foods and in tobacco smoke; radiation is a physical carcinogen; and a biological carcinogen may be a virus or a mold. The process by which a carcinogen causes cancer is called carcinogenesis.

Carcinoma: A cancer that arises in the epithelial tissues of the body. These tissues are found in the skin, the lungs, the stomach, and the intestines and colon, the breasts, the cervix, the pancreas, and the thyroid gland.

Cocarcinogen: A substance that increases the effect of a carcinogen.

Complete carcinogen: A carcinogen that can act as both the initiator and the promoter of the cancerous process.

Comutagen: A nonmutagenic substance that can either increase the activity of a mutagen or convert a nonmutagenic substance into a mutagenic one.

Contaminant: A chemical or biological substance that may or may not have carcinogenic properties, and which has not been intentionally added to foods or animal feed.

Delaney Clause: Congressional legislation passed in 1958 that forbids the

417

addition to food of any additives that have been shown to be carcinogenic in any species of animal or in humans.

Diet: The total composition of ingested food including all nutrients, naturally occurring contaminants, additives, and fiber.

Dietary Factors: Nutrient and nonnutrient substances that are present in the diet. Nutrients include protein, fat, carbohydrate, vitamins, and minerals. Nonnutrients include carcinogens, anticarcinogens, mutagens, antimutagens, additives, contaminants, and fiber. Some methods of cooking can create carcinogens and mutagens.

Environment: Anything that is external to the human body. In practice, this means anything that can react with the human body. The major influences are life-style, contaminated air, radiation exposure, ingested food, chemicals, and drink.

Epidemiology: The study of the distribution of diseases and their causes in human populations. Often such study provides information about local environmental influences.

Dietary fiber: This name describes the part of fruit, vegetables, and cereals that cannot be digested. Several types of fiber exist. Fiber reduces cancer risk by increasing stool bulk, reducing the effect of bile acids, and reducing fat absorption. Some fibers can lower cholesterol.

Food additive: Any substance that is added to food either directly or indirectly.

Food disappearance data (per capita intake):   Crude estimates of the amount of food or nutrients available for consumption by a specified population. These estimates may be based upon imports, exports, food production, food sales, etc. They are inevitably overestimates because of wastage and spoilage that cannot be avoided.

Free radicals: These are unstable chemical substances that can damage normal cells and activate carcinogens. They are formed from oxygen, unsaturated fats, certain metals, radiation, sunlight, ozone (smog) and alcohol. They can be neutralized by antioxidants.

Genotoxic: This describes something that damages the genetic material in cells. This effect could lead to mutations, to cancerous change, or to the death of the cell. Radiation, for example, is genotoxic.

Gut transit time: The time taken for food to pass completely through the gastrointestinal system.

Hyperplasia: An increase in the number of cells in an organ or a tissue of the body.

Incidence: This is the number of new cases of a disease expressed as a rate. This rate is calculated by dividing the number of persons in a specified population who develop a disease during a certain time period, by the total number of persons at risk of developing the disease during the same time period.

Initiator: An external stimulus or agent that changes a cell so that it can become malignant (cancerous) under certain conditions, often many years later. Initiating events are thought to be irreversible.

Latency period: This usually means the time between the first exposure to a carcinogen and the appearance of cancer.

Leukemia: This term refers to cancers of the blood-forming organs in which the white blood cells grow uncontrollably.

Life-style: Particularly, factors in daily living that can influence your health. Some examples are occupation, diet, drinking, exposure to pollution, and geographic location.

Lipotrope: An agent that acts on fat metabolism by hastening the removal, or decreasing the deposit, of fat in the liver.

Lymphoma: A form of cancer that arises in cells of the immune system. This usually occurs in the lymph nodes, but can also involve other organs.

Malignant tumor: This is another way to describe a cancer.

Melanoma: This is a cancer of pigment cells that usually occurs in the skin, but can also, rarely, occur in the eye and other sites.

Menarche: The age at which menstruation begins.

Metastasis: A growth of cancer cells in a part of the body that is distant from the original site of the cancer. Cancer cells detach from the original tumor and then are transported in the bloodstream or in the lymphatic circulation until they find a favorable site for growth.

Modifier: A substance that can alter the course of carcinogenesis. Potential modifiers include vitamin A (beta-carotene), folic acid, vitamin C, vitamin E, selenium, and a low-fat diet.

Morbidity: The condition of being diseased, or the incidence of a particular disease. The morbidity rate is equivalent to the incidence rate.

Mortality: The total number of deaths, or deaths from a specific disease, usually expressed as a rate. The number of deaths from a disease in a given population during a specified period is divided by the number of people at risk of dying from that disease during that time period.

Mutagen: A chemical or physical agent that interacts with the DNA to cause a change in the genetic material of a cell. Unless the cell repairs the damage, or is so badly damaged that it cannot replicate itself, the genetic damage is passed on to daughter cells when the cell divides. This genetic damage may or may not lead to the development of a cancerous change.

Multiple myeloma: A malignant tumor of plasma cells that usually arises in the bone marrow.

Neoplasm: A new growth of cells or tissue which may be benign or malignant.

Nutrient: A component of food such as protein, fat, carbohydrate, vitamins, and minerals. Nutrients provide nourishment for the growth and maintenance of the body.

Nutrition: This describes all the chemical processes by which the body utilizes food for the growth, structural integrity, and maintenance of all cells in the body.

Osteoporosis: A condition in which calcium is lost from bones. It leads to weakness and a tendency to fracutre easily. It is common among the elderly and those past menopause.

Per capita intake: A rough estimate of the amount of a particular substance such as a nutrient or a contaminant that is ingested by each member of the population over a given period of time.

Permissible residue: The amount of a residue such as a pesticide in a food crop that is allowed to remain in that food when it is consumed.

Precancerous lesions: An abnormality in some part of the body that has a significant possibility of developing into a cancer later.

Prevalence: The number of existing cases of a disease, usually expressed as a proportion of the population known to be at risk.

Promotor: An agent that causes a cell that has been previously exposed to an initiator to become malignant—usually after prolonged exposure. These late-stage promotional events in "initiated" cells are often reversible. If exposure to a promotional agent is discontinued, there is a good chance that the appearance of a malignant tumor will be prevented. Since dietary fat can act as a tumor promotor, a reduction in fat intake should reduce your risk of developing cancer.

Recommended Dietary Allowance (RDA): The level of intake of certain essential nutrients that is adequate to meet the basic nutritional needs of most healthy people. Usually, these amounts are calculated on the basis of what is needed to avoid any signs of deficiency. These estimates reflect the judgment of the Committee on Dietary Allowances of the Food and Nutrition Board, The National Research Council.

Risk: This term refers to the probability of the occurrence of a disease in a given population or individual.

Relative risk: An estimate obtained by dividing the incidence of a disease (cancer) in the exposed population group by the incidence in a corresponding unexposed or control group.

Synergism: This describes a situation in which two or more substances enhance each other's effects, producing more than the sum of their individual effects. For example, synergism may occur when certain drugs are combined.

Threshold dose: A dose of a substance below which exposure is safe and without risk.

Tolerance level: The maximum level of concentration of a drug or chemical that is permitted in or on food at a specific time during its gathering, processing, storage, and marketing up to the time of its final consumption.

Transformed cell: A cell that has undergone both initiation and promotion and has the potential to develop into a cancer cell.

Tumor: Although this word originally meant swelling, it is now used to describe a growth of tissue that may be either benign or malignant.

Unintentional residue or contaminant: The residue of a compound in the feed or food that is acquired during any phase in its growth, production, processing, or storage. This definition deliberately excludes contamination with substances used to protect the food against attack by parasites or infection.

Index

Paul, A. A., 130
Pauling, Dr. Linus, 153
Peanut butter, 196
Peanuts, 195
Pectin, 121, 124
Pellagra, 142
Pesticides, 63, 191–92
Pharynx, cancer of, 56
pH balance, 92–93
Phenols (chemicals), 198
Phosphorus, 178, 183
Phytic acid, 113
Phyto-estrogens, 205
Pickled foods, 233
Plants, 114
Pleura, cancer of, 28
Pneumonia, 49
Pollution, 49–51
Polo, Marco, 169
Polysaccharides, *see* Complex carbo-
    hydrates
Polyunsaturated fats, 75, 77, 83, 244
Popcorn, 116
Potatoes, 61, 108, 110, 111–12, 186,
    231, 240, 243
    see also French fried potatoes
Pots, 243
Pott, Percival, 48
Poultry, 346–51
    Chicken Cacciatore, 350–51
    cooking, 243–45
    low-fat, 257
    Marinated Chicken, 348–49
    Salad of Turkey with Oranges and
        Grapes, 346–47
Preservatives, food additives as,
    187–90
Preserves, 261
Pressure cooking, 243
Promotors, 31
Prostate cancer, 55, 80–81, 96, 176,
    210
Protease inhibitors, 198
Protein, 16, 64, 90–104, 224, 226,
    234, 278
    animal vs. vegetable, 102, 104
    and calories, 209
    and cancer, 93–98
    and carbohydrates, 107
    function of, 92–93
    need for, 98–101
    sources of, 103

and vitamin A, 134
see also Amino acids
Pyridoxine, *see* Vitamin B$_6$

Racial differences, 52–53
Radiation, 26, 44–45
Raspberries
    Strawberries with Raspberry
        Puree, 341
Ratatouille, 320–21
Recipes, 300–355
    breads, 302–9
    cereals, 310–19
    fish, 352–55
    fruit, 338–45
    poultry, 346–51
    soups, 334–37
    vegetables, 320–33
Rectal cancer, 16, 17, 55, 79, 80,
    94–95, 198, 210, 228
Red dye no. 3, 190
Red meats, 232, 237
Refined carbohydrates, 112–13
Refined sugars, 117, 226
Regional variations, in food, 61
Reheating, 243
Respiratory system, 36
Retinol, 133
Riboflavin (vitamin B$_2$), 141–42, 160
Rice, 115–16, 243, 249, 250
    Rice and Zucchini, 318–19
    see also Brown rice
Rickets, 132, 156
Roasting, 244
Royal Medical Society, 145
Russia, 176, 177
    see also Soviet Union
Rye flour, 113

Saccharin, 61, 63, 187, 189
Salads, 266
    Salad of Turkey with Oranges and
        Grapes, 346–47
Salt, 179, 200–201, 291
    see also Sodium
Saturated fats, 62, 75, 77, 83, 244,
    291
Scrotum, cancer of, 28
Scurvy, 32, 131, 149
Seeds, 114
Selenium, 167–71, 179, 180, 226, 235,
    292, 293, 294

About the Author

Oliver Alabaster, M.D., received his medical training in England at the University of London, graduating in 1966. In 1974 he accepted a two-year clinical and research fellowship at the National Cancer Institute, which is part of the prestigious National Institutes of Health in Bethesda, Maryland. While at the National Cancer Institute, he developed a profound interest in research and stayed on to continue his work.

In 1980, he moved to the George Washington University Medical Center as Associate Professor of Medicine and Director of Cancer Research. He now directs the Cancer Research Laboratories at the university and also practices as a medical oncologist. Although most of his research is directed toward improving cancer treatment, he is convinced that the solution to the cancer problem lies in prevention as well as in cure.